THE NEW HEALTH PROFESSIONALS

Nurse Practitioners
and Physician's Assistants

Edited by
ANN A. BLISS and EVA D. COHEN
Yale University School of Medicine

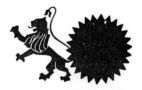

ASPEN SYSTEMS CORPORATION
GERMANTOWN, MARYLAND
1977

Library of Congress Catalog Card Number: 76-46831
ISBN:0-912862-35-1

Printed in the United States of America.
2 3 4 5

To

Bill, Ben, Daniel and Martin

Table of Contents

Contributors

Helen Aikins, RN
formerly Associate Director of Nursing
Medical Clinic
Peter Bent Brigham Hospital
Boston, Massachusetts

Elizabeth A. Allen, RN, PhD
Director, Continuing Education
University of Michigan School of Nursing
Ann Arbor, Michigan

Joseph Alpert, MD
Associate Professor of Medicine
Harvard Medical School
Boston, Massachusetts

Barbara J. Andrew, PhD
Director, Department of Research and
Development
National Board of Medical Examiners
Philadelphia, Pennsylvania

Len Hughes Andrus, MD
Professor and Chairman
Department of Family Medicine
University of California-Davis
Davis, California

Benjamin D. Berger, PA
Coordinator, PA Program
Department of Medicine
Kaiser Health Services System
Portland, Oregon

Alan Berkowitz, MD
Medical Advisor
System Sciences, Inc.
Bethesda, Maryland

Robert H. Blomquist, MD
Internist and Coordinator, P.A. Program
Department of Medicine
Kaiser Health Services System
Portland, Oregon

Elaine S. Bursic, MA
Department of Economics
University of Chapel Hill
Chapel Hill, North Carolina

Harriet D. Carroll, RN, MN
Division of Nursing, P.H.S.
Department of Health, Education, and
Welfare
Bethesda, Maryland

Earl M. Coffee
Accountant
Cooperative Health Services
Albuquerque, New Mexico

Phin Cohen, MD
Senior Associate in Medicine
Peter Bent Brigham Hospital
Boston, Massachusetts

John V. Dervin, MD
Associate Director
Family Practice Residency Program
Community Hospital of Sonoma County
Santa Rosa, California

Christine Thurber Ervin
formerly Research Assistant
Rochester Medical Program
Rochester, New York

Alvan R. Feinstein, MD
Professor of Medicine and
Director, Robert Wood Johnson Foundation Clinical Scholar Program
Yale University School of Medicine
New Haven, Connecticut

Donald W. Fisher, PhD
Executive Director
American Academy of Physician's Assistants
Washington, D.C.

Clifton R. Gaus, ScD
Director, Division of Health Insurance Studies
Office of Research and Statistics
Social Security Administration
Washington, D.C.

J. William Gavett, PhD
Associate Professor
Department of Preventive Medicine and Community Health
and Graduate School of Management
University of Rochester
Rochester, New York

Michael Gent, MSc
Chairman and Professor
Department of Clinical Epidemiology and Biostatistics
McMaster University
Hamilton, Ontario

David L. Glazer
Executive Director
National Commission on Certification of Physician's Assistants
Atlanta, Georgia

Karen A. Gordon, MPH
Research Associate
Frontier Nursing Service
Hyden, Kentucky

Virginia C. Hall, JD
Attorney
Ropes and Gray
Boston, Massachusetts

O. Marie Henry, RN, DNSc
Nurse Consultant
Division of Nursing, P.H.S.
Department of Health, Education and Welfare
Bethesda, Maryland

Susan M. Horowitz, MPH
National Coordinator
Physician's Assistant Training Program
Health Resources Administration, P.H.S.
Department of Health, Education and Welfare
Bethesda, Maryland

Arnold Hurtado, MD
Chief, Department of Medicine
Kaiser Foundation Health Services Research Center
Portland, Oregon

Gertrude Isaacs, DNSc, MPH
Education Director
Frontier Nursing Service
Hyden, Kentucky

Arthur R. Jacobs, MD, MPH
Director, Health Care Studies
Department of Community Health and Ambulatory Care
New England Medical Center Hospital
Boston, Massachusetts

David A. Jensen, MA
Vice President
American Health Management and Consultation Corporation, Inc.
Ardmore, Pennsylvania

Joyce Johnson, BA
Public Health Analyst
National Center for Health Services Research, P.H.S.
Department of Health, Education, and Welfare
Rockville, Maryland

Deloras Jones, RN, MS
Department of Pediatrics
Kaiser-Permanente Medical Center
San Francisco, California

Leona Judson, MSN, FNP
Lecturer
Department of Family Practice
School of Medicine
University of California-Davis
Davis, California

Robert L. Kane, MD
Associate Professor
Department of Family and Community Medicine
University of Utah Medical Center
Salt Lake City, Utah

David M. Kessner, MD
Professor
Department of Community and Family Medicine
University of Massachusetts
Worcester, Massachusetts

Philip C. Kissam, LLB
Associate Professor
School of Law
University of Kansas
Lawrence, Kansas

George Knox, BS
Director
Las Animas Huerfano County District Health Department
Trinidad, Colorado

Megan McDonald, BA
Health Services Analyst
System Sciences, Inc.
Bethesda, Maryland

Patricia McGrath, RN
Nursing Supervisor
Peter Bent Brigham Hospital
Boston, Massachusetts

Michael D. Miller, MD
Senior Partner
Department of Obstetrics and Gynecology
Kaiser Foundation Hospital
San Francisco, California

Stephen B. Morris, MRP
Social Science Research Analyst
Division of Health Insurance Studies
Office of Research and Statistics
Social Security Administration
Washington, D.C.

Joan E. O'Bannon, PhD
Economist
Kaiser Foundation Health Services Research Center
Portland, Oregon

Mary O'Hara-Devereaux, MS, FNP
Co-director FNP Program
Department of Family Practice
School of Medicine
University of California-Davis
Davis, California

Donna M. Olsen, PhD
Assistant Professor
Department of Family and Community Medicine
University of Utah Medical Center
Salt Lake City, Utah

John E. Ott, MD
Co-director
Child Health Associate Program
University of Colorado Medical Center
Denver, Colorado

Jane Cassels Record, PhD
Senior Economist
Kaiser Foundation Health Services
Research Center
Portland, Oregon

Robin Roberts, M Tech
Assistant Professor
Department of Clinical Epidemiology
and Biostatistics
McMaster University
Hamilton, Ontario

John W. Runyan, Jr., MD
Chairman
Department of Community Medicine
Professor of Medicine
University of Tennessee
Memphis, Tennessee

David L. Sackett, MD, MSc
Professor
Department of Clinical Epidemiology
and Biostatistics and Department
of Medicine
McMaster University Medical Centre
Hamilton, Ontario

Barbara Seigal, MS
Executive Director
Cooperative Health Services
Albuquerque, New Mexico

James Singer
Galt, California

David B. Smith, PhD
Associate Professor of Health Ad-
ministration
Temple University
Philadelphia, Pennsylvania

Carolyn K. Snow, MS
Staff Officer
National Academy of Sciences
Washington, D.C.

Gerald Sparer, MA
Associate Director for Demonstration
and Evaluation
National Center for Health Services
Research, P.H.S.
Department of Health, Education and
Welfare
Rockville, Maryland

Reynold Spector, MD
Associate Professor of Medicine
Harvard Medical School
Boston, Massachusetts

Walter O. Spitzer, MD, MHA,
MPH
Director
Division of Family Medicine
Montreal General Hospital
Montreal, Quebec

Barbara Stewart
Internal Auditor
I.T.T. Federal Electric Corporation
Paramus, New Jersey

Harry A. Sultz, DDS, MPH
Professor
Department of Social and Preventive
Medicine
State University of New York at Buffalo
Buffalo, New York

Collette Thomas
Administrator
Public Citizen's Health Research Group
Washington, D.C.

Barbara Ley Toffler, MA
Doctoral Candidate
School of Organization and Management
Yale University
New Haven, Connecticut

Mark J. Yanover, MD
Director, Newborn I.C.U.
Department of Pediatrics
Kaiser Permanente Medical Center
San Francisco, California

Foreword by:

Edmund D. Pellegrino, MD
Professor of Medicine
Yale School of Medicine and
Chairman of the Board of Directors
Yale-New Haven Medical Center,
  Inc.
New Haven, Connecticut

Foreword

The emergence of the "new health professions" in the last decade constitutes what may well turn out to be one of the most significant changes in the social structure of medicine and nursing. While the full implications are yet to be comprehended, they may hold for patients an importance approaching the feats of biomedical science.

It is already clear that many questions are posed which are fundamental to the future of how medical care is provided. Our traditional notions of the division of labor among physicians and other health professionals, the locus of authority and decision-making, and even the partitioning of resources between curative and curing medicine, have all been brought under new scrutiny.

Although the answers are far from final, a source book of this kind outlines with clarity abundant evidence that the previously closed precincts of the physician's activities are safely and competently being entered by other health workers. Physician's assistants and nurse practitioners are acting in the physician's stead as well as extending the range of services more properly part of their own traditions.

Currently, the field is beset by uncertainties. The roles and claims of all health professions are still rapidly shifting; there is frequent overlap of functions, and even some head-on collisions over perimeters of activity. It would be easy to dispose of the whole matter as rampant professionalism or unseemly territorial skirmishes. Disconcerting as they may be, these diversions must not obscure the social realities which gave impetus to the whole movement.

The new health professionals came into being to fill a variety of specific needs at a time, it must be remembered, when there was general agreement that the nation faced a shortage of physicians.* Physician's

---

*For example, in 1965-66 there were 87 medical schools in the U.S. admitting 9,012 students ("Medical Education in the U.S., 1975-76" *JAMA 1976 Annual Report* (Dec. 27, 1976) p. 2690); in 1975 there were 114 schools and 15,365 entering students (*JAMA* 198 (Nov. 21, 1966): 865).

assistants were conceived originally as alleviating this shortage by performing those tasks which would save the physician time and effort. These tasks were to be under close physician supervision and, generally, in highly structured hospital or clinic settings.

Thus, the first physician's assistants concentrated on the complicated tasks of tertiary care; the pediatric nurse practitioner focused on well baby care, parent education and prevention; and the clinical pharmacist extended his role as drug expert in hospital drug information centers. Each category permitted the physician to extend the range of his own practice, and presumably to spend more time on nontechnical and more professional tasks.

Almost simultaneously, however, public and governmental awareness of the existence of certain neglected areas in health care grew rapidly. Access, availability, and cost of "primary care"—however variously defined—took prominent place in discussions and in legislation. Soon, additional neglected needs like care for the chronically ill, prevention, patient education, and health maintenance were added to the list. The new health professions have begun to demonstrate their competence in these domains and there has been a resurgence of midwifery as well.

For a variety of reasons—geographical needs, public and physician acceptance, presumption of lower costs, and effectiveness—the new health professionals recently have become less tied to hospitals and structured settings. Close dependence on the physician still predominates in more narrowly technical tasks like those performed by assistants to clinical subspecialists. However, nurses and physician's assistants now raise the real possibility of increasingly independent practice in primary care, prevention, health maintenance, or the dispensing of medication.

The Carnegie Commission, which in 1970 proposed an elaborate national plan for easing physician shortages, in 1976 declared that we may face a surplus and that no new medical schools should be started. Even the previously unfavorable ratio of generalists to specialists has begun to change. Family practice departments in medical schools and family practice residencies now attract a large number of recent medical graduates; departments of internal medicine and pediatrics have discovered an interest in teaching primary care. Moreover, the conclusion is being reached widely that *more* medical care—more physicians, nurses, hospitals—may not result in *better* health for the nation.

The central issue now appears to bring some order to these conflicting movements, which at times seem to have become detached from their origins in social needs. What does the public perceive to be the need for these services? Who is to do what, and how will overlapping interests be resolved? What are the priorities of the services among the variety so eagerly offered by the new professions? How can the already evident tendencies to escalate education, costs, credentials and competition for choice tasks be neutralized?

The most vexing questions inevitably will be asked: to what extent can new health professionals replace the physician? And, to what extent can they provide primary care, preventive medicine or chronic care independently? If we were to build our health manpower system on significant numbers of new health professionals, how many physicians would we then need?

Unquestionably, more data on the effectiveness, safety and efficiency of using new health professionals would be desirable. But these data cannot alter the fact that the whole pattern of medical and health care by physicians has been brought under scrutiny. Manpower planning and education, professional remuneration, licensure, accreditation, and entry into the profession of medicine are already undergoing serious alteration.

It is important to emphasize that nursing, in particular, sees its extended roles as a logical development of its own special contributions to health care, and not an incursion into medicine. The new roles, they aver, are uniquely and properly part of nursing, especially in providing health rather than medical care. Extended nursing roles are conceived to be complementary and supplementary to physician care—not meant to substitute for it.

From the public viewpoint—and that of the majority of public policy decision-makers—these philosophical and professional distinctions are not so clear. They see the development of the new health professionals as a viable alternative to present patterns which have not resulted in universally available, reasonably priced, accessible, primary care—seven-days-a-week, twenty-four hours-a-day, at some convenient location near where most people live. This remains the underlying social reality which has motivated public and governmental support for a more optimal use of health manpower. It is expressed clearly as a national goal in the health planning legislation enacted in 1975 (P.L. 641). Despite compromises in the final version, this also was the source of much of the prolonged negotiation which delayed passage of the recent health manpower bill (P.L. 484).

In our society, access to primary medical care is assuming the character of a fundamental human need—one we all share when we become ill by our own definition of illness. At that moment of anxiety, most of us need access to someone readily accessible, to whom we can transfer some of our anxiety and to whom we can turn for advice. The logomachy about the meanings of *primary care* notwithstanding, it is the security of access to this first contact in the event of illness that concerns the public. What is wrong? Is it serious? Can it be cured? What will it cost? Will it hurt? Do I need to be in the hospital? Do I need a specialist? Can you treat me here? These simple questions must be dealt with as effectively, efficiently, promptly and humanely as the clinical situation allows.

The more comprehensive views of primary care—family medicine, health maintenance and prevention, continuity and comprehensiveness—are not to be deprecated. But for the majority of people in this country, they are secondary priorities when illness occurs. What is being sought is really another dimension of human security—the assurance of finding help, close-by, wherever one happens to be.

Primary medical care, then, is a human need first, and only secondarily a matter of economics, politics, professional prerogatives, or semantic debate. The urgency of the need is accentuated by the public's realization that it is not likely to be met by any of the traditional health professions, their patterns of practice or modes of education.

How the need for primary care is ultimately to be met, by what combination of health workers, by what reassignment of functions among them, and under what conditions, are matters forcefully placed before the public by the emergence of new health professions. This book describes some alternative health manpower demonstrations which should be useful to the wide audience that must wrestle with this problem.

My hope is that the reader will reflect frequently on the social origins of the new movement. The success or failure of the new health professions will be measured by the degree to which congruence is achieved between their professional aspirations and public need.

Edmund D. Pellegrino, M.D.
President, Yale-New Haven Medical Center, Inc.
Professor of Medicine, Yale University
New Haven, Connecticut

January 1977

Introduction

Nurse practitioners and physician's assistants have been categorized as "New Health Practitioners" (NHPs), a generic term referring to mid-level health practitioners who perform tasks which traditionally have been within the purview of physicians. Most NHPs are taught to elicit a complete history and perform a routine physical examination on all types and ages of patients. Additionally, NHPs can order diagnostic procedures, can interpret results and isolate abnormalities. They are also trained to carry out specific medical regimens under physician direction and take necessary, immediate action to preserve life in emergency situations. Some are trained to perform minor surgical services such as the removal of a foreign object from the eye, or minor suturing. Generally, when NHPs perform medical acts under physician supervision, the identified physician supervisor is legally responsible for their professional activity.

It has now been a little over ten years since the first program to train physician's assistants was initiated at Duke University. Similarly, programs to train nurses for extended roles have proliferated over the same decade. In 1976, there were approximately 7,000 NPs and 5,000 PAs who had completed training programs.* Both types of new health practitioner have been developed in response to health manpower shortages resulting from maldistribution of and an increase in specialization among physicians, resulting in a decrease in the number of primary care physicians. As Dr. Paul Beeson has pointed out, there are 70,000 generalists and 280,000 specialists in the United States in contrast to England where

---

*These figures on NPs have been extrapolated through 1976 from DHEW, Division of Nursing study findings on certificate and master's graduates as of 1974. The number of PAs is based on those candidates for the National Certification Examination for the Assistant to the Primary Care Physician who had graduated from formal training programs as of 1975 and an extrapolation of those data through 1976.

1

there are 22,000 generalists and 8,000 specialists.* Many NHP programs have been funded by the federal government and supported by private foundations in the hope that NHPs will help improve the access, distribution, supply, quality and efficiency of primary care.

This book is directed at medical, nursing, and physician's assistant educators; individual NPs and PAs; researchers; legislators and their staffs; health planners at all levels of government; administrators of health care institutions; professional associations; and the brave consumers who venture into the professional literature. The increasing volume of research on NHPs has been disseminated primarily through professional journals and government reports, many of which are unavailable to the reader without access to a well-stocked medical library. Thus, we have prepared a book which we hope will serve four purposes:

1. It is a *state-of-the-art document* about new health practitioners, variously referred to as Nurse Practitioners, Physician's Assistants and Associates, Medex, and Physician Extenders.

2. While there are many journal articles about NHPs, there are few books to date which can serve as a *single resource about the variety of NHPs.*

3. To date, studies have focused upon the types and amount of care which can be delegated safely and economically by physicians to trained NHPs. However, the impact of NHPs on the health status of individuals under their care is only beginning to be documented. In addition to providing an update on the different kinds of NHP personnel now practicing in different settings, the book *points to the clinical impact of NHPs and the importance of redirecting research to look at clinical outcomes.*

4. The place of NHPs in eventual national health insurance already is under serious consideration. The chapters herein are intended to provide as comprehensive *a data base as can reasonably be compiled in a book to be used for informed decisions* about the legitimate contribution of NHPs to the present and future system of health care.

Because of our work in the training and evaluation of NHPs during the last five years, we are frequently asked a variety of questions about NPs and PAs. Among the most common:

---

* Beeson, P. Jan. 1974. "Some Good Features of the British National Health Service," *Journal of Medical Education* 49, No. 1:43-49.

How many are there?

Where are they being trained?

How many and what types of programs are training NPs and PAs?

Where do they practice?

What do they do?

How much do they earn?

What are the legal boundaries of their practice?

Are there legal constraints?

Are they certified or licensed? Through what mechanism?

Are they acceptable to patients? To other health professionals?

Are there any differences between NPs and PAs? What are the differences?

Are they cost-effective? Can their services be reimbursed?

How much physician supervision do they require?

Do they make any clinical difference?

How does one measure the quality of their care?

What problems are inherent in evaluating NHPs?

In order to answer many of these questions, we have organized the book into five parts. Part I provides a demographic overview of Nurse Practitioners and Physician's Assistants. This part of the book is intended to provide the reader with a current state-of-the-art of new health practitioners (NHPs). In addition, Part I introduces the reader to a recent study revealing some of the obvious similarities and differences in NHP training and functions. While the editors are of the opinion that NPs and PAs are more similar than not, we are ready to acknowledge that there are some who would disagree with us. Some hold the view that PAs are technology and illness-cure oriented in the tradition of the medical profession which spawned them, and that NPs are health-care oriented in the finest tradition of nursing. Obviously, NPs bring a valuable foundation in nursing upon which their primary care skills are built. However, many other NHPs bring valuable health-related training and experience to their new role as well. In the editors' experience, many astute clinicians have been encountered among NPs who do an impressive job of diagnosis and management of common acute illness and chronic disease. Practicing PAs report considerable psychosocial counseling, health teaching, and follow-up in the care of their patients. Indeed, PAs are taught psychosocial skills during their training and find that counseling and health teaching are a prominent part of the National

Board of Medical Examiners "Examination for the Assistant to the Primary Care Physician." In any case, it remains to be documented by research whether significant differences among NHPs are real or merely a myth in the making.

In Part II certain major determinants of NHP practice have been identified as being crucial: enabling legislation for expanded medical delegation, certification, reimbursement, cost effectiveness, physician supervision, role development and evaluative research. While the impact of each separate determinant of practice is considerable, a determinant takes on even greater importance when it begins to interact with another. For instance, the law regulates certain forms of reimbursement which some NHPs now seek. Yet, third party payment for NHP services will likely be tied to certification as a competency assurance mechanism. In turn, regulatory state statutes may modify the nature of permitted medical delegation in such a way as to adversely affect the cost-effectiveness of NHPs. Finally, all of these major determinants of practice may stand on the success or failure of the role development of NPs and PAs, regardless of their real competence and cost benefits. Thus, the major determinants of practice appear to us to be so interrelated as to deserve considerable attention singly.

Parts III and IV are devoted to evaluative research, perhaps the most subtle and powerful determinant of NHP practice. It is our observation that the research data on NHP productivity, cost, task-competency, enabling legislation and acceptance continue to guide and direct the NHP professions more profoundly than is intended or may be wise.

In surveying the large and growing body of NHP research done to date, one finds a disappointingly small number of studies which measures the clinical impact of the NHP, or, in other words, asks the question, "What clinical difference does an NHP make?" The safety, competence and acceptance concerns about NHPs, certainly valuable questions at one time, have perhaps in part been answered. It is the purpose of the book now to focus attention on the clinical impact as well as on the nature of clinical decision making as fertile ground for new investigation. Then, motivation to hire, to create broad enabling legislation, to reimburse or to certify NHPs may be based on data which show the extent to which NHPs can improve the clinical outcomes of sick people, rather than improve the balance sheets of private physicians or financially beset Health Maintenance Organizations and hospital clinics. The present danger is that if research findings on NHP productivity and cost-effectiveness remain the primary motivation for hiring NPs and PAs, then NHPs will continue to be evaluated primarily in terms of cost-effectiveness. Perhaps many of the efforts to hire, reimburse, legislate and certify NHPs, while good, have not been as rightly motivated as based on the seductive nature of research findings.

Part V highlights where the NHP concept appears to be going, how it is getting there and who is paying the way. Most of the issues have been with the concept long enough to speak for themselves. However, firm conclusions about NHPs are a matter of present speculation which remains to be tested by the events and research of the future.

Finally, a word of dismay about the generic term "New Health Practitioners." It is simply inadequate to speak of professions developed ten years ago as "New." Will they still be called "New" fifty years from now? Nor does the term "health practitioners" by itself seem descriptive enough. However, some of the other terms applied to NHPs are even less satisfying. "Primary Care Associate" and "Assistant to the Primary Care Physician" suffer on two counts. First, primary care is as yet a loosely-defined word which obscures rather than clarifies. Second, the notion of being an assistant to a physician offends many nurses and does not accurately reflect the comprehensiveness of services provided by both NPs and PAs. "Physician Extender" is a term which even physicians find hard to accept. Perhaps the Johns Hopkins' "Health Associate" comes closest to describing broadly the role of NHPs, but to date it remains the label of a single program to designate its graduates. Throughout the book, we reluctantly use the generic term NHP but believe the concept still is in search of a more fitting and proper name.

Part I

New Health Practitioners

Continued public and private support has allowed programs for the training of nurse practitioners and physician's assistants to increase rapidly over the last decade, and one of the purposes of this book is to present an update on the evolution of these programs. While programs have been permitted to develop without major attempts to standardize their content, data from the American Academy of Physicians' Assistants and the Division of Nursing lend credence to our suggestion that there are more similarities among overall program goals and objectives than differences.

The first two chapters provide an overview of the two major types of New Health Practitioners that have emerged—nurse practitioners and physician's assistants. Sultz, Henry and Carroll are conducting a longitudinal study of NP programs and graduates. Their thorough overview is based on the findings about NP programs from the first phase of their study. Fisher and Horowitz, who have been involved with the organization and funding of the PA concept from its inception, describe the current status of PA programs and the demographic characteristics of PA programs and graduates.

The third chapter presents a statewide comparison of employed NPs and PAs in Connecticut. Toffler's study sheds light on several possible differences between the orientation of PAs and NPs as to care, practice patterns and attitudes about their respective roles.

These chapters are intended primarily to acquaint the reader with the selection, training and practice of NPs and PAs. The aim is to inform about both professions rather than to advocate either one.   ·

Chapter 1

Nurse Practitioners: An Overview of Nurses in the Expanded Role

Harry A. Sultz, O. Marie Henry and Harriet D. Carroll

In the last decade, nursing practice has evolved in response to society's changing health needs to incorporate a variety of expanded roles for nurses. Programs designed to prepare nurses for expanded roles have proliferated and a number of their graduates are now functioning in the new roles. Referred to in general as nurse practitioners, these personnel are also identified by a variety of other titles which indicate their areas of specialization such as pediatric, family, adult, medical or geriatric nurse practitioner or associate, nurse clinician, or clinical specialist. The programs preparing nurse practitioners generally combine the theory and practice involved in history taking, diagnosis and treatment, interpretation of tests, and provision of supportive services to restore health. Emphasis is also placed on health maintenance, prevention, health education and counseling as integral parts of most programs.

The interest of the Department of Health, Education, and Welfare in nurse practitioners developed in the early 1970s when federal funds became available for their training. The department's Division of Nursing contracted with the Research Foundation of the State University of New York at Buffalo for a study to obtain baseline information for the further development and support of nurse practitioner education and practice, and to evaluate program efforts related to nurses in expanded roles.* Planned as a longitudinal study, the first phase sought to obtain information on the education and preparation of nurse practitioners. Subsequent phases will link these findings with data obtained in the employment setting. This chapter highlights some of the findings of the first phase of the study—information on the educational programs and the students.[1]

---

*Project performed under Contract No. N01 NU-34064 with the Division of Nursing, Bureau of Health Manpower, Health Resources Administration, PHS, DHEW.

PLAN AND METHOD

Phase I involved the collection of data on the number and type of nurse practitioner educational programs, entrance requirements, program lengths, contents of curricula, types of faculty and degree of responsibility for which graduates are prepared. Student variables included prior background and preparation, previous work experience and income, function and satisfaction in previous nursing role, motivation to enter nurse practitioner programs, and expectations of the nurse practitioner role. Phase I data were obtained by means of mailed self-administered questionnaires addressed to directors of all programs engaged in nurse practitioner training and to the students of one class in each program. An overall response rate of 97 percent was attained from the programs and 85 percent from the students.

Phase II will be concerned with determining the types of agencies and facilities that provide nurse practitioner employment, the manner in which nurse practitioners are utilized in the provision of health care, the role they establish in the hierarchy of health care providers, the salaries they earn, and the expectations of both nurse practitioners and employers as to their functions in patient management. In addition, this component of the study will address some of the potential problems of employment, particularly as they relate to ethical and/or legal problems, physician understanding and patient acceptance. Phase II data will be obtained from mailed self-administered quexvnaires to the cohort of NPs identified as students in Phase I, and their employers.

PROGRAMS

Those programs included in the study, which were identified from an original list numbering more than 200, used these criteria in the selection of programs:

1. They must offer a formal curriculum, as opposed to in-service training for their own employees.

2. They must have started instruction with enrolled students by January 1, 1974.

3. They must provide preparation in extended nursing roles, i.e., primary care skills such as history taking, physical examination, ordering laboratory tests, and assuming responsibility for medical management of selected cases with emphasis on primary care.

4. They must require that students be registered nurses in order to enroll.

Geographic Distribution

The distribution of the programs meeting study criteria by specialty and by certificate and master's degree for each of four geographic regions designated by the National League for Nursing is shown in Table 1:1. There are greater concentrations of certificate programs in the Northeast and South than in the Midwest and West. The greater proportion of master's programs in the Northeast and South is largely because of the maternity and family programs.

TABLE 1:1

Geographic Distribution of Responding NP Programs, by Region,[1] Specialty, and Type of Program

Region and specialty	Type of program					
	Certificate		Master's		Total	
	Number	Percent	Number	Percent	Number	Percent
West						
Pediatric	9	11	1	2	10	8
Midwifery	1	1	1	2	2	1
Maternity	1	1	0	0	1	1
Family	5	6	2	5	7	5
Adult	3	3	1	2	4	3
Psychiatric	NA	NA	2	4	2	2
Subtotal	19	22	7	15	26	20
Midwest						
Pediatric	11	12	3	7	14	11
Midwifery	0	0	2	5	2	1
Maternity	2	3	0	0	2	2
Family	3	3	1	2	4	3
Adult	2	3	2	4	4	3
Psychiatric	NA	NA	0	0	0	0
Subtotal	18	21	8	18	26	20
Northeast						
Pediatric	11	13	2	5	13	10
Midwifery	1	1	2	4	3	2
Maternity	1	1	4	9	5	4
Family	3	3	5	11	8	6
Adult	5	6	2	5	7	5
Psychiatric	NA	NA	1	2	1	1
Subtotal	21	24	16	36	37	28

[1] Regions are those designated by the National League for Nursing.
"NA" in table indicates "not applicable."

TABLE 1:1 (Continued)

Geographic Distribution of Responding NP Programs, by Region,[1] Specialty, and Type of Program

| Region and specialty | Type of program | | | | | |
| | Certificate | | Master's | | Total | |
	Number	Percent	Number	Percent	Number	Percent
South						
Pediatric	11	13	2	4	13	10
Midwifery	3	3	1	2	4	3
Maternity	3	3	3	7	6	4
Family	6	8	4	9	10	8
Adult	5	6	3	7	8	6
Psychiatric	NA	NA	1	2	1	1
Subtotal	28	33	14	31	42	32
Total	86	100	45	100	131	100
Pediatric	42	48.8	8	17.8	50	38.2
Midwifery	5	5.8	6	13.3	11	8.4
Maternity	7	8.1	7	15.5	14	10.7
Family	17	19.8	12	26.7	29	22.1
Adult	15	17.5	8	17.8	23	17.6
Psychiatric	NA	NA	4	8.9	4	3.0
Total	86	100.0	45	100.0	131	100.0

[1] Regions are those designated by the National League for Nursing.
"NA" in table indicates "not applicable."

Students in the programs meeting study criteria graduated between May 1974, and June 1975. The Northeast accounts for the largest number of students although the programs having the largest number of students per program (an average of 12 to 13) are in the West. Programs in the South and Midwest average eight to nine students. There are also fewer master's students per program than certificate students per program, 8 versus 11 on the average.

Specialty, Type, and Length

The distribution of the responding programs by specialty preparation and whether they lead to a certificate or master's degree is seen in the totals of Table 1:1. About one-third of the NP programs lead to a master's degree. Half of certificate programs prepare pediatric NPs. The

TABLE 1:2

NP Programs, by Length, Specialty, and Type of Program

Specialty	Length (in months) and type of program							
	3-5	6-8	9-11	12-14	15-17	18-20	> 20	Total
	Certificate							
Pediatric	13	13	9	5	1	0	1	42
Midwifery	0	2	2	1	0	0	0	5
Maternity	4	1	2	0	0	0	0	7
Family	1	3	3	7	1	2	0	17
Adult	5	3	2	4	1	0	0	15
Total	23	22	18	17	3	2	1	86
	Master's							
Pediatric	0	0	0	2	1	5	0	8
Midwifery	0	0	1	0	1	3	1	6
Maternity	0	0	1	3	1	2	0	7
Family	0	0	0	5	4	3	0	12
Adult	0	0	0	4	1	3	0	8
Psychiatric	0	0	0	1	2	1	0	4
Total	0	0	2	15	10	17	1	45

four existing psychiatric programs are on the master's level and more than one-quarter of the master's programs prepare family NPs.

The total program length in months by type and specialty is seen in Table 1:2. As might be expected, the master's programs are much longer than the certificate programs. The average length for the certificate programs is 8.4 months and the range is from 3-24 months as compared to the master's programs which average 15.3 months and range from 10-21 months.

The average length of certificate programs with and without preceptorships is presented in Figure 1:1. The classroom didactic is the formal portion in which a specified curriculum is taught using lectures and self-instruction materials, and the clinical didactic includes the concurrent relevant clinical observations and experiences. The preceptorship is a specified period of supervised clinical practice in patient assessment and management, and is a requirement for completion of the program. This is distinct from and follows the clinical experience offered concurrently with the didactic portion. The presence of a preceptorship almost doubles the overall length of the programs. The average length of certificate pro-

FIGURE 1:1

Average Length of Certificate NP Programs With and Without Preceptorship, by Specialty

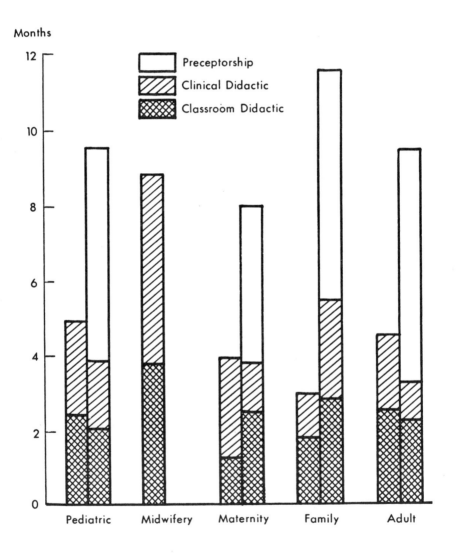

FIGURE 1:2

Average Length of Master's NP Programs With and Without Preceptorship, by Specialty

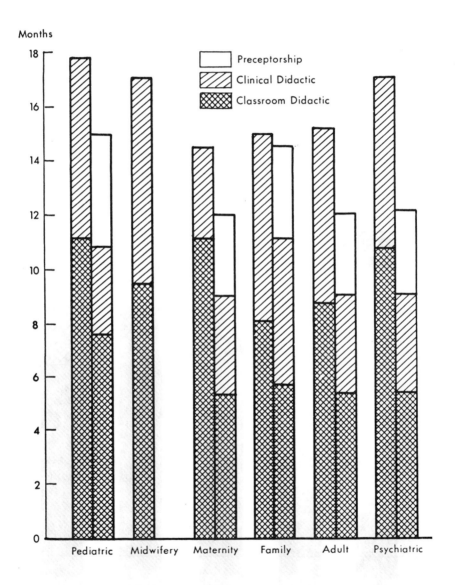

FIGURE 1:3

NP Graduates Per Year, by Specialty and Type of Program

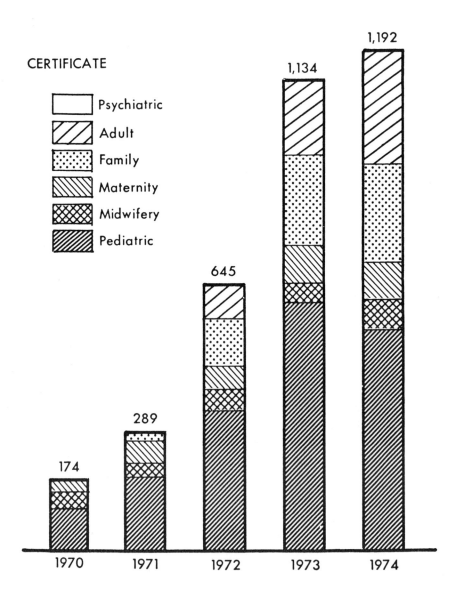

FIGURE 1:3 (Continued)

NP Graduates Per Year, by Specialty and Type of Progam

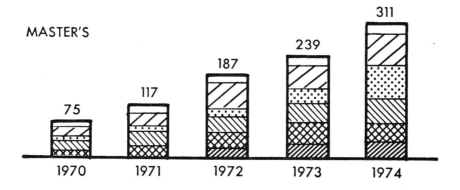

grams which do not include a preceptorship is 5.4 months, whereas the average length of those which do include a preceptorship is 10.2 months. Master's programs are very different from certificate programs in that those without preceptorships are longer than those with preceptorships, as can be seen in Figure 1:2. For master's programs, the average length of programs which do not include preceptorships is 15.8 months, whereas the average length of programs which do include preceptorships is 14.0 months. It should be noted that neither certificate nor master's mid-wifery programs includes preceptorships.

Admissions and Graduation

The first NP program, defined according to the criteria of this study, was instituted in 1965 at the University of Colorado. Since then there has been an impressive increase in the number of programs preparing nurse practitioners in a variety of specialty areas with 1972 marking the greatest growth spurt for both certificate and master's programs. Over-all, there has been a steady increase in both the number of students ad-mitted and graduated. Not only have the totals increased, but the average number of students admitted and graduated also has increased. As seen in Figure 1:3, the number of graduates per year for all types of programs has increased fivefold over the five years ending in 1974. Adult and family programs have shown the greatest increase, and it is evident that the number of both certificate and master's degree students has grown. While pediatric preparation constituted a large share of NP certificate programs in 1970, master's programs only began graduating pediatric NPs in 1972. The first certificate adult NPs graduated in 1972.

Tests

Of great interest in the development of NP programs is the use of standardized tests. The number of programs that use tests and the types used, primarily in connection with the admissions process, is seen in Table 1:3. Certificate and master's programs differ in their use of tests. Less than half of the certificate programs use tests of any kind. The certificate programs that do use tests are more interested in personality measures as is evidenced by the fact that about two-thirds of them use personality tests only. Master's programs' use of tests is very different. Eighty-four percent (38 out of 45) use tests of some kind. Of these 38 programs that utilize standardized tests, 32 programs use aptitude tests only, two use personality tests only, and four programs used both aptitude and personality tests.

Tuition

Another area of interest to those concerned with NP preparation is tuition. As can be seen in Table 1:4, 32 of the certificate programs have no tuition and the tuition for master's programs on the whole is more expensive than the tuition for certificate programs. The fact that a program charges no tuition does not appear to be related to sponsoring institution, or for that matter, length of program. Those five master's programs which charge tuition of more than $5,000 range in length from 13 to 19

TABLE 1:3

NP Programs, by Test[1] Used for Student Evaluation and Type of Program

Test	Type of program			
	Certificate		Master's	
	Number	Percent	Number	Percent
Aptitude test only	5	5.8	32	71.1
Personality test only	19	22.1	2	4.4
Both aptitude and personality tests	6	7.0	4	8.9
Neither aptitude nor personality test	56	65.1	7	15.6
Total	86	100.0	45	100.0

[1] This presentation does distinguish between tests given prior to acceptance and those used after entrance into the program.

months. This does not represent a departure from the average overall length of all master's programs of 15.3 months.

Faculty

Data on faculty of NP programs were analyzed with respect to specialty. The average number of NP program staff teaching personnel in selected disciplines by specialty and type of program is presented in Table 1:5. Nurses and nurse practitioners play the prominent role in teaching both certificate and master's students. An interesting difference between the certificate and master's programs is that the certificate programs depend somewhat less on nurses as teachers than do the master's programs and also that physicians account for more of the teaching in the certificate programs than in the master's programs. The staffing pattern for the midwifery programs is different from that of all the other programs in that there are more staff teaching personnel in midwifery programs and they are more likely to be NPs. The ratio of faculty to students is much higher for master's programs than for certificate programs.

TABLE 1:4

NP Programs, by Amount of Tuition Charged to Students, Sponsoring Institution, and Type of Program

Tuition charged to students (in dollars)	Type of program and sponsoring institution							
	Certificate						Master's	
	University/ college		Hospital		Other[1]		University/ college	
	No.	Pct.	No.	Pct.	No.	Pct.	No.	Pct.
0	23	34.8	5	55.6	4	66.6	—	—
1-500	24	36.4	3	33.3	1	16.7	7	17.1
501-1,000	14	21.2	1	11.1	1	16.7	7	17.1
1,001-2,000	5	7.6	—	—	—	—	12	29.2
2,001-3,000	—	—	—	—	—	—	—	—
3,001-4,000	—	—	—	—	—	—	7	17.1
4,001-5,000	—	—	—	—	—	—	3	7.3
> 5,000	—	—	—	—	—	—	5	12.2
Total[2]	66	100.0	9	100.0	6	100.0	41	100.0

[1] "Other" includes three programs sponsored by departments of health; one by a coordinated home health facility; one by an outpatient facility; and one by a regional medical program.

[2] Five certificate programs and four master's programs did not supply information on tuition.

TABLE 1:5

Average Number of NP Program Staff Teaching Personnel[1] in Selected Disciplines, by Specialty and Type of Program

| Specialty | Number of programs | Discipline and type of program | | | | |
		NP	Nurse	Physician	Other[2]	Total
		Certificate				
Pediatric	42	1.4	.2	.6	.1	2.3
Midwifery	5	4.9	—	.9	—	5.8
Maternity	7	1.3	.7	.4	.1	2.5
Family	17	2.3	.4	1.0	.4	4.1
Adult	15	1.3	.3	.7	.1	2.4
Total	86	1.7	.3	.7	.1	2.8
		Master's				
Pediatric	8	1.1	1.2	.4	.1	2.8
Midwifery	6	4.4	.1	—	.1	4.6
Maternity	7	1.5	.5	.3	.1	2.4
Family	11	1.7	.8	.8	.1	3.4
Adult	8	1.4	.7	.2	.1	2.4
Psychiatric	4	2.7	.6	.4	.3	4.0
Total[3]	44	2.0	.7	.4	.1	3.2

[1] "Staff teaching personnel" excluded guest lectures. Staff teaching personnel is presented in terms of full-time equivalents and was based on estimated percentage of total work time provided.

[2] "Other" was not specified.

[3] One family master's program did not supply information on number of staff teaching personnel.

Guest lecturers appear to provide a very substantial amount of the teaching in NP programs. As seen in Table 1:6, there are a reported 2,733 guest lecturers. Half of these guest lecturers are physicians teaching in certificate programs. In general, the certificate programs have a greater number of guest lecturers per program than the master's program.

The kind of preceptorship supervision available is shown in Table 1:7. There are 31 certificate programs out of 86 (36 percent) and 33 master's programs out of 45 (73 percent) with no preceptorship. NPs account for a very small number of preceptors. Not shown on this table is the fact that 67 percent of all programs report that practicing NPs are usually or always available for clinical consultation during the preceptorship.

TABLE 1:6

Guest Lecturers[1] in NP Programs, by Discipline, Specialty, and Type of Program

Specialty	Discipline and type of program							
	Nurse		Physician		Other[2]		Total	
	No.	Average no. per program	No.	Average no. per program	No.	Average no. per program	No.	Average no. per program
				Certificate				
Pediatric	209	5.2	588	14.7	233	5.8	1,030	25.7
Midwifery	12	2.4	33	6.6	22	4.4	67	13.4
Maternity	17	2.4	48	6.9	31	4.4	96	13.7
Family	136	8.0	462	27.2	85	5.0	683	40.2
Adult	89	5.9	254	16.9	34	2.3	377	25.1
Total[3]	463	5.5	1,385	16.5	405	4.8	2,253	26.8
				Master's				
Pediatric	19	2.4	37	4.6	15	1.9	71	8.9
Midwifery	28	4.7	38	6.3	10	1.7	76	12.7
Maternity	7	1.0	6	.9	5	.7	18	2.6
Family	37	3.7	124	12.4	42	4.2	203	20.3
Adult	33	4.1	49	6.1	11	1.4	93	11.6
Psychiatric	5	1.7	10	3.3	4	1.3	19	6.3
Total[3]	129	3.1	264	6.3	87	2.1	480	11.4

[1] "Guest lecturers" were not considered to be staff teaching personnel.
[2] "Other" was not specified.
[3] Two pediatric certificate programs, two family master's programs and one psychiatric master's program did not supply information on guest lecturers.

STUDENTS

The distribution of students by program type and specialty area is shown in Table 1:8. A total of 1,101 students is included in the study and 72 percent of them are in certificate programs. The greatest concentration of certificate students is in pediatric programs, whereas the higher proportion of the master's students is in family practitioner programs.

Demographic Characteristics

The demographic characteristics of the students are presented in Table 1:9. Both certificate and master's students overwhelmingly are female

TABLE 1:7

NP Programs, by Discipline of Students' Supervisor During Preceptorship and Type of Program

| Discipline of students' supervisor during preceptorship | Type of program | | | |
| | Certificate | | Master's | |
	No.	Pct.	No.	Pct.
NP and/or physician	14	26.4	9	75.0
NP only	1	1.9	1	8.3
Physician only	38	71.7	2	16.7
Total[1]	53	100.0	12	100.0

[1] Two certificate programs did not supply information on discipline of supervisor during preceptorship.

TABLE 1:8

NP Students, by Specialty and Type of Program

| Specialty | Type of program | | | | | |
| | Certificate | | Master's | | Total | |
	No.	Pct.	No.	Pct.	No.	Pct.
Pediatric	351	44.2	30	9.8	381	34.6
Midwifery	26	3.3	54	17.6	80	7.3
Maternity	60	7.6	30	9.8	90	8.2
Family	185	23.2	100	32.6	285	25.8
Adult	172	21.7	66	21.4	238	21.6
Psychiatric	NA	NA	27	8.8	27	2.5
Total	794	100.0	307	100.0	1,101	100.0

and white. The majority of certificate students are married as are almost half of the master's students. Certificate students are in general somewhat older than master's, their median age being 33 compared to 31 for the master's students.

Professional Characteristics

Differences of professional characteristics between NP students in certificate and master's programs are revealed in Table 1:10. Compared to students in master's programs, students in certificate programs are less frequently members of ANA. Additionally, certificate students have

TABLE 1:9

NP Students, by Selected Demographic Characteristics and Type of Program

Demographic characteristic	Type of program					
	Certificate		Master's		Total	
	No.	Pct.	No.	Pct.	No.	Pct.
Sex						
Male	16	2.0	6	2.0	22	2.0
Female	778	98.0	301	98.0	1,079	98.0
Total	794	100.0	307	100.0	1,101	100.0
Race						
White	695	88.4	286	93.8	981	89.9
Black	65	8.3	10	3.3	75	6.9
Other[1]	26	3.3	9	2.9	35	3.2
Total[2]	786	100.0	305	100.0	1,091	100.0
Marital Status						
Unmarried	337	43.0	148	49.2	485	44.7
Married	446	57.0	153	50.8	599	55.3
Total[3]	783	100.0	301	100.0	1,084	100.0
Age (in years)						
< 25	29	4.0	4	1.5	33	3.3
25-34	355	49.5	174	63.7	529	53.4
35-44	176	24.5	83	30.4	259	26.2
45-54	128	17.8	11	4.0	139	14.0
> 54	30	4.2	1	.4	31	3.1
Total[4]	718	100.0	273	100.0	991	100.0
Average	36.2		32.5		35.2	
Median	33		31		33	

[1] Includes oriental, American Indian, Mexican American, Puerto Rican, and Latin American.

[2] Eight certificate and two master's students did not supply information on race.

[3] Eleven certificate and six master's students did not supply information on marital status.

[4] Seventy-six certificate and 34 master's students did not supply information on age.

spent a median of eight years in professional nursing, and the credential from their prior education was most likely to have been a diploma. The master's students, on the other hand, had spent a median of five years in professional nursing, and the majority were prior recipients of baccalaureate degrees. The previous employment setting for the largest

TABLE 1:10

NP Students, by Selected Professional Characteristics and Type of Program

Professional characteristics	Type of program					
	Certificate		Master's		Total	
	No.	Pct.	No.	Pct.	No.	Pct.
ANA membership						
Member	309	39.1	189	61.8	498	45.4
Nonmember	481	60.9	117	38.2	598	54.6
Total[1]	790	100.0	306	100.0	1,096	100.0
Years in professional nursing						
0	23	2.9	4	1.3	27	2.5
1-5	233	29.7	159	51.8	392	35.9
6-10	228	29.1	72	23.4	300	27.5
11-15	118	15.1	48	15.6	166	15.2
16-20	96	12.2	18	5.9	114	10.5
> 20	86	11.0	6	2.0	92	8.4
Total[2]	784	100.0	307	100.0	1,091	100.0
Average	10.3		7.0		9.4	
Median	8		5		7	
Prior nursing preparation						
Hospital diploma	370	46.7	11	3.6	381	34.7
Associate degree	70	8.8	2	.6	72	6.5
Baccalaureate degree	299	37.7	287	93.8	586	53.3
Master's degree	54	6.8	6	2.0	60	5.5
Total[3]	793	100.0	306	100.0	1,099	100.0
Previous employment setting[4]						
Hospital outpatient service	92	12.0	19	6.3	111	10.4
Hospital inpatient service	215	28.0	172	57.1	387	36.2
Health center	133	17.3	16	5.3	149	13.9
Extended care facility	16	2.1	2	.7	18	1.7
Fee-for-service physician	54	7.0	1	.3	55	5.2
Prepaid group practice	12	1.6	—	—	12	1.1
Community/home health agency	148	19.3	40	13.3	188	17.6
School	53	6.9	8	2.7	61	5.7
Teaching	25	3.2	35	11.6	60	5.6
Other[5]	20	2.6	8	2.7	28	2.6
Total[6]	768	100.0	301	100.0	1,069	100.0

[1] Four certificate and one master's student did not supply information on ANA membership.

[2] Ten certificate students did not supply information on the number of years in professional nursing.

[3] One certificate and one master's student did not supply information on prior nursing preparation.

[4] Twenty-three certificate and four master's students had not been previously employed.

[5] Includes settings within state and federal agencies including the armed services, inservice education, and social agencies as well as combined inpatient/outpatient settings.

[6] Three certificate and two master's students did not supply information on previous employment setting.

single group of both certificate and master's students—more than one-quarter of the certificate students and more than one-half of the master's students—was hospital inpatient service. The second most frequently reported previous employment setting was community/home health agency. This is further borne out in Table 1:11. The length of time respondents spent in the job held just prior to entering the NP program is presented in Table 1:12. The majority of NP students had spent less than three years in the job just prior to entering the NP program. Certificate students had spent more time in the job just prior to entering NP programs than master's students. More than 10 percent of the certificate students entered NP programs after they had been in a job for more than 10 years.

Factors Influencing Students to Become NPs

An important question for the first phase of this study was why nurses chose to enter NP programs. The factors cited are presented in Table 1:13. Both certificate and master's NP students most frequently cited the desire to have a greater influence on patient care. The second most important factor was the desire for additional learning opportunities, and the third was the challenge of the work. Among the less important reasons for entering NP programs were increased salary, increased status and opportunity for collaboration with physicians. This subject will be dealt with in greater detail later.

Anticipated Employment

Data on the students' knowledge of their future employment are presented in Table 1:14. It should be noted that 52 of the 86 certificate programs required their applicants to have guaranteed employment at completion of the program. Students in those programs are excluded from the presentation in Table 1:14. Of those students in programs which do not require guaranteed employment, 65 percent of certificate students and 55 percent of master's students had knowledge of their future employment. As might be expected, since most of these NP students come from hospitals, community agencies and health centers, which are often located in urban areas, the majority reported that they expected to serve inner-city populations (Table 1:15).

TABLE 1:11

Percent of NP Students, by Previous Employment Setting, Specialty, and Type of Program

Previous employment setting[1]	Specialty and type of program							
	Pediatric	Midwifery	Maternity	Family	Adult	Psychiatric	Total Pct.	Total No.
	Certificate							
Hospital outpatient service	11	4	7	12	18	NA	12	92
Hospital inpatient service	25	61	31	35	21	NA	28	215
Health center	9	8	19	18	33	NA	17	133
Extended care facility	1	—	3	1	6	NA	2	16
Fee-for-service physician practice	6	—	5	10	6	NA	7	54
Prepaid group practice	1	—	2	3	1	NA	2	12
Community/home health agency	26	11	31	14	8	NA	19	148
School	15	—	—	1	1	NA	7	53
Teaching	4	8	—	2	4	NA	3	25
Other[2]	2	8	2	4	2	NA	3	20
Total pct	100	100	100	100	100	NA	100	
Total no.[3]	332	26	58	181	171	NA		768
	Master's							
Hospital outpatient service	7	2	14	11	—	8	6	19
Hospital inpatient service	77	59	45	40	71	72	57	172
Health center	3	4	7	6	5	8	6	16
Extended care facility	3	—	—	1	—	—	1	2
Fee-for-service physician practice	—	—	—	1	—	—	3	1
Prepaid group practice	—	—	—	—	—	—	—	—
Community/home health agency	—	21	10	25	1	4	13	40
School	7	—	—	3	3	4	3	8
Teaching	3	7	24	10	19	4	12	35
Other[2]	—	7	—	3	1	—	3	8
Total pct.	100	100	100	100	100	100	100	
Total no.[3]	30	53	29	97	66	26		301

[1] Twenty-three certificate and four master's students had not been previously employed.

[2] Includes settings within state and federal agencies including the armed services, in-service education and social agencies as well as combined inpatient/outpatient settings.

[3] Three certificate and two master's students did not supply information on their previous employment settings.

TABLE 1:12

NP Students, by Number of Years in Job Just Prior to Entering NP Program, and Type of Program

Number of years in job just prior to entering NP program	Type of program					
	Certificate		Master's		Total	
	No.	Pct.	No.	Pct.	No.	Pct.
< 2	179	23.7	107	36.4	286	27.2
2	190	25.2	94	32.0	284	27.0
3-5	182	24.1	53	18.0	235	22.4
6-10	125	16.5	29	9.9	154	14.7
11-15	57	7.5	9	3.0	66	6.3
16-20	13	1.7	2	.7	15	1.4
> 20	10	1.3	NA	NA	10	1.0
Total[1]	756	100.0	294	100.0	1,050	100.0
Average	4.5		3.0		4.1	
Median	3		2		2	

[1] Twenty-eight certificate and nine master's students were not employed just prior to entering an NP program. Ten certificate and four master's students did not supply information on the number of years in job just prior to entering NP program.

TABLE 1:13

NP Students by the Most Important Factor Influencing Them to Become NPs, by Type of Program

Factor	Type of program			
	Certificate		Master's	
	No.	Pct.	No.	Pct.
Greater influence on patient care	235	30.7	82	27.4
Additional learning opportunities	199	26.0	72	24.0
Challenge of the work	163	21.3	38	12.7
Frustration of former work	53	7.0	31	10.4
More independence	30	3.9	34	11.4
More responsibility	30	3.9	12	4.0
Collaboration with physicians	7	.9	2	.7
Salary increase	5	.6	5	1.7
Increased status	2	.3	5	1.7
Other[1]	41	5.4	18	6.0
Total[2]	765	100.0	299	100.0

[1] Includes to provide better patient care, for personal benefits such as time and pay, to prepare for a specific job, and because it was recommended by someone else.

[2] Twenty-nine certificate and eight master's students did not supply sufficient information on factors influencing them to become NPs to be included in this distribution.

TABLE 1:14

NP Students, by Whether or Not They Have Knowledge of Future Employment,[1] Specialty, and Type of Program

Specialty	Future employment and type of program					
	Known		Unknown		Total	
	No.	Pct.	No.	Pct.	No.	Pct.
	Certificate					
Pediatric	91	62.8	54	37.2	145	100.0
Midwifery	16	61.5	10	38.5	26	100.0
Maternity	13	50.0	13	50.0	26	100.0
Family	77	73.3	28	26.7	105	100.0
Adult	—	—	—	—	—	—
Total	197	65.2	105	34.8	302	100.0
	Master's					
Pediatric	18	60.0	12	40.0	30	100.0
Midwifery	33	62.3	20	37.7	53	100.0
Maternity	18	60.0	12	40.0	30	100.0
Family	44	44.0	56	56.0	100	100.0
Adult	41	62.1	25	37.9	66	100.0
Psychiatric	15	55.6	12	44.4	27	100.0
Total[2]	169	55.2	137	44.8	306	100.0

[1] Those programs which do not require guaranteed employment are the basis for this presentation. Thirty-four certificate and all 45 master's programs do not require guaranteed employment.

[2] One master's midwifery student did not supply information on whether she had knowledge of future employment.

The study respondents did not rate salary increases as a primary motivating factor to enter NP programs. However, a substantial number of NP students expected an increase. Some differences between certificate and master's students in terms of salary expectations are revealed in Figures 1:4 and 1:5. Only 45 percent of certificate students expected salary increases. Far more master's students (75 percent) expected salary increases. Master's students also had much higher expectations for salary increases than certificate students (an average annual increase of $3,336 compared to $1,358), somewhat more positive expectations regarding salary, and less uncertainty about future salary.

In addition to the positive factors that these students felt had motivated them to enter NP training, the amount of dissatisfaction among

TABLE 1:15

Percent of NP Students, by Anticipated Patient Population, Specialty, and Type of Program

Specialty	Anticipated patient population and type of program					
	Inner city only	Rural only	Both	Other[1]	Total	
					Pct.	. No.
	Certificate					
Pediatric	56.2	22.6	15.1	6.0	100.0	345
Midwifery	53.8	19.2	19.2	7.7	100.0	26
Maternity	43.3	23.3	25.0	8.3	100.0	60
Family	33.0	42.9	18.1	6.0	100.0	182
Adult	49.4	22.0	12.2	16.4	100.0	164
Total[2]	48.3	27.1	16.1	8.5	100.0	777
	Master's					
Pediatric	69.0	10.4	3.4	17.2	100.0	29
Midwifery	63.5	11.5	15.4	9.6	100.0	52
Maternity	65.5	20.7	3.5	10.3	100.0	29
Family	53.1	26.5	10.2	10.2	100.0	98
Adult	53.1	15.6	23.5	7.8	100.0	64
Psychiatric	70.4	7.4	18.5	3.7	100.0	27
Total[2]	59.2	17.7	13.4	9.7	100.0	299

[1] Includes populations such as those in the military, suburban settings, nursing home for retired nuns, technical institute, school for deaf students.

[2] Seventeen certificate and eight master's students did not supply information on anticipated patient population.

respondents in their employment situations before they entered NP training and their expectations following graduation were considered. To obtain this information, the study subjects were asked to respond to eight questions concerned with different aspects of job satisfaction. The job characteristics taken from a questionnaire designed by Arnold Bellinger and the responses from both certificate and master's students are shown in Table 1:16. The characteristics relate primarily to independence, autonomy or authority in planning, decision making and carrying out nursing activities. It is clear from this table that prior job dissatisfaction in regard to these characteristics was common to nurse practitioner students. First, the characteristics were rated very highly in importance, greater than six on a scale of seven. Second, there was a difference of approximately one and one-half for certificate programs and two for

FIGURE 1:4

NP Certificate Students, by Anticipated Salary as an NP

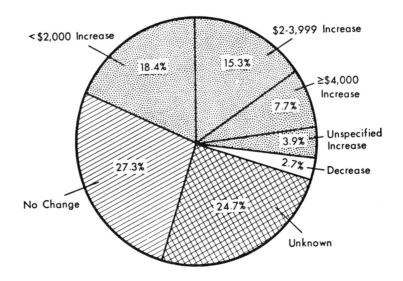

FIGURE 1:5

NP Master's Students, by Anticipated Salary as an NP

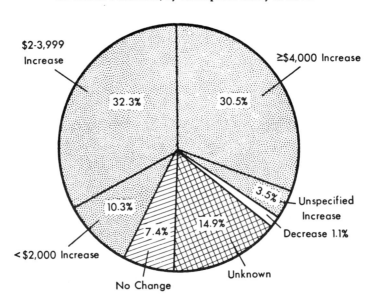

FIGURE 1:6

NP Students' Job Dissatisfaction and Expected Improvement, by Type of Program[1]

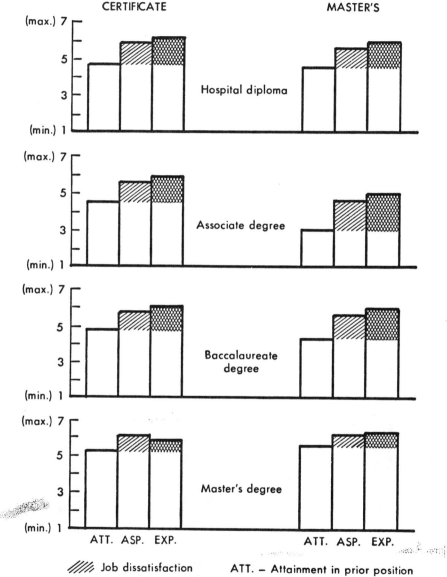

Job dissatisfaction   ATT. — Attainment in prior position
Expected improvement   ASP. — Aspiration in prior position
       EXP. — Expectation as NP

[1]Based on responses to a questionnaire designed by Arnold C. Bellinger, Ph.D., Wayne State University.

TABLE 1:16

Average Response of Students to Selected Job Characteristics in Terms of Attainment and Aspiration in Prior Nursing Position, Importance to the Student, and Expectation in the NP Role, by Type of Program[1]

Job characteristic[2]	Job satisfaction variables and type of program[3]			
	Prior Position		Importance	Expectation as NPs
	Attainment	Aspiration		
Certificate				
Opportunity for planning and organizing your own work routine	4.91	5.81	6.20	6.02
Opportunity to use your own initiative	5.14	6.19	6.44	6.37
On-the-job freedom in your nursing position	4.82	5.77	6.17	6.01
Opportunity for independent thought and action	4.87	6.05	6.38	6.23
Opportunity for participating in the setting of goals	4.60	6.02	6.29	6.18
Opportunity to participate in the decision making process	4.43	5.97	6.34	6.01
Opportunity for participating in determining methods and procedures	4.36	5.83	6.10	5.92
Authority connected with your position	4.47	5.52	5.78	5.72
Overall average	4.70	5.90	6.21	6.06
Standard deviation	1.36	.75	.64	.78
Master's				
Opportunity for planning and organizing your own work routine	4.46	5.64	6.33	6.08
Opportunity to use your own initiative	4.61	6.14	6.54	6.43
On-the-job freedom in your nursing position	4.22	5.61	6.32	6.00
Opportunity for independent thought and action	4.50	6.07	6.55	6.35
Opportunity for participating in the setting of goals	4.23	6.08	6.47	6.25
Opportunity to participate in the decision making process	3.96	5.92	6.43	6.22

TABLE 1:16 (Continued)

Average Response of Students to Selected Job Characteristics in Terms of Attainment and Aspiration in Prior Nursing Position, Importance to the Student, and Expectation in the NP Role, by Type of Program[1]

Job characteristic[2]	Job satisfaction variables and type of program[3]			
	Certificate			
	Prior Position		Importance	Expectation as NPs
	Attainment	Aspiration		
Opportunity for participating in determining methods and procedures	3.92	5.72	6.07	5.96
Authority connected with your position	3.94	5.40	5.83	5.75
Overall average	4.22	5.80	6.32	6.13
Standard deviation	1.35	.81	.57	.73

[1] Fifty-eight certificate and 14 master's students did not supply information on the selected job satisfaction characteristics, so that this presentation is based on responses from 736 certificate and 293 master's students.

[2] The job characteristics are taken from a questionnaire designed by Arnold C. Bellinger, Ph.D., Wayne State University.

[3] The scale used to measure these job satisfaction characteristics ranged from 1 (minimum) to 7 (maximum).

TABLE 1:17

Average Number of Months NP Programs Spend on Specific Functions Within the Didactic Component, by Specialty and Type of Program

Function	Type of program and specialty										
	Certificate					Master's					
	Pedi-atric	Mid-wifery	Mater-nity	Family	Adult	Pedi-atric	Mid-wifery	Mater-nity	Family	Adult	Psychi-atric
1. Taking health and social history; performing physical examination	1.4	1.6	1.1	1.4	1.2	2.4	2.8	2.0	2.3	3.8	2.9
2. Surveillance of essentially well individuals and management of care of the ill	1.1	3.8	1.1	1.7	1.1	2.5	4.6	1.9	2.7	3.2	2.4
3. Teaching, counseling and support of patients/families	1.0	1.5	.8	.9	.7	2.5	2.5	2.5	1.7	2.5	2.2
4. Planning, developing and implementing group educational programs	.2	.8	.2	.2	.3	1.1	1.6	1.2	1.1	1.3	1.3
5. Assessment of quality and effectiveness of nursing practice; use of demographic, social and health data regarding community and population groups to identify high-risk subgroups	.3	.6	.2	.4	.3	1.3	1.3	1.0	1.4	1.2	1.1

TABLE 1:17 (Continued)

Average Number of Months NP Programs Spend on Specific Functions Within the Didactic Component, by Specialty and Type of Program

Function	Certificate					Master's					
	Pedi-atric	Mid-wifery	Mater-nity	Family	Adult	Pedi-atric	Mid-wifery	Mater-nity	Family	Adult	Psychi-atric
6. Other[1]	.4	.7	.6	.6	.2	4.5	4.3	4.4	4.0	1.9	5.1
Total[2]	4.4	9.0	4.0	5.2	3.8	14.3	17.1	13.0	13.2	13.9	15.0

[1] "Other" for certificate programs included role reorientation, understanding the legal aspects of extended roles, and developing cultural sensitivity; and for master's programs, research and scholarly efforts, teaching, supervision, and social, psychological and philosophical issues.

[2] Two pediatric, one midwifery and one family certificate program did not supply information on specific functions. One maternity and one adult master's program did not supply information on specific functions.

TABLE 1:18

Average Percent of Time NP Programs Spend on Specific Functions Within the Didactic Component, by Specialty and Type of Program

Function	Type of program and specialty									
	Certificate				Master's					
	Pedi-atric	Mid-wifery	Mater-nity	Family Adult	Pedi-atric	Mid-wifery	Mater-nity	Family	Adult	Psychi-atric
1. Taking health and social history; performing physical examination	30.8	18.5	27.2	27.0	16.5	16.8	14.8	18.1	25.1	18.9
2. Surveillance of essentially well individuals and management of care of the ill	25.6	37.4	26.1	30.0	18.1	26.6	13.5	21.4	23.2	17.3
3. Teaching, counseling and support of patients/families	22.4	17.7	20.8	16.7	16.9	14.8	18.6	12.7	17.0	14.5
4. Planning, developing and implementing group educational programs	4.6	9.5	6.2	5.2	7.9	9.2	9.5	7.9	10.2	8.6
5. Assessment of quality and effectiveness of nursing practice; use of demographic, social and health data regarding community and population groups to identify high-risk subgroups	6.4	7.1	4.4	8.1	9.1	7.6	8.1	10.0	9.4	7.7

TABLE 1:18 (Continued)

Average Percent of Time NP Programs Spend on Specific Functions Within the Didactic Component, by Specialty and Type of Program

Function	Type of program and specialty										
	Certificate					Master's					
	Pedi-atric	Mid-wifery	Mater-nity	Family	Adult	Pedi-atric	Mid-wifery	Mater-nity	Family	Adult	Psychi-atric
6. Other[1]	10.2	9.8	15.3	13.0	4.4	31.5	25.0	35.5	29.9	15.1	33.0
Total[2]	100.0	100.0	100.0	100.0	100.0	100.0	100.0	100.0	100.0	100.0	100.0

[1] For certificate programs this included role reorientation, understanding the legal aspects of extended roles, and developing cultural sensitivity; and for master's programs, research and scholarly efforts, teaching, supervision, and social, psychological and philosophical issues.

[2] Two pediatric, one midwifery and one family certificate program did not supply information on specific functions. One maternity and one adult master's program did not supply information on specific functions.

master's programs between the students' attainment in their prior position and their expectation for their next position as nurse practitioners (Figure 1:6). Interestingly, the certificate and master's students both appeared to have about the same levels of aspiration and expectation. Since master's students were slightly less satisfied with their attainment, however, their expected improvement is slightly greater.

Content

The preparation of NP students to perform specific tasks was also studied (Tables 1:17 and 1:18). Although master's programs spend considerably more time on most of these functions than do certificate programs, the proportion of total time is smaller.

Program Evaluation

An area of very great interest was the evaluation of the programs. Unfortunately not every program in this study submitted to an extensive evaluation of its components. Only 63 (73 percent) of certificate programs and 20 (44 percent) of master's programs evaluated themselves. On Table 1:19, five characteristics are shown which were of interest for purposes of evaluation. Both certificate and master's programs placed primary importance on the competence of their graduates, the degree of

TABLE 1:19

NP Programs, by Characteristic Evaluated and Type of Program

Characteristic evaluated	Type of program			
	Certificate		Master's	
	Number	Percent[1]	Number	Percent[1]
Effect of the graduates' employment on the availability of health care	22	34.9	4	20.0
Effect of the graduates' employment on the cost of health care	8	12.7	1	5.0
Competence of the graduates	40	63.5	13	65.0
Degree of independence with which the graduates function	50	79.4	10	50.0
Match of the graduates' functions and responsibilities with those for which they were trained	50	79.4	12	60.0

[1] This presentation is based on the 63 certificate programs and 20 master's programs which evaluated their programs.

independence with which their graduates function and whether their graduates could do what they were prepared to do. It is apparent that the programs' own evaluations were directed toward assessing the adequacy of their educational efforts.

CONCLUSIONS

As in most ventures into uncharted territory, a variety of approaches to NP preparation has occurred naturally. The development of nurse practitioner preparatory programs reflects the broadest possible range of professional judgment as to length, content, faculty, and so forth. It would be inconceivable that the programs under study which vary so much can produce nurse practitioners of equal competence and probability for successful careers. On the other hand, it is quite possible that the factors that determine NP preparation are completely outweighed by the characteristics of the employment setting as the major determinant of future success.

The data presented here provide the first half of the information necessary to answer these questions. The data being collected regarding NP employment will complete the information necessary to judge the relative effects of NP preparation, characteristics and setting, as well as factors affecting subsequent NP roles and functions. Whereas the Phase I information permits comparison of programs, subsequent phases of study will allow for standards of success to be included in such comparisons.

Note

1. See Harry A. Sultz and Louis Kinyon, "Longitudinal Study of Nurse Practitioners: Phase I," HEW, Division of Nursing Bureau of Health Manpower, Health Resources Administration (March 1976), HRA-76-43 for the results and complete data.

Chapter 2

The Physician's Assistant:
Profile of a New Health Profession

Donald W. Fisher and Susan M. Horowitz

HISTORICAL EVOLUTION

The history of the concept, training and utilization of the mid-level health professional known as a physician's assistant (PA) began in 1965 when Dr. Eugene A. Stead, Jr., instituted a two-year training program for the assistant to the primary care physician at Duke University in Durham, North Carolina. Dr. Stead's program to train physician's assistants followed his unsuccessful attempt with Thelma Ingles, RN, in the late 1950s and early 1960s, to train master's degree nurse practitioners at Duke University. The program was denied accreditation on three occasions by the National League for Nursing, which is the accrediting agency for degree-granting nursing programs, on the basis that the assumption of medical tasks by nurses was at least inappropriate and perhaps dangerous. Failure to achieve accreditation necessitated phaseout of the nurse practitioner program and caused Dr. Stead to turn his attention to training ex-military corpsmen as physician's assistants.

In 1969, Dr. Richard A. Smith began a one-year MEDEX program at the University of Washington, Seattle, to augment the training of former independent-duty military medical corpsmen who it was felt could help meet the demand for physician services, especially in rural areas. Soon thereafter, Stanford University Medical Center in California initiated a two-year program. About the same time, a four-year college-based physician's assistant training program was started at Alderson-Broaddus College in Phillippi, West Virginia, and a five-year Child Health Associate Program was begun by Dr. Henry Silver at the University of Colorado in Denver.[1] These demonstration programs soon attracted interest and intellectual support from other innovative physician educators throughout the nation. By 1972, thirty-one programs were in operation: twenty-one of the programs were federally supported from agencies such as the Office of Economic Opportunity, the Model Cities Program, the Veterans Ad-

40

ministration, the Public Health Service, the Department of Defense, and the Department of Labor, while the remainder were financed by private foundations and institutional sources.

In June 1972, the Bureau of Health Manpower, Health Resources Administration, DHEW, mandated by Section 774a of The Public Health Service Act as amended by PL 93-157, "The Comprehensive Health Manpower Training Act of 1971," assumed responsibility for twenty-four of the thirty-one programs and initiated contracts with sixteen developing programs. This federal support represented an investment in experimental programs to test the hypothesis that mid-level health professionals could provide many physician-equivalent services in primary and continuing care. Under the Bureau's direction, the programs were designed to carry out the intent of Congress to relieve problems of geographic and specialty maldistribution of health manpower and to improve access to primary health care for large urban and rural populations through the efficient utilization of health manpower. This intent was reflected in the contract process which required each PA program to emphasize three major objectives in its demonstration: (1) train for delivery of primary care in ambulatory settings; (2) place graduates in medically underserved areas; and (3) recruit residents of medically underserved areas, minority groups and women. Each program was free to devise various curricula and methods of instruction, but the above three requirements were held constant to carry out the intent of Congress.

It is worthy of note that the Comprehensive Health Manpower Training Act of 1971 did not restrict the training of physician's assistants to medical schools. Rather there was an attempt to foster the concept that basic and clinical sciences necessary for preparation as a physician's assistant could be adequately provided in academic settings other than medical schools. It was also conjectured that programs whose parent institution was located in or adjacent to medically underserved areas might best fulfill the intent of Congress by orienting students toward the primary ambulatory care needs of these areas. This was a deliberate attempt to contrast the emphasis medical schools placed on specialty in-patient care given in teaching hospitals. Finally, it was hoped that the diverse educational and health care experience of the students might be more easily accepted in a nontraditional medical academic center. All programs were encouraged to develop educational pathways which would build on a student's individual academic and prior health experience, and to devise a choice among such credentials as a certificate or an academic degree.

The total number of programs has remained fairly constant. Since the summer of 1972, ten new programs have begun, four programs have closed,* and it is expected that four more will terminate upon graduation of their current students.** Reasons for closing have varied, but for the most part involved economic support problems, graduate placement difficulties within the confines of the geographic catchment area of the program, and lack of adequate support for the physician extender concept by other health care providers.

LOCATION OF TRAINING PROGRAMS

The 56 primary care assistant programs currently matriculating students are located in 30 states and the District of Columbia. Figure 2:1 depicts the number of primary care programs by U.S. Census Region. Continued federal investment in the physician's assistant concept is anticipated. Currently Congress has included the authority for further support of training programs for the assistant to the primary care practitioner within the general scope of health manpower legislation.

CURRICULUM CONTENT AND STRUCTURE

Physician's assistants are trained to be interdependent practitioners under physician supervision. This is in contrast to some nurse practitioners, who view themselves as independent practitioners in the expanded role of nursing. This interdependent nature of the physician's assistant is evidenced in the structure and content of program curricula.

Throughout the development process there have been essentially three basic types of physician's assistant programs:

- The MEDEX program, originally designed for former independent-duty military corpsmen, requires 12-15 months of study. This usually involves three months of intensive didactic work in basic and clinical sciences at a university medical center followed by a preceptorship with a practicing physician for 9-12 months. The student, upon completion, receives a certificate.

- The university medical center-based program consists of a two-year training period beginning with 9-12 months of didactic work in basic and clinical sciences followed by 12-15 months of various clinical rotations in tertiary care centers and preceptorships in private practice settings. Upon completion, students receive a certificate and/or a baccalaureate degree.

---

*University of California, San Diego; University of Mississippi; University of North Dakota MEDEX; Dartmouth MEDEX.

**Indiana University; University of Alabama (Medical); University of Cincinnati (Urologic); U.S. Army, Fort Sam Houston, Texas.

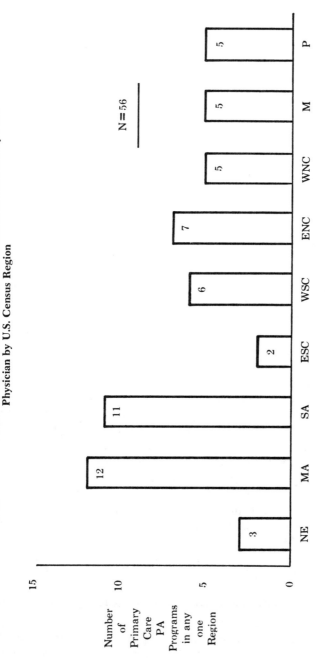

FIGURE 2:1

Geographical Distribution of Training Programs for the Assistant to the Primary Care Physician by U.S. Census Region

Census Regions of the United States[1]

[1] NE = New England; MA = Middle Atlantic; SA = South Atlantic;; ESC = East South Central; WSC = West South Central; ENC = East North Central; WNC = West North Central; M = Mountain; P = Pacific

- The college or university program in a nonmedical school setting requires about two years of training beginning with 9-12 months of basic and clinical didactic work followed by 10-15 months of clinical rotations in an affiliated teaching hospital and local community-based preceptorships. These programs result in a certificate, or an associate or baccalaureate degree for those students completing the program.[2]

Selection criteria of programs and the varied backgrounds of the candidates have influenced the length of the programs. Today, programs range from 12-42 months with the majority of programs being 24 months in length.

Curricula for physician's assistant programs were developed around five fundamental functions which establish the parameters of practice of a physician's assistant, namely the ability: (1) to elicit a comprehensive health history, (2) to perform a comprehensive physical examination, (3) to perform simple diagnostic laboratory determinations and to understand their values, (4) to perform basic treatment procedures for common illnesses, and (5) to make an appropriate clinical response to commonly encountered emergency care situations.[3]

To provide the student with an understanding of the theoretical concepts of disease process, the didactic curriculum includes such basic science courses as anatomy, physiology, pathology, microbiology and pharmacology, as well as courses in behavioral sciences and medical ethics. The clinical curriculum provides students with an opportunity to apply basic science knowledge to the needs of the patients they encounter in both inpatient and ambulatory settings. The clinical curriculum includes courses in clinical diagnosis and rotations in clinical medicine, surgery, pediatrics, ob-gyn and psychiatry. The care of patients commonly encountered in primary care practice is stressed.

The most important element of the training process is the preceptorship phase. Fee-for-service sites, solo and group practices, university medical centers, health maintenance organizations or prepaid groups, public health departments, prisons, specialty hospitals, and military installations provide a broad experience which orients the student toward primary, ambulatory care. No comparative studies have been conducted at this time from which conclusions could be drawn about the relative merit of any one setting over another.

As physician's assistant programs evolved, it became apparent that in addition to the essential elements of clinical medicine it was necessary to introduce the caring and preventive health concepts physician's assistants would be required to use in their practice. Questions were raised as to whether programs would be of adequate caliber if located outside the confines of the academic medical center and whether the traditional basic medical science courses could be compressed within the short length of program in order to augment the varied educational backgrounds of students. This new orientation in primary care content and presentation sought the active participation of private community practitioners in addition to the clinical faculty. The private practitioners' identification of the essential elements of the daily delivery of primary care guided the development of behavioral objectives for both basic and clinical sciences. In many schools the resultant interaction created a dialogue between medical academicians and practicing physicians, and may have been a precursor of the current methods used to orient medical students to general and family practice. As one might expect, these educational innovations presented a distinct challenge and burden for program directors and administrators who were faced with a need to use untested educational theories and to raise the faculty's consciousness about the concept so that they could teach relevant material. In addition, the program staff had to evaluate carefully the impact of this new orientation on students.

Today, the faculty of physician's assistant programs is a combination of university and community physicians. Program directors bring them together frequently in an attempt to increase their awareness of students' needs relative to their previous educational and practical experience. The PA program faculty must also keep informed about the evolving role of the physician's assistant in the health care delivery system and inform students of the many different approaches to health care.

Accompanying the need for an atypical medical curriculum for the physician's assistant has been the development of audiovisual and computer-based educational techniques. In many programs, economic necessity initiated the use of these techniques, but it has become apparent that they do provide instruction and self-assessment for the student as well as a familiar mechanism by which the PA can pursue lifelong learning through continuing medical education.

This new presentation of clinical medicine content has resulted in an elaborate program accreditation mechanism which seeks the answers to specific questions. Does the program employ a full-time academic coordinator and a medical director? Are there adequate course outlines with specific objectives available for each unit? Is there a well-defined feedback or follow-up method used for curricular coordination and test development? How many full-time and part-time faculty members are there and do they provide the students with effective evaluations? What is the faculty's relationship to the community? What self-tutorial and self-assessment techniques are available for the student? Lastly, does the program have routine faculty meetings to draw together the clinical and basic science faculties with the program administrators and physician preceptors?

SELECTION OF CANDIDATES

Only a limited number of students may be enrolled each year. Consequently, the physician's assistant selection process is highly competitive. It is estimated that there are generally 1,000 applicants for each class, the average enrollment of which is 35 students. The evolution of the current selection criteria for PA programs has been guided by the successes and failures of traditional medical school selection processes. A recent recommendation put forth from a conference sponsored by the Teachers of Preventive Medicine at the Fogarty International Center called for medical schools to reexamine their admission procedures as well as to recruit future physicians who will work in health care teams.[4] Today, the primary consideration in the selection of physician's assistant students is the role of the physician's assistant in the delivery of care in the United States. Program admissions committees endeavor to select individuals who can function as interdependent practitioners in the team delivery of health care.

Each physician's assistant program admissions committee is composed of faculty, staff and student members. This committee seeks information which will allow its members to gain a better understanding of each applicant's background and motivation for wanting to become a physician's assistant. Each candidate's application is carefully reviewed to determine his or her patient care experience, academic achievement (especially in math and science), college entrance examination results (Scholastic Aptitude Test, American College Test, Miller Analogies Test and others), personal references and the applicant's personal statement of his or her future role as a physician's assistant. Following this review, but prior to final selection, those applicants most qualified in the opinion of the admissions committee, are requested to visit the program for an interview. At this time the applicant meets with program administrators, affiliated practicing physicians, program faculty and physician's assistant graduates and students. The interview process is mutually beneficial because it not only permits the admissions committee to gain a better understanding of the applicant, but gives a prospective student an opportunity to learn about the program. During the interview many programs require the candidate to complete specific psychological tests such as the Minnesota Multiphasic Personality Inventory and the Sixteen Personality Factors Test. Preliminary data from an ongoing study of PA program selection processes indicate that the interview is the most crucial component of the selection process for those candidates who are academically qualified.[5]

TUITION

Studies of training costs indicate that the tuition charged to the PA student does not cover actual costs. Variant costs among programs appear to be attributable to geographic location, managerial structure of the parent institution, use of teaching hospitals, and services of clinical faculty and preceptors, among other factors.[6]

Current data from the Association of Physician Assistant Programs show that thirty-three programs for the assistant to the primary care physician require students to assume tuition and fees in addition to their room and board. Here are the estimated first-year expenses for the 1976-77 academic year:[7]

Expense	Range	Average	Median
Tuition	$160-3,800	$1,400	$1,000
Resident	160-3,900	1,954	1,800
Nonresident	800-4,000	2,166	2,100
Room and Board (Minimum)	1,900-4,000	2,950	3,000

Decreasing federal support and rising costs of higher education for all health professions will continue to necessitate a greater financial investment on the part of students.

DEMOGRAPHIC CHARACTERISTICS OF GRADUATES AND STUDENTS

A proliferation of training programs since 1972 has resulted in an increase in the number of graduates in recent years. The first graduating class of physician's assistants in 1967 were, with one exception, all white males. Since then there has been an increase in the graduation of minority physician's assistants and a gradual decline in the number of male graduates. The 1975 and 1976 graduating classes reported 25 percent of the graduates being female. Also, as one might expect, the average age of physician's assistants at graduation has generally declined since 1970, the average age at graduation now being thirty years.[8] These trends have been supported further by a recent survey of physician's assistants who were graduated prior to 1975.[9] The average age of respondents was 32.5 years; 6 percent of the respondents were Black, 3.6 percent Chicano/Mexican American and 3.6 percent American Indian and Oriental. A large number (71 percent) of graduates were married, 16.6 percent single, and 3.8 percent divorced.

Most program admissions criteria require that an individual has demonstrated competence either at a high level of education such as college or in related health experiences. Ninety-nine percent of those admitted to PA programs hold a high school diploma and 92 percent have had prior health experience, with the majority of those having a combination of three years of college and more than three years of health related experience. Consequently, for many applicants entry into a physician's assistant program appears to be a change of career from medical technology, pharmaceutical sales, respiratory therapy, nursing, and so forth. By no means should it be deduced that one's ability to meet the minimum basic competencies to practice as a physician's assistant requires this combination of college and health related experience. To date there have been no definitive studies to draw any conclusions about the merits of prior college or health experience background.

PRACTICE PROFILE

A recent study of 1,250 physician's assistants who graduated prior to 1975 indicated that: 23 percent are in family practice, 22 percent in general medicine, 15 percent in internal medicine, 5 percent in pediatrics, and 2 percent in obstetrics/gynecology.[10]

If one considers that these clinical specialties deliver the bulk of primary care, the conclusion might be drawn from Figure 2:2 that as of 1975, 67 percent of graduates were employed in primary care. Only 8 percent are practicing for specialists identified by the respondents as surgeons. The remaining 25 percent are in nonprimary care categories such as emergency medicine, education, administration and clinical research.

More than 42 percent of the graduates are located in non-metropolitan counties with populations between 10,000 to 50,000. As seen in Table 2:1 PAs have gone to areas with sparse health care resources, which is especially significant when considering the percent of nonfederal physicians practicing in these areas. Table 2:1, however, should be interpreted with caution, since the data tabulated for Total Population, Total Nonfederal Physicians and Total PAs and Medex were collected from different years.

FIGURE 2:2

Practice Setting of 1,250 PA Graduates in 1975

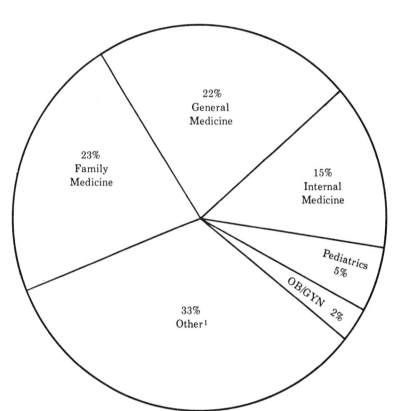

22%
General
Medicine

23%
Family
Medicine

15%
Internal
Medicine

Pediatrics
5%

OB/GYN 2%

33%
Other [1]

[1] Program administration and education 20%; surgery 8%; clinical research, specialty practices, emergency medicine, 5%

The highest concentration of PAs exists in the southern and Pacific regions of the United States, as indicated in Figure 2:3.

No conclusions should be drawn between the location of programs by census region as displayed in Figure 2:1 and the concentrations of practicing PAs in these regions as seen in Figure 2:3, because of the fluidity of employment and the variations in enabling legislation by state for physician's assistants.

A study conducted in 1975 by the Association of Physician Assistant Programs indicates that the annual compensation for all graduates

FIGURE 2:3

Percent of Distribution of Physician's Assistants and Medex by Census Region

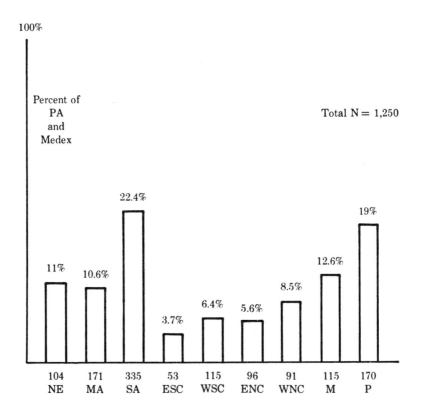

averages $14,300, which has been substantiated in the more recent Scheffler study. However, this average salary should be qualified as the majority of respondents were only in their first or second year of employment. Table 2:2 shows the average annual salary of PAs by type of employer, and indicates that average salary does not differ substantially among various practice settings.

Tables 2:3 and 2:4 exhibit the total annual compensation of a sample of 556 graduates by year of graduation. In 1974, forty percent of the graduates were paid an annual compensation of more than $15,000. Of these, 10 percent earned more than $20,000. Also, the majority of graduates in the survey had been employed less than two years. Displayed in Table 2:4 is annual compensation shown as a function of the year of graduation. All of the 1968 graduates earned more than $15,000 and sixty-eight percent of the 1971 graduates earned more than $15,000. The percentage of graduates earning more than $15,000 diminished by 1974.

ISSUES AFFECTING THE FUTURE OF THE CONCEPT

Continued federal investment in the education of physician's assistants is anticipated in new health manpower legislation. In addition, many state legislatures have recognized the benefit of training physician's assistants to augment the delivery of health care to the residents of their states. As a result, the future fiscal support for programs will be tied firmly through legislative action to identified state health manpower needs and state institutional capacities for training.

However, there are issues for consideration which portend problems for continued support of the physician's assistant concept. Reimbursement, malpractice insurance and interprofessional conflicts are well known possible impediments to the future of the PA concept; but then these problems threaten the rest of the health care delivery system as well.

Less talked about, but equally germane to program continuation, are issues related to the education of physician's assistants. For instance,

TABLE 2:1

Distribution of PAs and Medex by Demographic County Classification, with % of Total
U.S. Resident Population, and % of Distribution of Nonfederal Physicians

Demographic County Classification[1]	% Total U.S. Resident Population as of 12/31/72	% Total Non-federal Physician Population	% Total PAs and Medex Population[2]
Nonmetro 10,000	2.2	.7	7.8
Nonmetro 10,000-24,999	7.2	2.6	8.9
Nonmetro 25,000-49,999	7.6	4.0	10.6
Nonmetro 50,000	7.7	5.3	15.6
Potential SMSA 60,000	2.0	1.3	1.2
Metro 499,999	18.6	16.9	19.5
Metro 500,000-999,999	13.2	13.5	11.4
Metro 1,000,000-4,999,9999	29.9	37.4	18.8
Metro 5,000,000	11.5	17.4	6.0

[1] Distribution of Physicians in the United States, 1972, AMA Center for Health Services Research and Development.

[2] Survey Results: Project on the Status of Physician's Assistants and Medex, Richard M. Scheffler, Ph.D., University of North Carolina, Chapel Hill, N.C., February 1976.

TABLE 2:2

Average Annual Salary of PAs & Medex by Type of Employer—1975

Type of Employer	PAs	Medex
Private Solo Practice	$15,141	$14,019
Partnership or Group	15,000	14,396
Clinic	13,736	15,078
Nonprofit Hospital	14,442	15,875
Government Hospital	13,071	14,115
Nursing Home	14,505	12,000
Other Hospital	14,706	*
Other Institution	15,955	17,367
Average All Types	14,342	14,555

* Too few observations for calculating purposes.

TABLE 2:3

Total Annual Compensation Paid In 1974

Salary	Percent of Graduates
< $10,000	7
$10,000—$15,000	53
$15,000-$20,000	30
> $20,000	10

TABLE 2:4

Total Annual Compensation by Year of Graduation

Year of Grad.	Number of Graduates	Compensation Paid			
		< $10,000	$10,000-$15,000	$15,000-$20,000	> $20,000
'68	9			56%	44%
'69	8			63%	37%
'70	8		50%	25%	25%
'71	25	12%	20%	52%	16%
'72	77	2%	40%	45%	13%
'73	181	3%	54%	33%	10%
'74	248	7%	65%	23%	5%
Totals	556	4%	54%	32%	10%

Average Compensation All Graduates: $14,300

there continue to be variations in the type and duration of their education. It is not known yet whether individual differences in institutional approaches to training produce graduates with dissimilar competencies.

In many institutions, the introduction of a new educational program has produced a strain on existing medical faculty and departmental commitments. As a result, some students are being placed in medical school classes which may not be appropriate for the role for which they are being trained. Because the PA is not trained as an independent practitioner, his/her ultimate practice role and acceptance by physicians is dependent in part upon effective clinical models in PA and medical education programs. To date, there are too few graduate PAs who can serve as role models.

Finally, the economic reality of limited federal, state, and institutional resources accentuates the competitiveness for funds needed for program initiation, development, and continuation. The fiscal needs of medical and nursing schools to maintain or expand class size and to initiate innovative forms of existing education, present formidable barriers to those educators who desire to begin new PA training programs. State educational budgets place similar restraints on community colleges eager to start PA programs in response to community needs and student interest. All PA programs are required continually to undertake cost control efforts in response to the intense auditing of resources being directed toward PA training and education.

While these issues are constraining forces in some parts of the nation, they are accepted challenges for changing the health care system in other parts. The influence of these issues on the national expansion of new programs for training PAs should be considered in the context of the rapid development of this educational program and the positive impact it already appears to have had on medical education and the health care delivery system.

Notes

1. U.S. Department of Health, Education and Welfare, *The Training and Utilization of Assistants to the Primary Care Physician: An Overview*, an unpublished working paper, Division of Medicine, January 1976.

2. *Ibid.*

3. L.M. Detmer, *1975 Physician's Assistants—Education, Accreditation, and Consumer Acceptance*, prepared for the 25th Annual Group Health Institute of the Group Health Foundation, June 23, 1975, Chicago, Illinois.

4. U.S. Department of Health, Education and Welfare, *New Health Practitioners*, Robert L. Kane, ed. Presented at a conference sponsored by The John E. Fogarty Interna-

tional Center for Advanced Study in the Health Sciences and the Association of the Teachers of Preventive Medicine, May 1974 Pub. No. (NIH) 75-875.

5. Eugene Schneller, 1975 Duke University, Physician's Associates' Careers. DHEW contract, HRA N01-MB4416, in process.

6. System Sciences, Inc., "Physician Extender Training and Deployment Study," in process (1976), DHEW/HRA 230-75-0198.

7. Association of Physician Assistant Programs 1976-1977, *National New Health Practitioner Program Profile.* 2nd ed. (1976), Washington, D.C.

8. *Ibid.*

9. Richard M. Scheffler, "Factors Affecting the Training and Employment Demand for Physician's Assistants," in process, University of N.C., Chapel Hill, North Carolina (1975), DHEW, HRA N01-MB44184.

10. T. Aschenbrenner and S. Horowitz, "Working Papers," BHM, HRA, DHEW, Division of Medicine, Bethesda, Maryland (1976).

Chapter 3

A Comparative Study of New Health Practitioners in Connecticut

Barbara Ley Toffler

In July 1975, a study of New Health Practitioners (NHPs) in Connecticut was initiated under the aegis of the Center for the Study of Health Services at Yale University. This research represented a multidisciplinary project involving members of the Medical School, the Physician's Associate Program, the School of Nursing, the School of Organization and Management, the University Health Services and the Community Health Care Center Plan. The focus of the study was the investigation of specific activities performed and attitudes held by NHPs toward self and job during their first six months post-training work experience. The study further examined NHP supervisors' reports of the impact of NHPs on patient load and time spent with patients.

Questionnaires were distributed by mail to 107 practitioners, who were either (1) members of the 1975 graduating classes of the Yale School of Nursing and the Yale Physician's Associate Program, or (2) Physician's Assistants, Nurse Practitioners and Nurse Midwives practicing in Connecticut who had graduated from other NHP training programs since 1972. Sixty-six NHPs returned completed questionnaires.* Table 3:1 shows the number of respondents in each NHP role. The Physician's Assistant category included graduates of both two-year PA programs and twelve month MEDEX programs; the Nurse Practitioner category included both two-year masters degree graduates and short-term program certificate recipients. The Nurse Midwife category represented a more biased sample than either of the other two groups, inasmuch as all Nurse Midwives were graduates of the Yale School of Nursing and eight of the thirteen midwife respondents were employed in a Yale facility. With the agreement and cooperation of the respondents, questionnaires

---

*Of the 29 1975 Yale PA and YSN program graduates contacted, 8 did not respond; 7 of these nonrespondents were practicing out of state. Of the 78 NHPs practicing in Connecticut who were contacted, 33 did not respond; two-thirds of these nonrespondents were graduates of programs other than Yale.

were also distributed to their supervisors. Fifty of the 66 supervisors contacted had responded by the time data analysis was initiated. The breakdown of supervisors according to type of role supervised is also found in Table 3:1.

TABLE 3:1

Participants in Study

New Health Practitioners		Supervisors	
Physician's Assistant	24	PA Supervisors	15
Nurse Practitioners	29	NP Supervisors	22
Nurse Midwives	13	NMW Supervisors	13
	66		50

The mean age of each group of participants in the study is presented in Table 3:2. On the average, NHPs in this study were about nine years younger than the individuals who supervised them.

TABLE 3:2

Age of NHPs and Supervisors

	mean	s.d.		mean	s.d.
PA	30.2	5.13	PA Supervisors	42.86	8.30
NP	34.93	7.29	NP Supervisors	40.90	9.29
NMW	30	3.96	NMW Supervisors	38.38	3.28
Total Group Mean:	31.38		Total Group Mean:	40.71	

A tally of NHP roles and supervisors by sex is seen in Table 3:3.

TABLE 3:3

Sex of NHPs and Supervisors

	Male	Female		Male	Female
PA	18 (75%)	6 (25%)	PA Supervisors	13 (87%)	2 (13%)
NP	2 (7%)	27 (93%)	NP Supervisors	17 (77%)	5 (23%)
NMW	0 (100%)	13 (100%)	NMW Supervisors	5 (38%)	8 (62%)

As this table indicates, each type of NHP role tended to be characterized by a single sex: proportionately more PAs were male while more NPs and NMWs were almost entirely female. On the other hand, both PA and NP supervisors tended to be male, while NMW supervisors were predominantly female. While most PAs and NPs reported their supervisors to be physicians, NMWs seemed to find some difficulty in identifying a supervisor and ultimately reported a senior nurse midwife as the principal supervisor.

The types of practice settings in which the NHPs in this study were working are seen in Table 3:4. "Hospital" included university, community and VA hospitals as well as schools of nursing; "private practice" included both solo and group settings; "HMO" included primary care clinics and prepaid health plans; and the fourth category was made up of alcoholism and methadone clinics, Planned Parenthood and family planning clinics, Visiting Nurse Associations, and state or municipal health departments.

TABLE 3:4

Type of Practitioner in Each Type of Practice Setting

	PA	NP	NMW
Hospital (includes nursing school)	10 (42%)	10 (34%)	12 (93%)
MD's and Private Practice	5 (21%)	2 (6%)	1 (7%)
HMO	7 (29%)	10 (34%)	0
Clinic, VNA, State or City Health Dept.	2 (8%)	7 (26%)	0
	24 (100%)	29 (100%)	13 (100%)

As shown, almost half of the entire NHP sample was employed in a hospital setting. However, while both PAs and NPs were represented in all types of health organizations, NMWs were primarily hospital-based with only a single member of this group employed in a private practice setting.*

---

*Midwife employment settings in Connecticut appear to be changing, however. Subsequent to the collection of these study data, two midwives formerly employed in hospital settings reported recent job changes to HMOs.

The percentage of increase in patients served as a result of employment of each type of NHP is seen in Table 3:5. Included in the table is the range of percentages reported by the supervisors.

TABLE 3:5

Percent Increase in Patient Population Served
(as reported by Supervisors)

		mean	range
PA	(N = 15)	11.4%	3-20%
NP	(N = 22)	26	2-100
NMW	(N = 13)	24.5	10-100

As can be seen, supervisors of PAs reported their increase in patient population to be less than half of that reported for NPs and NMWs. Further, the range among PA supervisors was considerably narrower than among the other two groups—differences which may reflect the variety of practice settings and types of task activities performed or possibly a lack of clarity or convergence of opinion among supervisors as to the amounts of responsibility and autonomy which an NPH can or should assume.

Difference of supervisor perceptions of the NHP role can be seen in Table 3:6.

TABLE 3:6

Role of NHP (as reported by Supervisor)

Percent of supervisors who see NHP as substitute for physician	25%
Percent of supervisors who see NHP as complement to physician	61%
Percent of supervisors who see NHP as both	14%

Among supervisors who viewed NHPs as *substitutes* for the physician, were PA and NP supervisors who worked in hospital, family planning, or planned parenthood settings. Supervisors of NMWs and supervisors of PAs and NPs in private practice settings viewed the NHP as a *complement* to the physician.

The amount of time spent by the NHP per patient unit, as reported by supervisors, is presented in Table 3:7. The range of time reported within each group is also given.

TABLE 3:7

Time in Minutes Spent by NHP Per Patient Visit
(as reported by Supervisors)

		mean	range
PA	(N = 15)	20.5 minutes	1-30 minutes
NP	(N = 22)	34	10-90
NMW	(N = 13)	21.9	15-30

The major difference to emerge was between the NPs and the other two groups. According to their supervisors, NPs spent an average of one and one-half times as long as the other two groups per patient visit and, in addition, demonstrated a wider range of time spent per patient visit than either PAs or NMWs. This may reflect a wider diversity in practice settings and task activities among the NPs.

TABLE 3:8

Tasks PAs Tend to do More than NPs or NMWs

Task	Percent of Reporting NHPs Who Do (D) Each Task and Percent Who Are Required (R) To Do Each Task					
	PAs (N=24)		NPs (N=29)		NMWs (N=13)	
	D	R	D	R	DR	
Decided drug therapy based on clinical judgment outside standing orders	87.5%	71.4%	57.7%	50.0%	18.2%	18.2%
Debride and Suture Lacerations	86.4	80.0	0	0	25.0	12.5
Remove Foreign Objects	86.4	65.0	22.7	14.3	25.0	12.5
Draw Arterial Blood	61.9	52.6	26.3	21.1	40.0	20.0
Supervise Staff Nurses	60.0	44.4	47.8	34.8	20.0	20.0
Start Blood Infusion	57.1	52.6	0	0	22.2	22.2
Aspirate Joints and/or Inject Medication into Joints	52.4	57.9	0	0	0	0
Do Cutdown	38.1	47.4	0	0	0	0
Do Lumbar Puncture	35.3	33.3	0	0	0	0
Do Sigmoidoscopy	26.3	41.2	0	0	0	0
Do Thoracentesis	12.5	28.6	0	0	0	0
Do Paracentesis	6.3	28.6	0	0	0	0

TASK ACTIVITIES

Questionnaires distributed to both NHPs and supervisors included a list of 51 specific task activities. Analyses of task list data from the NHP questionnaires suggested that for each NHP role there was a set of tasks which members of that role tended to perform more than members of other NHP roles. Further analyses also revealed discrepancies between required and tasks actually done, i.e. some practitioners reported that their job descriptions required performance of tasks which they were not, in fact, actually doing. Those tasks which PAs did more than NPs or NMWs are listed in Table 3:8. It also indicates the percent of NHPs who *actually did* each task, in contrast to the percent who were required to do each task.

Data in Table 3:8 indicate that PAs performed procedures—particularly invasive procedures—requiring technical skill more than either NPs

TABLE 3:9

Tasks NMWs Tend To Do More Than PAs or NPs

Task	Percent of Reporting NHPs Who Do (D) Each Task and Percent Who Are Required (R) To Do Each Task					
	NMWs (N=13)		PAs (N=24)		NPs (N=29)	
	D	R	D	R	D	R
Deliver Baby	100.0%	100.0%	20.0%	20.0%	0	0
Insert IUD	100.0	91.7	30.8	18.2	26.3	21.1
Do Episiotomy and Episiotomy Repair 1°	100.0	100.0	40.0	30.0	0	0
Do Developmental Counseling	91.7	83.3	55.6	35.3	73.1	65.4
Do Abortion Counseling	91.7	83.3	58.8	40.0	65.2	60.9
Do Vaginal Smears	91.7	83.3	52.9	33.3	56.5	31.8
Do HCT	90.9	90.9	42.3	46.7	29.4	34.6
Take History Using Only Algorithm or Printed Form	80.0	70.0	45.5	60.0	45.5	34.8
Do Internal Fetal Monitoring	75.0	66.7	10.0	11.1	0	0
Do Episiotomy and Episiotomy Repair 2°	75.0	58.3	10.0	10.0	0	0
Do Episiotomy and Episiotomy Repair 3°	58.3	16.7	0	0	0	0
Do Episiotomy and Episiotomy Repair 4°	33.3	16.7	0	0	0	0

or NMWs. The data also suggest that PAs performed activities demonstrating a high level of responsibility and autonomy, as indicated by the percentage of PAs who "decide drug therapy based on clinical judgment outside standing orders" and who "supervise staff nurses." It is important to note that this table does not include data on amount of supervision required for each task. The actual doing of the above tasks does *not* indicate that they were performed without supervision, i.e., the amount of autonomy indicated by performance of a specific task is modified, differentially, by the amount of supervision required for its performance.

Those tasks which NMWs did more than PAs or NPs are shown in Table 3:9. NMWs performed tasks which related specifically to their obstetrics/gynecology specialty.

Those tasks which NPs did more than PAs or NMWs are indicated in Table 3:10.

TABLE 3:10

Tasks NPs Tend to Do More than PAs or NMWs

Task	Percent of Reporting NHPs Who Do (D) Each Task and Percent Who Are Required (R) To Do Each Task					
	NPs (N=29)		PAs (N=24)		NMWs (N=13)	
	D	R	D	R	D	R
Do Socioeconomic Counseling (e.g. financial considerations of care, household management)	88.0%	81.5%	52.4%	61.1%	75.0%	50.0%
Make Referrals to New Health Practitioners	57.1	53.6	20.0	22.2	50.0	33.3

The large number of NPs doing socioeconomic counseling may reflect the types of practice sites (e.g., community family planning clinics) and the socioeconomic status of their patient population. Of the three NHP groups, NPs were likely to refer patients to other new health practitioners. While only a slightly smaller percentage of NMWs than NPs made such referrals, over 50 percent of the NPs were required to do this as part of their job, while just over 30 percent of the NMWs and 20 percent of the PAs indicated that such was their case. In sum, the task list data from the NHP questionnaires suggest that sets of tasks such as technical procedures, obstetrical activities, and specific types of counseling may serve as discriminating variables among the NHP roles.

JOB ATTRIBUTES

In the NHP questionnaire, participants were asked to report objectively on several characteristics, or attributes, of their jobs. The means, standard deviations and F-ratio* for the three groups of NHPs on five job attributes are presented in Table 3:11. All groups saw their jobs as challenging and as offering the opportunity to use personal initiative and judgment in doing the work. Differences among the groups appeared in three of the job attributes. NMWs held jobs which offered significantly (< .001 level) less frequent and helpful evaluation than either PAs or NPs; PAs reported significantly (< .05 level) greater opportunity for salary renegotiation than either NMWs or NPs; NPs held jobs which offered significantly (< 0.5 level) greater opportunity for independence and freedom in the work done.

ATTITUDE MEASURES

Several measures of NHP attitudes about themselves and their jobs were administered in the questionnaires. The means, standard deviations, and F-ratios for the three groups are presented in Table 3:12. Most

TABLE 3:11

Means, Standard Deviations and F-Ratios on Job Attributes[1]

Job Attribute	PA	NP	NMW	F-Ratio
1. Very challenging job	5.96 1.30	6.66 0.67	6.00 1.53	n.s.
2. Job offers opportunity to use personal initiative or judgment in carrying out work	6.17 1.86	5.97 1.74	5.75 1.55	n.s.
3. Job offers frequent and helpful evaluation	4.75 2.13	5.35 1.82	2.92 1.75	7.1367[3]
4. Job offers opportunity for salary renegotiation	5.42 1.93	3.83 2.19	3.85 2.48	4.1073[2]
5. Job offers opportunity for independence and freedom in how work is done	5.21 1.87	6.21 1.21	5.15 1.46	3.6282[2]

[1] Measured on 7-point scale: 1 = not at all true, 7 = very true.
[2] Significant at < .05
[3] Significant at < .001

---

*An F-ratio is a test of the significance of the difference between and among sample means; the level of significance indicates the likelihood that such difference will occur by chance, i.e., significance at .05 level = occurrence by chance 5 times out of 100.

striking in these results was the similarity of attitudes among the groups of NHPs. All groups demonstrated high growth need strength (desire for challenge and learning, for example) and moderately high levels of confidence in themselves. All reported moderately low need for independence which suggested that these NHPs were able to work interdependently in a team and experienced moderately low intersender conflict, i.e. low receipt of different and incongruent messages or "orders" from those with whom they work. Members of all three NHP groups reported very low personal-role conflict, which suggests that these NHPs found their general view of their roles to be compatible with the view of the role as prescribed by the organization in which they were employed. On only two attitude measures was there evidence of differences among NHP groups. The first of these was status concerns on the job. Although all NHPs appeared low on this attitude, NMWs were significantly ($<$ .10 level) higher than NPs, and higher, although not significantly, than PAs. It is interesting to compare this to general concerns about status on which the practitioners did not differ significantly: all NHPs reported feeling slightly

TABLE 3:12

Means, Standard Deviation and F-Values on Attitude Scales[1]

Attitude Measure	PA	NP	NMW	F-Ratio
General Self-confidence	5.31	5.19	4.64	1.1334
	1.26	1.31	1.46	
General Concerns About Status	3.20	3.40	3.37	0.2217
	1.05	1.13	1.28	
Growth Need Strength	6.71	6.77	6.87	0.8282
	0.42	0.35	0.19	
Status Concerns on the Job	2.66	2.15	3.00	2.3603[2]
	1.42	0.90	1.61	
Person-Role Conflict	2.83	2.48	2.83	0.6737
	1.34	1.08	1.27	
Need for Independence	3.47	3.58	3.98	1.0193
	1.13	1.02	0.99	
Intersender Conflict	3.47	3.67	4.51	2.0838
	1.65	1.51	1.24	
Perceived Job Ambiguity	2.28	2.61	3.22	3.4824[3]
	0.89	1.12	1.13	

[1] Measured on 7-point scale: High # = High on attitude
[2] Significant at $<$ .10
[3] Significant at $<$ .05

higher general concerns about status than they felt in their specific work situations, which suggests that the actual work setting may operate to satisfy, and thus alleviate, status needs. The second area of difference among practitioners was perceived job ambiguity. On this measure, NMWs reported significantly (< .05 level) greater feelings of job ambiguity than did either NPs or PAs.

JOB SATISFACTION MEASURES

Several measures of job satisfaction were taken on the NHP questionnaire. The results appear in Table 3:13. All groups reported moderate satisfaction with pay and with control of their own time on the job, and moderately high satisfaction with job security and social relationships on the job. NPs reported significantly higher (< .10 level) satisfaction of growth needs than PAs and NMWs, and NMWs reported a significantly lower (< .10 level) satisfaction with supervisors than NPs and PAs. Responses of all groups on general job satisfaction suggest that NHPs in these studies enjoyed their work and found their jobs satisfying.*

FUTURE PLANS

Practitioners were asked about opportunities for advancement in their present organizations, in other organizations and in other geographical locations. The results are presented in Table 3:14. It is unclear as to whether these data present the NHPs' accurate appraisal of their employment opportunities or, in fact, simply a "grass-is-greener" outlook. Practitioners were also asked about plans for further education. See Table 3:15 for results. More than half of the total sample planned to pursue further formal education: in general, PAs to seek admission to medical school, NMWs to work toward a Ph.D. degree, and NPs were divided among plans to pursue bachelor degrees, master's degrees and doctorates.

While this study focused on the New Health Practitioners' satisfactions with their jobs and did not investigate, at length, the supervisors'

---

*A 1974 study of 658 workers in a cross section of blue-collar, white-collar and professional occupations which used the same general satisfaction scale as utilized in this study, resulted in a national mean on general job satisfaction of 4.62. In comparison, the mean of the three groups in this study is 5.57. (Richard J. Hackman and Gregory R. Oldham, "Development of the Job Diagnostic Survey," *Journal of Applied Psychology* 1975, 60:159-170.)

TABLE 3:13

Means, Standard Deviation and F-Values on Satisfaction Measures[1]

Satisfaction Measure	PA	NP	NMW	F-Ratio
General Satisfaction	5.57	5.83	5.31	0.6487
	1.21	1.48	1.58	
Job Security Satisfaction	5.15	5.03	5.12	0.0416
	0.97	1.70	1.52	
Pay Satisfaction	4.56	4.48	4.87	0.2343
	1.58	2.02	1.49	
Satisfaction with Control of Time Use	4.63	5.07	4.31	0.8850
	2.06	1.68	1.63	
Growth Need Satisfaction	5.46	6.06	5.45	2.4120[2]
	1.26	0.94	1.19	
Social Satisfaction on the Job	5.35	5.74	5.10	1.7054
	1.26	0.95	1.12	
Satisfaction with Supervisor	5.54	5.69	4.93	2.6442[2]
	1.19	0.89	0.81	

[1] Measured on 7-point scale: High # = High Satisfaction
[2] Significant at < .10

TABLE 3:14

Opportunities for Advancement

Percent of NHPs Who See Opportunity for Advancement in:

	Present Organization	Other Organization	Other Geographic Location
PA	59%	89%	90%
NP	37.5	80	81
NMW	60	87	100

TABLE 3:15

Number of NHPs Seeking Further Formal Education

	BA/BS	MA/MS	Ph.D.	M.D.	Other	Total
PA	2	1	0	6	0	9
NP	4	6	4	1	1	16
NMW	0	1	7	0	1	9
Total	6	8	11	7	2	34

satisfactions with the NHPs, one piece of data was collected from supervisors on that issue: When asked if they planned to continue working with New Health Practitioners, 98 percent of responding supervisors answered *yes.*

CONCLUSION

This report describes several demographic characteristics, task activities, job attributes, attitudes about self and job, and job satisfactions of a sample of NHPs employed in Connecticut. To summarize these data:

1. Typically, PAs are male, while NPs and NMWs are female.

2. Although almost half of all NHPs in this study are employed in hospital settings, PAs and NPs can be found in all types of health care settings while NMWs are situated only in hospitals and private practices.

3. The use of NHPs has increased the number of patients served, an average of 11 to 25 percent.

4. Sets of task activities appear to discriminate between types of NHPs: PAs perform more technical procedures than do others; NMWs perform activities related to their area of specialty more than do others; and NPs do specific kinds of counseling and referral more than do other NHPs.

5. On job attributes: PAs hold jobs which offer greater opportunity for salary renegotiation than others; NPs report greater opportunity for independence in their work than do other NHPs; NMWs hold jobs which offer them less evaluation than is offered other NHPs.

6. Attitudes for all NHPs are relatively similar, with NMWs demonstrating slightly higher status concerns on the job and perceiving their work situation to hold greater ambiguity than is held by other NHPs.

7. All NHPs appear to be generally satisfied with their jobs.

8. More than half of NHPs plan to pursue further formal education.

One final comment is essential: The findings reported here are descriptive *only* of this group of employed NHPs studied in Connecticut; they are not meant for generalization to NHPs employed elsewhere and to do so might lead to inaccurate conclusions. The value of these results lies in (1) describing a specific sample of NHPs and (2) providing data on which to build hypotheses which may be tested within the broader population of NHPs and their supervisors elsewhere in the country.

EXHIBIT 3:1

Task Inventory on Questionnaire
Administered to NHPs in Connecticut°

1. Screen patient for appropriate initial disposition (triage).
2. Pull and file patient records. Do clerical work with patient billing.
3. Take history using only algorithm or printed form.
4. Do complete physical examination including:
   a. breast
   b. male genitalia
   c. female genitalia
   d. pelvic examination for complete pelvic/uterine assessment
   e. pelvic examination for CA screening
   f. assessment of heart and lungs
   g. sigmoidoscopy
5. Develop and/or revise diagnostic problem list or formulate a clinical impression.
6. Order diagnostic procedures.
7. Interpret lab test results.
8. Decide drug therapy based on clinical judgment outside standing orders.
9. Decide drug therapy based on clinical judgment within standing orders.
10. Make majority of referrals without physician's approval:
    a. to specialist physicians
    b. to other New Health Practitioners
    c. to community agencies
11. Get majority of consultations without physician's approval.
12. Do counseling:
    a. nutritional
    b. socioeconomic (e.g. financial considerations of care, household management)
    c. sexual
    d. anticipatory guidance (e.g. preparation for surgery, childbirth)
    e. psychological (e.g. life crises; interpersonal problems)
    f. developmental
    g. abortion
13. Follow own case load.
14. Supervise staff nurses.
15. Supervise ancillary personnel (technician, orderly, clerical personnel).
16. Debride and suture lacerations.
17. Episiotomy and episiotomy repair Extension 1°
18. Episiotomy and episiotomy repair Extension 2°
19. Episiotomy and episiotomy repair Extension 3°
20. Episiotomy and episiotomy repair Extension 4°
21. Removal of foreign objects.
22. Deliver baby.
23. Do cutdown.
24. Start IV.
25. Draw arterial blood.

*Charles Heikkinen, Charlotte Houde, Paul Moson, Donald Patrick, Donald Riedel, Gerrit Wolf, and John Wolfer participated in constructing research instruments.

26. Start blood infusion.
27. Do lumbar puncture.
28. Do internal fetal monitoring.
29. Do thoracentesis.
30. Do paracentesis.
31. Aspirate joints and/or inject medication into joints.
32. Insert intrauterine devices.
33. Do WBC.
34. Do HCT.
35. Do urine.
36. Do vaginal smears.

Part II

Major Determinants of Practice

A number of factors work singly or together to determine how NPs and PAs practice. One such determinant of practice is the credentialing process—accreditation of programs and certification or licensure of the practitioner—traditionally important in the evolution of any new profession. This process is particularly important in the health care professions, since components of credentialing often determine whether third party payment will be made for the practitioner's services.

For PAs, the American Medical Association House of Delegates in December 1971 adopted standards for educational programs preparing assistants to primary care physicians implemented by the AMA Council on Medical Education. In reviewing PA programs for accreditation, the AMA examines: curriculum content, faculty, facilities, student selection, mechanisms for evaluating student competence and preceptorships, among other components. (*Essentials of an Approved Program for the Assistant to the Primary Care Physician* is provided in Appendix A.) As of January 1976, the Council had accredited fifty-two programs for assistants to primary care physicians and two for surgeons' assistants.

HEW guidelines require that nurse practitioner programs fulfill specific criteria promulgated with the passage of the Nurse Training Act of 1975. (A copy of these guidelines is included in Appendix B.)

The National League for Nursing, as the accrediting agency for nursing education programs, applies its baccalaureate and higher degree criteria to degree programs which prepare NPs. These criteria include the organization and administration of the program, student selection, faculty, curriculum, resources, facilities, and services. (The NLN *Criteria for the Appraisal of Baccalaureate and Higher Degree Programs in Nursing* is provided in Appendix C.)

For nondegree granting nurse practitioner programs, which award a certificate, the American Nurses Association has placed itself in the role of accrediting agency. Elizabeth Allen gives a detailed overview of the

development of the ANA accreditation mechanism for continuing education NP programs to date and also includes a brief description of NP certification programs recently unveiled by the ANA. Nursing's professional
organization only relatively recently responded to the desirability of providing national certification programs for NPs. However, to date, these
programs require that the applicant practice for two years before becoming eligible for certification. This still leaves most beginning NPs uncertified, although licensed broadly to practice as registered nurses.

The collaborative development of the certification examination for the
assistant to the primary care physician is outlined by David L. Glazer.
Designed to be a national certification mechanism for PAs, this collaboration by representatives of fourteen health professional associations who comprise the National Commission on Certification of Physician's Assistants continues to develop proficiency examination of PAs
both at the entry level and at regular intervals throughout their practice.

Barbara J. Andrew of the National Board of Medical Examiners presents an overview of the certification examination for PAs and the test
results from the first three years of its administration. She emphasizes
the role of the examination as a proficiency assessment, the success of
which depends on its capacity to be predictive of the examinee's competence as a practitioner.

Another important determinant of NHP practice is the law. Virginia C.
Hall and Philip Kissam provide detailed analyses of the changes in nurse
practice acts and medical practice acts to accommodate the new and expanded roles of NPs and PAs. Terminology problems inherent in defining
the expanded role and the outer boundaries of task delegation are discussed in both papers, and model statutes proposed by Kissam who presents his reasons for recommending them. (Legislative changes in nurse
practice acts to provide for the expanded role in nursing, and in medical
practice acts to allow expanded medical delegation, are presented in Ap-
pendices D and E, respectively.)

Reimbursement for NHP services is discussed by Stephen B. Morris in
a report on the Social Security Administration Physician Extender
Reimbursement Study. He cites the reasons for undertaking this am-
bitious experiment in reimbursement and outlines the hypotheses to be
tested in the study.

Cost-effectiveness of NHPs is addressed in the three subsequent chapters. Mary O'Hara Devereaux and her colleagues, examining the practice
patterns of family nurse practitioners relative to those of physicians and
the economic feasibility of FNP care, conclude that FNPs result in a net
income gain to the practice.

Barbara Seigal and her co-authors, in a discussion of FNP versus MD-staffed clinics, outline the factors which place rural health clinics at financial risk and identify the role of current reimbursement policies as a deterrent to the efficient use of NHPs.

The important issues of scope and cost of PA supervision are addressed by Jane C. Record and her collaborators. The longitudinal evaluation of physician supervision of PAs at Kaiser-Permanente focuses on several issues: the legal determinants of supervision as required by state statutes, the patterns of PA consultation, and the cost of supervision. Record et al. speculate on the optimal qualities of the supervisor—another important determinant in the cost-effectiveness of new health practitioner utilization.

A final chapter by Elaine S. Bursic reports on a very small subsample of PA and MEDEX respondents to a recent study. Problems encountered in their practice, barriers to career and geographic mobility, and a measure of the varying degrees of frustration experienced in the new role are among the topics discussed. Her chapter lends testimony to the courage and confidence with which the PA profession has placed itself under scrutiny. Even though her study represents a small fraction of PAs and MEDEX, it underscores the impact of determinants such as the credentialing process, enabling legislation, third party reimbursement, and the public's lack of understanding of the capabilities of many new health practitioners.

Chapter 4

Credentialing of Continuing Education Nurse Practitioner Programs

Elizabeth A. Allen

The nursing profession has long accepted the responsibility delegated by the public to professions to establish and implement standards for the education and practice of its members. Assurance to the public that standards have been met and maintained has been achieved through various methods of credentialing.*

First however, the terms "credential," "approval" and "accreditation" must be defined: (a) "Credential" is based on the word "credence" which means "mental acceptance, belief; something that gives a title to, credit or confidence; testimonials showing that a person is entitled to credit or has a right to exercise official power." (b) "Approval" implies a favorable opinion of something and may suggest esteem or admiration. (c) "Accreditation" implies official endorsement attesting to conformity to set standards.

This chapter focuses on two components of credentialing: (1) the accreditation process as it applies to short term continuing education programs which prepare nurses for expanded nursing roles; and (2) the certification of NP graduates. This process can be understood best if considered within the context of other credentialing processes within nursing. There will not be a discussion here of the conflicts between nursing and medicine, or between the American Nurses' Association and the National League for Nursing which accredits degree granting programs, nor of the pros and cons of special licensure for nurse practitioners in expanded roles.

One basic aspect of credentialing is accreditation of a school of nursing. This school may or may not have accreditation by the NLN but must be approved or accredited by the State Board of Nursing. NLN accreditation is a voluntary process whereas the state board accreditation is man-

*Much of the information presented in this chapter is taken from *Accreditation of Continuing Education in Nursing,* American Nurses' Association, 2420 Pershing Road, Kansas City, Missouri 64108, 1975.

datory. A major difference between the two processes is that the National League for Nursing is limited to baccalaureate and master's degree programs excluding doctoral programs, whereas the State Board of Nursing may have the prerogative to accredit or approve any nursing education program within its jurisdiction.

Another form of credentialing is licensure of the nurse. Licensure is granted for the successful passing of the state board examination following completion of an approved and/or accredited educational program. The examination, although administered through the State Boards of Nursing, is the property of the Council of State Boards of Nursing, a constituent of the American Nurses' Association. The examination is graded and recorded, and the applicant is notified of the results by the National League for Nursing. Thus, this examination serves in essence as a form of national licensure. An applicant who passes the examination in one state may be recognized as a registered nurse in any other state.

Yet another component of credentialing is certification of the nurse, which may be either legal or voluntary. This discussion of certification is defined by the American Nurses' Association as a voluntary process of recognition for excellence in a specific area of nursing practice.

EVOLUTION OF ANA ACCREDITATION

Credentialing of NPs has been discussed and implemented over the past several years in an atmosphere beset with emotionalism reflected in questions such as: "Who should set standards of nursing education and practice?" "Is a nurse practitioner different from a physician's assistant?" "Is the nurse practitioner practicing medicine or nursing?" "Who should accredit nondegree granting educational programs?" And even more basic is the question: "Is the nurse practitioner different from a well prepared practicing nurse?" None of these questions has been answered to the satisfaction of the many persons concerned with the issue of the nurse practitioner. This section outlines the events which led to the development of a system of accreditation for continuing education programs preparing nurses for expanded roles and discusses that system.

In 1965, a program for nurses in expanded roles was started by Loretta Ford, RN, Ed.D. and Henry Silver, MD at the University of Colorado. Since that time nearly 150 programs have been developed which purport to prepare nurse practitioners. Housed in every type of institution, from doctor's offices to universities, these programs range from four weeks to two years and grant anything from no official recognition to a master's degree. The proliferation of these educational programs was not unnoticed by accreditation bodies in nursing but the opinion appeared to be: "If we don't notice them, they will go away." However, they did not go away; on the contrary, the number of programs increased over time.

In 1973, a letter was sent from the Department of Accreditation and Institutional Eligibility, Bureau of Post Secondary Education of the U.S. Office of Education to the American Medical Association and the National League for Nursing, requesting the two organizations to consider accreditation of nurse practitioner programs. Neither organization accepted the responsibility, perhaps rightly. The continuing education NP programs were neither medical nor degree granting.

In 1972, the American Nurses' Association and the American Academy of Pediatrics issued a joint statement, "Guidelines on Short-term Continuing Education Programs for Pediatric Nurse Associates." This was the first of a series of statements to identify content standards for the various areas in which nurses function in expanded roles. It was also the first such statement to categorize the programs as continuing education. Since this initial publication, there have been several statements of standards for specialties, including geriatrics, school nurses, college health, community health and neonatal nurses, among others.

The definition of these educational programs as continuing education and nondegree granting allowed the American Nurses' Association to explore the development of a system of accreditation for continuing education programs preparing nurses for expanded roles.

Several events occurred in 1973 which set the stage for the development and implementation of such a system. The Interim Executive Committee of the ANA Council on Continuing Education outlined three major functions for the council:

(1) Revision of standards of continuing education in nursing.

(2) Development of a system of accreditation for continuing education in nursing.

(3) Development of a record system facilitating interstate transferability.

The Interim Executive Committee and the Task Force on the Model Practice Act of the Congress on Nursing Practice developed at the same time the document "Continuing Education Guidelines for State Nurses' Associations," which was approved for publication in the fall of 1973 by the ANA Commission on Nursing Education and published in January 1974.

By this time, the ANA Ad Hoc Committee for the Development of a System of Accreditation had determined that the magnitude of the task was too great for one committee. At their request, the Interim Executive

Committee appointed a subcommittee to develop the system of accreditation. The last major hurdle in the development of the system was surmounted at the 1974 ANA convention. The ANA House of Delegates passed a resolution which directed the Association "to move ahead in the development of a system of accreditation for continuing education in nursing." The resolution signified a major move in the history of nursing—the visible assumption by its professional association of the responsibility for quality in one segment of its educational process. Let it be stressed that this move also activated much confusion within the nursing profession.

NATIONAL ACCREDITATION BOARD FOR CONTINUING EDUCATION

Organizational Structure

The overall authority and responsibility for reviewing and revising the accreditation mechanism, approval of criteria, and implementing, regulating, and evaluating the accreditation process rests with the National Accreditation Board for Continuing Education which works through five Regional Accrediting Committees and a National Review Committee. These relationships are delineated in Figure 4:1. The standards of continuing education and policies governing the accreditation process for continuing education programs in nursing are developed by the ANA Council on Continuing Education and approved by the ANA Commission on Nursing Education. This Commission has the responsibility to provide overall recommendations on the direction of educational programs in view of changing health care needs and practice, as well as encouraging research on nursing practice. In addition, its functions include the formulation of policy and recommendations on legislation affecting nursing education.

Periodic reports of the activities of the National Accreditation Board are submitted to the ANA Council on Continuing Education, the ANA Commission on Nursing Education, the ANA Board of Directors and the ANA House of Delegates. Recommendations standards of continuing education and/or policies governing the accreditation process may be forwarded by the National Accreditation Board to the ANA Council and Commission.

A monitoring group of seven persons will be established to evaluate the effectiveness of the National Accreditation Board for Continuing Education. This group will function for a minimum of five years and will be accountable to the ANA Commission on Nursing Education. The monitor-

FIGURE 4:1

Accreditation of Continuing Education in Nursing

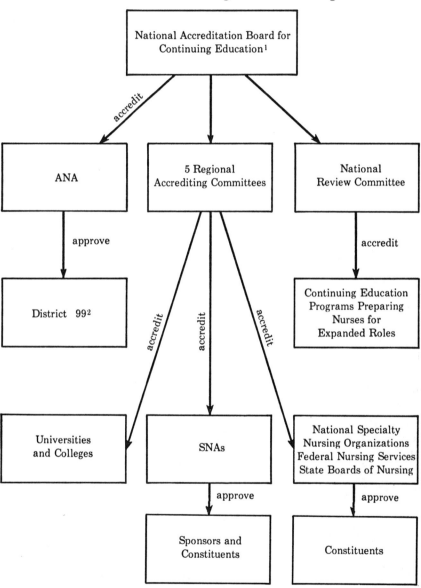

[1] A monitoring group will be established to evaluate the effectiveness of the National Accreditation Board for a minimum of five years.

[2] Nurses registered in the United States who are functioning overseas.

ing group will consist of three persons designated by the Commission on Nursing Education, three designated by the Executive Committee of the Continuing Education Council, and one representative not affiliated with either.

Purpose and Functions

The purpose of the National Accreditation Board is to act as the governing body for the national accreditation process for continuing education for the nursing profession. Its functions are to:

1. Establish and regulate the ANA Regional Accreditation Committees and the National Review Committee.

2. Serve as a final appeal mechanism for the Regional Accrediting Committees and National Review Committee.

3. Review, evaluate, and revise criteria for accreditation and approval consistent with the Standards of Continuing Education developed by ANA.

4. Serve in an advisory capacity on accreditation policy matters to the Commission on Nursing Education at its request.

5. Review ANA's approval process and program of continuing education for purposes of accreditation.

6. Approve the continuing education program or offerings of District No. 99 if ANA is not accredited.

Composition

The Board is composed of fourteen members, at least eight of whom are registered nurses. The members of the Board must represent the following groupings: five from nursing education (at least two of whom must be involved in continuing education and one in staff development), three from nursing practice, two from credentialing groups, two representatives of the public, and two members-at-large. The Board is managed by an elected chairperson who serves without vote except in the case of a tie.

There were approximately 250 applicants for the 14 positions filled by the Commission. The criteria for selecting Board members included, among others, evidence of commitment to the principles of excellence in nursing practice and to the role of nursing in health services delivery. Members must be able to evaluate continuing education programs and have thorough understanding of the components of the credentialing process.

Appointment of members to vacancies are made by the National Accreditation Board. Members serve four-year terms. No member may serve two consecutive terms. For continuity, terms are staggered. Initial appointments are for two-, three-, and four-year terms. The regional committees were also selected from names submitted to the Commission.

REGIONAL ACCREDITING COMMITTEES

Organizational Structure

The five Regional Accrediting Committees are responsible to the National Accreditation Board for Continuing Education. (See Figure 4:1.)

Purpose and Functions

The purpose of the Regional Committees is (1) to establish and implement a process for accrediting continuing education programs in nursing within universities and colleges and (2) to accredit state nurses associations (SNAs), national specialty nursing organizations, federal nursing services, and state boards of nursing to offer programs and to approve such offerings.

The Regional Committees' functions are to:

1. Review and evaluate applications for accreditation from universities and colleges, SNA, national specialty nursing organizations, federal nursing services, and State Boards of Nursing according to the accreditation criteria.

2. Conduct site visits as necessary.

3. Act on applications.

4. Notify applicants in writing of the decision.

5. Establish an appeal mechanism.

6. Review and update evaluation criteria periodically.

7. Approve the continuing education program or offerings of an SNA which is not accredited and those of sponsors which would apply to the SNA if they were accredited.

8. Approve the continuing education programs or offerings of those sponsors within the state if the SNA is not accredited.

Composition

Each Regional Accrediting Committee is composed of 10 members, at least 7 of whom are registered nurses. All Committee members reside within that particular region. The chairperson is a member of the Committee and is elected by the Committee. Membership on the Regional Committee consists of four nurses with expertise in nursing education (at least two of whom are involved in continuing education and one in staff development), three nurses with expertise in nursing practice, one representative with expertise in the area of credentialing, one representative of the public, and one member-at-large. The criteria for selecting members of the Regional Committees are essentially the same as those for the National Accreditation Board, with emphasis on a commitment to nursing practice and to the role of nursing in the provision of care.

NATIONAL REVIEW COMMITTEE

The National Review Committee for Accreditation of Expanded Role programs was originally appointed by the Commission on Nursing Education. Names for consideration were solicited from state nurses' associations, specialty nursing organizations, specialty medical societies, federal nursing services, state boards of nursing, among other sources. The National Review Committee was expected to be the most plagued by vested interests, and so it was. No group believed it had enough representation. Some of the conflicts were medicine vs. nursing, nursing vs. nursing, specialty vs. specialty, education vs. practice. The variable composition of this group and the nature of accreditation itself contributed to the conflicts.

Organizational Structure

The National Review Committee is responsible to the National Accreditation Board for Continuing Education. (See Figure 4:2.)

Purpose and Functions

The purpose of the National Review Committee is to establish a process for accrediting nondegree granting continuing education programs preparing nurses for expanded roles. This task is accomplished with the help of review teams selected for the type of practitioner program to be accredited (Figure 4:2).

Its functions are to:

1. Appoint review team according to designated practice areas.

2. Review and evaluate programs of applicant agencies according to the criteria for accreditation of continuing education programs preparing nurses for expanded roles, taking into account the recommendations of the review teams.

FIGURE 4:2

Accreditation of Continuing Education Programs Preparing Nurses for Expanded Roles

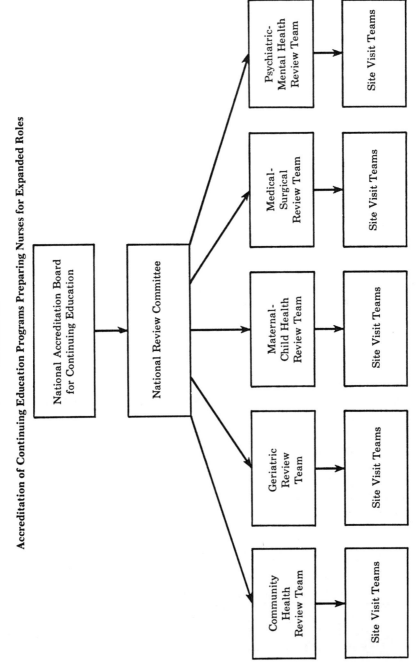

3. Act upon application for accreditation.

4. Notify applicant in writing of decision.

5. Establish an appeal mechanism.

6. Review and update evaluation criteria periodically.

7. Send periodic reports to the National Accreditation Board for Continuing Education.

Composition

The National Review Committee is composed of 11 members, at least seven of whom are registered nurses. The National Review Committee is made up of individuals who represent the same groups as those comprising the membership of the Regional Accrediting Committees, i.e., nursing education and practice, credentialing, the public, and members-at-large.

The criteria for membership on the National Review Committee are similar to those required for membership on the National Accreditation Board and the Regional Committees.

Appointment of members will be made by the National Accreditation Board for Continuing Education from persons whose names have been solicited from ANA's Division on Nursing Practice, Council on Continuing Education, Commission on Nursing Education, and Commission on Nursing Services, and from state nurses' associations and other appropriate groups. Initially, appointment to the National Review Committee will be made by the ANA Commission on Nursing Education. Members will serve four-year terms. No member may serve two consecutive terms. For continuity, terms will be staggered. Initial appointments will be for two-, three-, and four-year terms. The National Review Committee for Expanded Roles has a shared chairpersonship.

The accreditation mechanism was activated in September 1975. The activation was far from smooth. Many people wanted to know what its significance would be. The potential danger in the activity is certainly obvious with its large and cumbersome organization and its expensive mobilization. However, despite these problems, its major assets are that:

1. It forces interaction between education and service.

2. It allows for the involvement of many people.

3. It forces participation at the local level.

4. It provides for the interaction between ANA and specialty nursing organizations.

5. It provides for the interaction of nursing and medicine in the accreditation process.

Whether or not the system works will depend by and large on the willingness of the involved groups to work cooperatively. The vested interests of every group involved could slow down or potentially stop progress.

It is true that the American Nurses' Association has not historically been involved in the educational accreditation process. However, the ANA, through its Commission on Nursing Education, has "the responsibility to enunciate standards for nursing education and devise methods for their implementation." Accreditation is one such mechanism.

CERTIFICATION

The ANA Divisions on Practice formed the Interdivisional Council on Certification in early 1976, to "coordinate certification activities and to establish definitions, administrative policies and procedures, and guidelines for recognition of specialties and relationships with other organizations in regard to certification." [1] Membership on this Council is made up of the chairpersons of the divisions and the certification boards. The separate divisions will continue to develop the certification criteria as well as the certification examination content.

As of July 1, 1976, a new ANA program took effect which provides for two types of recognition for professional achievement. Adopted by the Interdivisional Council on Certification of the ANA, April 15, 1976, the definitions and basic eligibility requirements for these two types of "recognition of professional achievement and excellence in practice" are as follows:

CERTIFICATION (for competence)

Definition: Certification is the process by which an ANA division on nursing practice grants recognition to an individual registered nurse who has met predetermined qualifications for competency in a designated area of nursing practice, and predetermined qualifications for continuing competency.

Eligibility Requirements:*
1. Current licensure as a registered nurse.
2. Two years of practice as a registered nurse in a designated area of nursing practice immediately prior to application, up to one year of which may have been in an organized program of

---

*There are basic eligibility requirements common to all divisions on nursing practice. Other eligibility requirements may be developed as appropriate by each division.[2]

study in an institution of higher learning or in a continuing education program.

3. The applicant must be currently engaged in the practice of nursing in the ANA division in which certification is sought.

AMERICAN COLLEGE OF NURSING PRACTICE (for excellence)

Definition: Membership as a diplomate is recognition granted to a certified nurse who has met predetermined qualifications for excellence in a designated area of practice and predetermined qualifications for continuing diplomate status. Criteria and qualifications for excellence are determined by the ANA divisions on nursing practice.

Eligibility Requirements.*

1. Current ANA certification in the designated area of nursing practice.

2. Current practice in the area in which membership is sought.

3. Two years of practice in the area of specialization post master's.

4. A master's degree in nursing or a related field from an accredited educational institution.

The purpose of these two types of recognition for professional achievement, as noted in the announcement of their availability, is to "provide a mechanism which attests to competence in practice as well as continuing to provide recognition of excellence."[3]

The two new approaches to certification were reported to have been adopted in response to ANA members' demands for more accessible competence certification. Practice of nursing as an eligibility requirement constitutes "involvement in the nursing process in a clinical setting, where the nursing actions and judgments are focused on a particular individual, family, or group of individuals, and where there is professional responsibility and accountability for the outcome of these actions."[4] The eligibility requirement for both types of certification includes two years of nursing practice; thus the certification process is not intended to certify the new graduate of a training program.

The purpose of these new certification procedures is to provide a credentialing mechanism which enhances career and geographic mobility

---

* There are basic eligibility requirements common to all divisions of nursing practice. Other eligibility requirements may be developed as appropriate by each division.[2]

and, in addition, the prospect of third party reimbursement for nursing services.

Notes

1. ANA, "ANA Divisions on Practice: Recognition of Professional Achievement and Excellence in Practice," *The American Nurse*, 8, No. 9 (June 1, 1976), p. 1.
2. Ibid., p. 3.
3. Ibid., p. 1.
4. Ibid, p. 1.

Chapter 5

National Commission on Certification of Physician's Assistants: A Precedent in Collaboration

David L. Glazer

The National Commission on Certification of Physician's Assistants (NCCPA) is a model of unprecedented collaboration among a group of health professional organizations. One has only to read carefully the list of member organizations to appreciate the significance of this collaborative effort:

American Academy of Family Physicians
American Academy of Pediatrics
American Academy of Physicians' Assistants
American College of Physicians
American College of Surgeons
American Hospital Association
American Medical Association
American Nurses' Association
American Society of Internal Medicine
Association of American Medical Colleges
Association of Physician Assistant Programs
Federation of State Medical Boards of the U.S.
National Board of Medical Examiners
U.S. Department of Defense

NCCPA's major charge is to help assure the public of the entry level and continued competency of physician's assistants. This is accomplished through various mechanisms, including entry-level examination, certificate reregistration based on acquisition of continuing medical education (CME), and recertification examinations. Individual states, of course, retain the authority concerning who may and may not practice as

86

PAs. However, NCCPA receives requests from a number of states to advise them concerning PA enabling legislation, rules and regulations. Many state agencies still are not aware of precisely what PAs are, what they can do, or how the profession relates to others in the health system. In fact, many states continue to group all health professionals otherwise uncategorized as "physician's assistants." NCCPA, by virtue of its fourteen member organizations and its independence from control by any single professional organization, is not viewed by states as representing a vested interest. Rather, states have begun to see NCCPA as having a similar goal as their own—competency assurance in the public interest.

HISTORY

With the proliferation of PA training programs during the early 1970s, it became clear that a mechanism was necessary to accredit programs in order to assure the quality of the educational process. The result was the advent of what is now known as the Joint Review Committee on Educational Programs for Physician's Assistants in collaboration with the AMA Council on Medical Education. This committee, however, only reviewed the educational process and not the product of the programs. Simultaneously, PA graduates began to develop their professional organizations into what are now the American Academy of Physicians' Assistants (AAPA) and the Association of Physician Assistant Programs (APAP).

The next step, under the auspices of the federal government, AMA and private foundations with the blessing of AAPA and APAP was to develop a mechanism to evaluate the product of the training programs. Thus, the National Board of Medical Examiners' (NBME) Certifying Examination for Assistants to the Primary Care Physician was developed and first administered in December 1973. At the same time, nurse practitioner, nurse clinician and child health associate programs were gaining momentum; graduates of these programs were also eligible to take the examination. And, additionally, there was an unknown number working as PAs who had not graduated from formal programs. It was decided that the 1974 examination would be open to informally trained PAs who met certain eligibility criteria to be determined by a committee of NBME. NBME would also form a Standard Setting Committee to determine pass/fail levels.

These were new and uncomfortable roles for NBME whose traditional charge had always been confined to the developing, administering and scoring of examinations for physicians. With this in mind, AMA and

NBME worked to bring together representatives of twelve other professional groups in late 1973 to form a free-standing, independent commission to assure the PA profession, employers, state boards, and most important, patients, of the competency of this type of health professional. In February 1975, after being formally structured and organized, NCCPA opened a national office in Atlanta, Georgia.

Specifically, NCCPA has responsibility for the following functions:

1. Determine eligibility criteria for the National Certifying Examination.

2. Review applications to take the examination and register candidates.

3. Administer the examination under subcontract to NBME.

4. Determine pass/fail standards for the certifying examination for PAs.

5. Issue and verify certificates.

6. Periodically recertify PAs through the continued demonstration of competency.

7. Publish lists by state of PAs certified each year.

8. Assist state medical boards at their request to establish/modify PA enabling legislation, rules, and regulations as they pertain to national certification.

Eligibility Criteria

There are actually three ways an individual is eligible to sit for the examination:

- Formally trained PAs are eligible by virtue of their graduation from a program approved by the Joint Review Committee on Educational Programs for Physician's Assistants.
- Nurse practitioners are eligible provided they have graduated from a family or pediatric nurse practitioner/clinician program of at least four months duration, affiliated with an accredited medical or nursing school.
- Informally trained PAs may sit for the examination provided they can demonstrate that they have functioned for four out of the past five years as PAs in a primary care setting. Candidate applications and detailed employment verification by current and former employers provide the data for determination of eligibility.

Of the 1,411 candidates who took the 1975 examination, 1,034 attended formal PA programs, 151 were graduates of MEDEX, 152 were informally trained, and 74 had attended nurse practitioner programs.

Application Review

Each application undergoes a minimum of three separate reviews by independent raters. The sequential flow of the review process includes a preliminary in-house review, a second more detailed in-house review, and ultimate evaluation by the NCCPA Eligibility Committee.

Examination Administration

Beginning in 1975, the NBME, under subcontract from NCCPA, continued development, administration and scoring of the certifying examination. The examination consisted of one day of written testing, including both multiple choice and patient management problems, and two days of practical examination. Over 50 test sites were available in the United States, with an additional two sites in West Germany and Korea. The examination fee, $55 in 1973/74, was raised to $100 in 1975. Of the 1,411 people who sat for the 1975 examination, 1,260 were formally trained. The overall failure rate was 20 percent; the failure rate of the 151 informally trained candidates was 60.5 percent in contrast to the 14 percent failure rate for formally trained.

Standard Setting Committee

Each year, a Standard Setting Committee meets to review the examination and set pass/fail levels. The 1974 and 1975 examination had similar results and pass levels indicating that the examination had become consistent in its ability to differentiate competencies.

Certification

As of early 1976, approximately 3,000 PAs had received national certification and were designated PA-C. In 1973/74, prior to NCCPA operation, the $55 fee levied by NBME was solely to offset a portion of the examination costs and did not cover the issuance of a certificate. NCCPA certification was voluntary and required an application and a $15.00 fee.

Reregistration and Recertification

Part of the NCCPA's effort to ensure continued competency of physician's assistants will be the requirement of all certified PAs to engage in Continuing Medical Education (CME) activities in order for their certificate to remain valid. The present requirements are 100 hours of CME every 2 years, which will be verified and approved by AAPA. A certified PA need not be a member of the Academy to utilize that agency's resources in the acquisition of CME.

NCCPA also plans to develop recertification examinations, the first of which is expected to be administered in 1981, to those PAs whose certificate has been valid for the previous six years. The reexamination will consider certified PA deployment and role evolution, and it will utilize performance-based techniques. NCCPA seeks the ultimate development of an examination that will be both a learning experience and an evaluative tool. Emphasis will be on the identification of weaknesses in order that certified PAs can remedy those weaknesses, pass the recertification examination and assure themselves, their employing physicians and their patients of a high level of competency. Those who may fail the initial recertification examination will be allowed to study specific areas and retake the examination without losing certification during the interim.

Certified PA deployment and role evolution will be determined on the basis of various studies and reregistration application forms. NCCPA is committed to developing recertification examinations which are as relevant to certified PA practice as the entry level examination is to primary care PA training and utilization. If, for example, it is discovered that by 1981, 80 percent of the certified PAs are functioning *only* in adult medicine, then the recertification examination will necessarily address the requisite knowledge and skills attendant to such practice.

Directory

Beginning in mid-1976, a directory of certified PAs will be printed and available to bona fide requestors. The directory will include an alphabetical listing of certified PAs, certificate number, and date of expiration. A second section will list certified PAs alphabetically by state. One copy of the directory will be sent to each state medical board free of charge. Additional copies for state boards or other agencies will be available at a moderate fee to cover NCCPA printing costs.

State Board Activity

Another major activity of NCCPA has been to advise state boards of medical examiners concerning PA enabling legislation, rules and regulations. Many states are actively developing or modifying legislation, rules and regulations concerned with physician's assistant activities. Partially through NCCPA efforts, nearly 25 states now require a valid certificate from NCCPA as a prerequisite to employment of primary care PAs in those states.

NCCPA has played a vital role on behalf of both the public and PAs through the formation of its State Board Liaison Committee. A resolution, recently proposed and unanimously passed by the Federation of State Medical Boards of the United States (FSMBUS), urges state medical boards to seek legislation and formulate rules and regulations which would permit acceptance of the NCCPA certification in the authorization of physician's assistants in their respective states.

Specialist PAs

The current charge of NCCPA is directed toward the assistant to the primary care physician. However, there is a group of unknown size of PAs who are either graduates of specialty programs or are working in a non-primary care setting. Thus far, they have been ineligible to sit for the national certifying examination; further it is unlikely that they would be able to pass because of the examination's broad scope. Nonetheless, they do fit under the generic term, "physician assistant," by virtue of training and the functions they perform. NCCPA hopes eventually to develop specialty examinations. In the interim, a registry for specialized physician's assistants may be developed. Although unable to attest to the competency of these individuals, NCCPA could attest to the nature and level of their training and provide a certificate of registration. One group then would be certified as assistants to the primary care physician and another group would be registered (and ultimately certified in each state) as, for example, orthopedic physician's assistants.

SUMMARY

In conclusion, NCCPA's function is to certify the entry level and continued competency of PAs through the vehicles of testing, continuing medical education and periodic recertification evaluation. The uniqueness of the Commission's organization lies in its representation of 14 diverse health organizations, enabling it to serve the public and the PA profession. The Commission also serves as a resource for states, urging the acceptance of national certification and encouraging continued competency assurance in the best interest of patients. Simultaneously this assures the acceptance by states of PAs as a useful and professional addition to the health care field. Continued professional growth can be enhanced by the combined efforts of NCCPA in the public interest, AAPA in the profession's interest, and by demonstrations of the impact of the profession on improving health care delivery.

Chapter 6

National Examination for Assistants to the Primary Care Physician

Barbara J. Andrew

BACKGROUND

As the concept of new health practitioners gained acceptance by the public and the medical and nursing professions, state legislatures began to turn their attention to the formulation of statutes that could provide for the inclusion of these professionals within the framework of the health care delivery system. Particularly in those states where new health practitioners could practice only after their credentials had been evaluated by the appropriate state agency, the development of a nationally standardized mechanism for evaluating their proficiency seemed desirable. With this objective in mind and with the cooperation of the American Medical Association, the National Board of Medical Examiners began the development of a national certifying examination for assistants to the primary care physician in July 1972.

Two primary goals for this examination program were: (1) to identify the roles and responsibilities of the primary care physician's assistant, and (2) to develop a set of evaluation techniques that could be used to assess the knowledge and skills required to perform the functions of a physician's assistant.

The development of examinations for health care professionals had long been based upon curricular content: the subject matter presented and the way in which its presentation is structured in the curriculum. However, because of the goals of this examination program, an approach was devised which had not previously been used for national examinations of health care professionals. Instead of relying upon descriptions of the subject matter within the various programs, a task inventory consisting of several hundred health care functions was designed. These functions were compiled from several task analysis studies of physician and nonphysician activities. Once compiled, each health care function was classified under one of ten categories reflecting various components of the clinical problem-solving and management process. These categories are:

Data Gathering
—History Taking and Patient Records
—Physical Examination
—Laboratory Tests and Diagnostic Procedures
—Patient Monitoring
Analysis and Interpretation
—Consultation and Referral
—Diagnostic Acumen
Medical and Health Care Strategies
—Emergency Procedures
—Surgical and Technical Procedures
—Patient Management
—Patient Counseling

The resulting task inventory was distributed to each member of the National Board Advisory Committee on Physician's Assistants whose membership included physician's assistants, physicians who were training and utilizing them, and nurses involved with the nurse practitioner concept. They were asked to consider each of the 900 health care functions included in the inventory and to decide whether the health care function was one that a primary care physician's assistant should definitely, probably, probably not or definitely not be skilled in performing. Since the examination would be administered on a national basis to evaluate individuals trained in different types of educational programs, it was felt that the examination should be designed to measure those health care functions that a representative group of experts felt physician's assistants definitely should be skilled in performing. To identify the health care functions about which there was consensus, a frequency distribution of the judgments made concerning each health care function was tabulated. Each of the four rating categories was given a numerical value on a scale of one to four, and the arithmetic mean of these judgments was then computed for each health care function. Those functions receiving a mean value of 3.5 to 4.0 were considered those that a primary care physician's assistant definitely should be skilled in performing. Functions receiving a mean value of 3.40 to 3.49 were also reviewed at the meeting in which the results of the task inventory study were presented.

A review of the health care functions identified from this task inventory suggested that not all functions were equivalent in terms of their importance to a PA's proficiency. Moreover, the number of functions was so large that no examination could attempt to sample adequately the knowledge and skills related to all of them. For these reasons, a priority study was conducted using the same experts who had participated in the task inventory study. The purpose of the study was to establish the relative importance of the several hundred health care functions, so that those receiving high ratings would be given high priority in the development of the certifying examination.

Two dimensions were selected for determining the priority of each function: (1) the frequency with which the function would be performed in a primary care practice, and (2) its criticalness to optimum health care delivery. A frequency distribution of the judgments was made and the criticalness of each function tabulated. A mean value for each health care function on each dimension was calculated by assigning a numerical value of one to four to the intervals on each scale. The priority value assigned to each function was determined by using a formula in which the critical value was weighted more heavily than the frequency value. This was done because while some functions are performed infrequently (e.g., closed chest cardiac massage), they often carry life-and-death implications when they are required as part of health care.

The validity of an examination as an assessment of proficiency depends upon its capacity to evaluate the knowledge and skills required to carry out specific functions. Therefore, test committees were appointed to analyze related health care functions and to identify the knowledge and skill components related to each. These components were stated behaviorally to help select appropriate evaluation methodology and to serve as the performance criteria in assessing the proficiency of physician's assistants.

THE FIRST CERTIFYING EXAMINATION—1973

The first certifying examination was administered in December 1973 to 880 candidates at 38 test centers. Eligibility for the first examination was limited to graduates of physician's assistant training programs approved by the AMA Council on Medical Education, funded by the Bureau of Health Resources Development, or, in the case of family and pediatric nurse practitioners, programs of at least four months' duration within a nationally accredited school of medicine or nursing.

Candidate Population

Of the total number of eligible physician's assistants, 75 percent registered for this examination, while almost 100 percent of the eligible

Medex did so. Of the eligible nurse practitioners, approximately 10 percent registered.

In relation to the 880 candidates who took this examination, 62 percent had received their training in physician's assistant programs, 29 percent in Medex training programs and 9 percent in nurse practitioner programs.

Biographic data collected on each examinee indicated that 89 percent already had completed their formal training prior to the examination, and 81 percent already had acquired clinical experience as a physician's assistant or nurse practitioner. Table 6:1 summarizes the clinical experience of this examinee group. Of those examinees who had acquired experience as a new health practitioner, 88 percent had up to two years of clinical experience, while 12 percent had acquired more than two years of clinical experience.

In addition, 91 percent of the total examinee group had been involved in health care delivery prior to their training as a new health practitioner. Of those, 86 percent had direct patient contact as a nurse, military corpsman or physical therapist, while 11 percent had been involved in a technical capacity. These data indicate that the typical examinee for the 1973 Certifying Examination had completed a formal educational program and had acquired several months to several years of clinical experience. Moreover, prior to having been trained as a new health practitioner, the typical examinee had provided direct patient care for a period of two to four years.

Examination Format

The 1973 examination program consisted of a one-day written examination divided into two sections. The first section contained multi-

TABLE 6:1

Clinical Experience of First Examinee Group—1973

Biographic Data	Total Group N = 880	Yes Respondents
Completed an educational program	89%	
Clinical experience since training:	81%	
Up to 2 years clinical experience		(88%)
More than 2 years clinical experience		(12%)
Prior experience in health care delivery:	91%	
Patient contact		(86%)
Technical		(11%)
Other		(3%)

ple-choice and other objective questions presented in printed and pictorial form. These materials were designed to assess the candidate's knowledge and skill in applying knowledge related to high priority health care functions.

The afternoon section of the examination involved a programmed testing technique for patient management problems. The candidates were presented with a simulated clinical case and asked to make decisions regarding the appropriate diagnostic work-up and management of the patient as they would in an actual clinical setting. These patient management problems were designed to assess the candidate's skill in making appropriate clinical decisions in adult and pediatric medicine as well as emergency and nonemergency problems.

Validation Studies

In order to investigate the validity of this first examination, a number of studies were conducted. The first evidence of construct validity was provided by statistical analysis of examination performance in relation to biographic data. Examinees who had completed a training program and had clinical experience as a physician's assistant or nurse practitioner scored significantly higher on the examination than did examinees without such postgraduate clinical experience. This finding provided evidence of the construct validity of the examination since it appeared to be measuring knowledge and skills that increased with clinical experience and were, hence, relevant to practice. Since examinees with experience in patient care *prior to* training as a new health practitioner did not score significantly higher than individuals without such prior experience, this suggests that the examination measured competence specifically pertinent to the proficiency of a physician's assistant or nurse practitioner.

In addition to this internal evidence of validity, two external studies were also conducted, each focusing on somewhat different aspects of the examination's validity. Having found evidence to suggest that the examination was measuring knowledge and skills relevant to actual clinical practice, a study was conducted to determine whether or not the examination was measuring components of competence that could be attributed to the training process itself. If the certifying examination was measuring knowledge and skills that could be acquired only through a training program for physician's assistants and nurse practitioners, then one would expect examinees for the 1973 certifying examination to score significantly higher than those beginning a training program who, presumably, had not yet acquired the same level of proficiency.

Hence, the 1973 certifying examination was administered to groups just beginning training as physician's assistants, Medex or nurse practitioners. A stratified random sample was selected of 16 representative programs in which candidates for the 1973 examination had been trained. The 1973 certifying examination was administered to the group of trainees entering those 16 programs, using the same procedures.

The validation sample consisted of 357 examinees: 83 percent physician's assistants, 15 percent Medex and 3 percent nurse practitioners. The 1973 test group consisted of 880: 62 percent physician's assistants, 29 percent Medex, and 9 percent nurse practitioners. A statistical comparison of the performance of these two groups was done by performing t-tests on the total examination score as well as on scores obtained on the three components of the written examination. With respect to overall examination performance, the mean score of examinees from the validation sample was 374, while a comparable sample of 1973 examinees obtained a mean score of 497. This difference was highly significant (p < .001) and indicated that those who had completed their formal program scored significantly higher than those just beginning training. Similar differences in performance were also observed on each of the three components of the written examination.

A third validation study was conducted to estimate the concurrent validity of the certifying examination. This study was designed to investigate the relationship between performance on the various components of the certifying examination and ratings of clinical competence as provided by program faculty. A clinical competence rating form was developed consisting of 40 statements, each describing different aspects of the competency. These statements described behavior related to: (a) history taking, (b) physicial examination, (c) laboratory tests and diagnostic procedures, (d) management/treatment, (e) medical records, and (f) interpersonal relations. A clinical competence rating form for each of the 1973 examination registrants was mailed to the appropriate program director who was asked to identify a member of the faculty familiar with the candidate's clinical performance. The faculty rater was asked to read each statement contained in the rating form and decide at what level of competence the candidate performed. A scale consisting of five intervals was used with the end points labeled "minimum competence" and "optimum competence." An 86 percent response rate was obtained.

A factor analysis of items contained on the rating scale was performed to identify clusters of related items and the dimensions of clinical competence each cluster appeared to be measuring. The factor analysis yielded the following three dimensions: (1) data gathering and recording, (2) interpersonal skills, and (3) clinical judgment. The data gathering and recording factor consisted of rating items assessing competence in taking histories, performing physical examinations and recording patient data.

The interpersonal skills factor contained items pertinent to interactions between the new health practitioner and the patient, the patient's family and other members of the health team. The clinical judgment factor consisted of items pertinent to patient management. Analysis of the examination and rating scale data was performed by correlating an individual's clinical competence rating on each of the three factors with scores on the various examination components. To provide a more detailed analysis of the examination itself, items on the multiple-choice question portion were classified into one of four categories: (1) identification and classification of physical findings, (2) patient management, (3) knowledge of clinical procedures, and (4) interpersonal skills. Items on patient management problems (PMP) were classified into a data gathering or management/treatment scale.

Pearson product-moment correlation coefficients were computed to determine the direction and magnitude of the simple correlations between examination components and rating factors. In those instances where an examination component correlated significantly with more than one rating factor, step-wise multiple regression analyses were performed to identify the nature and magnitude of these complex relationships. Evidence for the construct validity of the certifying examination would be provided by the extent to which significant positive correlations were observed between those examination components and rating factors where it would be logical to expect such a relationship.

Candidate performance on multiple-choice questions dealing with the identification and classification of physical findings correlated significantly with ratings of data gathering and recording skills and clinical judgment. One would not expect performance on this examination component to correlate with ratings of interpersonal skills, and, in fact, such a relationship was not observed. Performance on multiple-choice questions related to patient management correlated significantly with ratings of clinical judgment, but not with ratings of data gathering and recording or interpersonal skills, a pattern of correlation which is consistent with the logical constructs of these examination and rating scale components.

Similarly for patient counseling and instruction, examination performance on these multiple-choice questions correlated significantly with ratings of interpersonal skills and clinical judgment. A significant relationship with ratings of data gathering and recording skills was not expected, and none was observed. Performance on the PMP data gathering section (which included history taking, physical examination, and selection of laboratory tests) correlated significantly with ratings of data gathering and recording skills, and clinical judgment. Since interpersonal skills were not measured on this component of the examination, one would not expect to find a significant relationship with ratings of interpersonal skills. This was observed to be the case. The four examination components thus far described were all found to correlate positively and significantly with the rating factors to which they bore the most logical relationship and not with rating factors that did not seem pertinent to the nature of the component. To this extent, the pattern of significant correlation provides evidence for the convergent and discriminant validity of the certifying examination.

Multiple-choice questions related to the knowledge of clinical procedures did not correlate significantly with any of the three rating factors. This, too, is consistent with the discriminant validity of the certifying examination since none of the rating factors dealt with a candidate's level of competence in performing clinical procedures. Thus, the absence of significant correlation is consistent with the logical constructs of the examination components and rating factors. The one examination component for which evidence of discriminant validity was not observed was that patient management problem component which dealt with management and therapy decisions. One would have expected to observe a significant correlation between this examination component and ratings of clinical judgment. Although the magnitude of the correlation coefficient between PMP management/therapy and ratings of clinical judgment was greater than that observed for the other two rating factors, it did not reach statistical significance. A further analysis of the statements contained on the clinical judgment rating factor indicated that behavior related to the selection and sequencing of appropriate diagnostic tests and procedures contributed a large number of the items included on this rating factor. However, the examination component labeled PMP management/therapy did not include patient management problems related to the selection and interpretation of diagnostic tests and procedures. Instead, these items were included in the PMP data gathering component. It is possible, therefore, that the lack of significant correlation was attributable to the incorrect classification of patient management problem items related to the selection of laboratory tests. The simple and multiple correlation coefficients are summarized in Tables 6:2 and 6:3. The magnitude of the multiple correlations is greater than that for the simple correlations because more than one rating factor is used to predict performance on a single examination component.

1974 CERTIFYING EXAMINATION

In addition to requiring graduation from an approved educational program, eligibility for the 1974 certifying examination was expanded to include those qualifying on the basis of work experience. They were required to have a high school diploma or an equivalency certificate and four years of medical clinical experience in primary care as a physician's assistant or nurse practitioner. The work experience outlined on each application form was verified by contacting the physicians whose names

TABLE 6:2

Simple Correlations Between Rating Factors and Components of First Examination
Performance—1973

Examination Component	Rating Factor		
	Data Gathering and Recording	Interpersonal Skills	Clinical Judgment
Identification and Classification of Physical Findings	.18[1]	.02	.25[2]
Patient Management	.08	.11	.21[1]
Patient Counseling and Instruction	.13	.23[1]	.23[1]
Knowledge of Clinical Procedures[3]	.04	.04	.16
PMP Data Gathering	.29[2]	.12	.25[2]
PMP Management/Therapy	.06	.07	.11

[1] Significant beyond the .05 level
[2] Significant beyond the .01 level
[3] Rating scale did not contain items that permitted faculty to indicate registrant's level of competence in performing clinical procedures.

TABLE 6:3

Complex Correlations Between Rating Factors and Components of First Examination
Performance—1973

Examination Component	Rating Factors	Multiple Correlation[1]
Identification and Classification of Physical Findings	Data Gathering Clinical Judgment	.29
Patient Counseling and Instruction	Interpersonal Skills Clinical Judgment	.33
PMP Data Gathering	Data Gathering Clinical Judgment	.37

[1] All correlation coefficients are significant beyond the .05 level of confidence.

and addresses were provided. Each physician was required to provide a detailed description and estimated frequency of the health care functions performed by the applicant. These details of an applicant's employment history were then evaluated in relation to specific criteria established in advance by an eligibility committee.

Announcements of the eligibility requirements were placed in the major primary care medical journals and newsletters. As a result, 550 completed application forms were received from individuals wishing to qualify on the basis of work experience. Of this number, 150 met the established eligibility requirements and 116 sat for the certifying examination. The most frequently encountered factors in failing to meet eligibility requirements were: less than the required four years of clinical experience and/or health care functions that did not include patient management decision-making.

The written component of the 1974 certifying examination followed the same format as in 1973, that is, a multiple-choice examination designed to assess the candidate's knowledge and skill applied to clinical material in printed and pictorial form, and management of simulated adult and pediatric clinical cases, designed to assess the candidate's skill in gathering pertinent information about patients and in making appropriate management decisions. The number of items included on both portions of the written examination was increased on the 1974 examination. In addition, multiple-choice questions using pictorial material required the identification and *interpretation* of physical findings instead of the identification and classification of findings as had been the case in the previous year.

In addition to the written component, candidates underwent assessment of their physical examination skills using standardized behavioral checklists that had been developed as part of an extensive research and development project. This assessment consisted of an evaluation of the candidate's proficiency in performing five components of the physical examination (i.e., heart, lungs, eyes, abdomen, and nervous system). Test centers were established on the two days following the written examination, and candidates were given individual appointments for assessment. The candidate performed three examination components on one patient while observed by a physician examiner and performed the remaining two components on another patient while observed by another physician examiner. The total assessment time for each candidate was approximately forty minutes.

Physician examiners were appointed by program directors at the various test centers. Prior to the examination, three regional orientation meetings were held to acquaint examiners with the assessment objectives, procedures and guidelines for patient selection. In addition, proctors were appointed for these special test centers to ensure the adequacy of the arrangements and to maintain the security of the procedure itself. Since written reports from the chief proctors and physician examiners did not disclose any problems that would jeopardize the integrity of this procedure, the physical examination component of the certifying examination was used for scoring purposes. Each of the five physical examination components was weighted equally, and performance on this part of the examination accounted for 25 percent of a candidate's total score.

The 1974 examination was administered to 1,303 candidates at 49 test centers. The statistical properties of the 1974 examination program closely paralleled those encountered in 1973. Although the number of candidates still enrolled in educational programs increased to 23 percent in 1974 as compared to 11 percent in 1973, the typical examinee had completed a formal program and acquired up to two years of postgraduate clinical experience. Seventy-five percent of the formally trained examinees received their training in programs from 13 to 24 months in length, and 92 percent had been involved in health care delivery prior to being trained as a physician's assistant or nurse practitioner. Of those examinees with prior experience in health care, 58 percent had more than four years of experience. These data are summarized in Table 6:4.

Statistical analysis of the 1974 examination indicated that the average difficulty level and reliabilities for the examination were comparable to statistics derived from the 1973 examination. The one exception was that average level of the 1974 multiple-choice questions was somewhat more difficult than in 1973. In 1973, the average difficulty level equaled .64; in 1974, this figure was .57. The composite reliability for all examination components increased from .89 in 1973 to .93 in 1974. This modest increase in reliability was attributable, however, to the larger number of items on the 1974 examination. An analysis of the intercorrelations among the various components yielded correlation coefficients ranging from .13 to .53. The correlations among the written portions ranged from .37 to .53, and closely resembled those encountered on the 1973 examination program. These modest correlations suggested that the various written portions measured different aspects of competence. As might be anticipated, the correlations between the written and the physical examination portions of the certifying examination were lower, ranging from .13 to .28. Given the magnitude of these intercorrelations, it was evident that one could not predict physical examination skills by knowing the candidate's score on the written portion of the examination. The variation in scores on the physical examination component indicated a wide range of proficiency among the 1,303 candidates who sat for the

1974 examination. This range of scores was greater than that observed for the written component.

In addition to the above analyses, a comparison was made of the performance of informally and formally trained candidates on all components of the certifying examination. In all instances, candidates who had not graduated from formal educational programs scored significantly

TABLE 6:4

Physician's Assistant Certifying Examination Description of Examinee Populations

	1973	1974	1975
Percentages of total respondents:	N=880	N=1303	N=1411
Current status			
Currently in educational program	11%	23%	—[1]
Currently employed or graduated	89	77	—
Type of training			
Physician's assistant/associate	62%	71%	73%
Medex	29	15	11
Nurse	9	5	5
Informally trained	—	9	11
Amount of experience			
None	19%	25%	—
0 - 2 years	72	62	—
More than 2 years	9	13	—
Percentage of respondents with formal training (informally trained candidates not included)	N=880	N=1187	—
Length of educational program			
4-12 months	12%	13%	—
13-24 months	65	75	—
25-36 months	10	7	—
More than 36 months	3	5	—
Experience in health care delivery prior to educational program			
Yes	91%	92%	—
No	9	8	—
Type of experience			
Technical	11%	12%	—
Patient contact	86	84	—
Other	3	4	—
Length of experience			
0-1 year	4%	4%	—
1-2 years	10	11	—
2-4 years	30	27	—
More than 4 years	56	58	—

[1]Only limited data on the 1975 examinee population have been tabulated by the National Commission on Certification of Physician's Assistants.

lower than did candidates who had been trained in formal educational programs. This trend was also observed on the 1975 examination.

1975 CERTIFYING EXAMINATION

In 1975, 1,411 candidates were tested. No significant changes were noted in the examinee population in 1975, and the examination statistics followed the same pattern as had been observed in 1974.

Beginning in 1975, the certification of physician's assistants and the examination program became the responsibility of the National Commission on Certification of Physician's Assistants. The National Board of Medical Examiners continues to develop the certifying examination under a contract with the Commission. It is anticipated that approximately 1,400 candidates annually will continue to be tested through this examination. At present approximately 25 states use the examination results as one component in their evaluation of qualifications for practice.

Chapter 7

The Legal Scope of Nurse Practitioners under Nurse Practice and Medical Practice Acts

Virginia C. Hall

Each of the 50 states and the District of Columbia has a nurse practice act,[1] a licensure statute governing the practice of professional and practical nursing. These statutes, typically passed from 1940 to the early 1950s, parallel a medical practice act which similarly licenses and regulates physicians, the only other generally recognized health professional until recent times. The overall structure of the various nurse practice acts is very much the same: minimum requisites for licensure as well as grounds for discipline of licensed nurses are stated; a board made up to a greater or lesser extent of nurses is created with authority to administer the licensing and disciplinary provisions; and the content of the practice of nursing is stated in a definition.*

In the "extended" or "expanded" nursing role, specially trained nurses perform acts of diagnosis, treatment or prescription which traditionally have been within the exclusive province of the physician and therefore improper and presumably illegal for a nurse. For this reason there has been an increasingly widespread effort to provide clear legal authorization through statutory amendment for a nurse practicing in such a role. These efforts have uniformly focussed on the definition of "professional nursing" in the nurse practice act, which is the obvious cornerstone although not the only determinant of the legal scope of nursing practice in a given state. The following summarizes the changes in the definition of nursing practice in the various states and how these changes have affected the legal scope of practice. Because of space limitations, other provisions in the nurse and medical practice acts which might bear on the legal scope of practice are summarized very briefly or omitted entirely.**

---

*Only two jurisdictions, Georgia and the District of Columbia, do not have a definition of nursing in their nurse practice act.

**Among the provisions not dealt with are those pertaining to specific nursing specialties, such as nurse anesthetists, and provisions for the performance of certain specific acts such as the prescription of drugs or procedures involving the drawing of blood. Such provisions may be significant not just for what they say about the limited subjects to which they are addressed, but also for the broader implications they may have for nurses not in the specialties covered or performing acts and procedures not specifically dealt with.

In addition, those provisions of the nurse practice acts which do not bear on the legal scope of practice are not addressed. These other provisions, although they admittedly make up the majority of the various acts, are more procedural than substantive and have remained largely unchanged.

LEGAL STATUS OF NURSE PRACTITIONERS UNDER NURSE PRACTICE ACTS

At the outset it is worth clarifying the legally significant difference between the traditional role of the nurse and that of the nurse practitioner or other nurse practicing in the extended role. The latter role involves many functions which were not traditionally performed by a nurse, but it is only in her performance of *medical* functions—diagnosis, treatment and prescription—that her role assumes a legal significance. Other new aspects of her role do not consist of functions which she traditionally has been prohibited from performing by custom as well as by law, whereas the medical aspects of her role at least arguably do. In making this point it should be stressed that it is not just the *types* of medical tasks that a nurse practitioner performs which arguably have been illegal for a nurse under the traditional nurse and medical practice acts, but also her performance of them—not so much under the supervision and direction of a physician as in collaboration with one or more physicians and other health care professionals.* The ideal amended nurse practice act therefore would recognize and legitimize both the types of medical tasks and their collegial performance with physicians, while imposing suitable safeguards to insure that nurses who are not qualified to act in this capacity are not permitted to do so.

DEFINITIONS OF PROFESSIONAL NURSING PRACTICE

Traditional Definitions

Twenty-seven states have retained without change or only minor change, a definition based on the American Nurses' Association (ANA)

---

* In this regard the extended role of the nurse is sharply distinguishable from that of the physician assistant, who likewise performs a rather wide range of medical tasks but whose role has been universally statutorily defined as involving physician supervision.

model definition formulated some years ago. As adopted by the ANA, and as it exists substantially verbatim in the nurse practice acts of 13 states, this definition is:

> The term "practice of nursing" means the performance, for compensation, of any acts in the observation, care and counsel of the ill, injured or infirm or in the maintenance of health or prevention of illness of others, or in the supervision and teaching of other personnel, or the administration of medications and treatments as prescribed by a licensed physician or a licensed dentist; requiring substantial specialized judgment and skills and based on knowledge and application of the principles of biological, physical and social science. The foregoing shall not be deemed to include acts of diagnosis or prescription of therapeutic or corrective measures.

Four states likewise follow the ANA definition, with the omission of the last sentence of prohibition. Several other states have variants of the ANA definition, substituting such phraseology as "supervision of the patient, observation of symptoms and reactions, and application of nursing procedures" or services "in the care of the sick, in the prevention of disease, or in the conservation of health."

Despite differences in phraseology, all these definitions share certain important features insofar as they purport to define the medical portion of nursing practice. Each contains broad, vague terms—"care and counsel of the ill," "application of nursing procedures," etc.—which could be interpreted as encompassing medical acts, including those performed by a nurse in the extended role. However, given the age of these definitions it is unlikely that these terms were intended to extend to anything beyond the traditional nursing role. It is significant in this regard that the only portion of them which clearly refers to medical acts, contrasted with the rest of the definitions, is emphatically specific. This portion is the phrase *"administration* of treatments and medications *prescribed* by a physician or dentist"* [author's italics], or similar words. In seventeen states, there is an outright prohibition of acts of diagnosis and prescription. In these states this prohibition precludes any broad interpretation of the vague terms of the definitions which encompass medical acts. Even without prohibition, the narrow reference to administration of prescribed treatments and medications carries a substantial inference that the definition was not intended to encompass the performance of other medical acts by a nurse nor the performance of such acts of treatment or prescription in other than the specified subordinate capacity.

The only change which has been made in any of these definitions in an attempt to accommodate them to the newer developments in nursing is to qualify the prohibition of diagnosis and prescription so as to apply only to acts of "medical" diagnosis and prescription. Such a qualification has been adopted by 11 of the states which otherwise have not changed their traditional definitions. However, since the legal problems of a nurse in the extended role arise precisely because of her performance of medical diagnosis and prescription, thus creating an overlap between her role and that of a physician to an extent which did not previously exist, this qualification would appear to serve little or no purpose.

New Approaches

Among the states which have made some major effort to modify the definition of nursing in their nurse practice act to make it consistent with new developments in the profession, two basic approaches may be discerned: The additional acts amendment and total redefinition.

The Additional Acts Amendment

The additional acts amendment, which has been adopted by 17 states, is generally added to a traditional form of definition which is not itself changed in any way; it can also, however, be found in conjunction with a total redefinition. Such an amendment is characterized by the omission of any attempt to characterize in substantive terms the acts which it encompasses. Rather, it refers to some other source to define and delimit those acts. Typically this other source is rules and regulations to be issued by the State Board of Nursing, often together with the State Board of Medicine, and/or professional nursing and medical opinion. In addition, the entire amendment is frequently made applicable only to nurses with "education and training," presumably in addition to that required for all professional nurses. Finally, a very few states directly or indirectly make the entire amendment hinge on delegation of the permitted acts by a physician.

As an approach to legitimizing the medical portion of the extended nursing role the additional acts amendment has a great deal to recommend it inasmuch as it avoids the semantic difficulties likely to arise from any attempt to deal with the content of the practice in substantive terms. In addition, it need not be amended again as the practice changes because rules and regulations can be changed with the practice without necessitating any change in the governing law. On the other hand, because rules and regulations cannot be predicted, especially in the long term, it is advisable to have professional opinion as an additional independent (as opposed to cumulative) determinant of legality under an additional acts amendment. This is because professional opinion will always exist and should at all times provide a meaningful test for the legality of any given act. Unfortunately, only two of the states which have adopted an additional acts amendment have followed this pattern. The others, if they refer to professional opinion at all, specify that the state *and* its rules and regulations shall determine the permitted additional acts.

Total Redefinition

Twelve states, of which seven also have adopted an additional acts amendment, have replaced their previous statutory definitions entirely with a new definition which bears little or no resemblance to the ANA definition quoted earlier. On closer examination, however, it is evident that these new definitions almost uniformly have incorporated the traditional concept of the role of the nurse in the medical sphere: i.e., as a dependent functionary who can make no independent decisions of her own, but who must act under the direction and supervision of a physician. In fact, in the case of some of the new definitions, this concept is at least arguably more explicit than it is in some of the vaguer variants of the traditional ANA definition.

New definitions have so far been adopted in three broad formats. By far the most common is based on New York's definition, which was adopted in 1972 as the first of the total redefinitions and widely hailed at the time as a major legislative break-through. The New York definition is:

> The practice of the profession of nursing as a registered professional nurse is defined as diagnosing and treating human responses to actual or potential health problems through such services as casefinding, health teaching, health counseling, and provision of care supportive to or restorative of life and well-being, and executing medical regimens prescribed by a licensed or otherwise legally authorized physician or dentist. A nursing regimen shall be consistent with and shall not vary any existing medical regimen.[2]

The terms "diagnosing," "treating," and "human responses" as used in the definition are in turn defined as follows:

> 1. "Diagnosing" in the context of nursing practice means identification of and discrimination between physical and psy-

chosocial signs and symptoms essential to effective execution and management of the nursing regimen. Such diagnostic privilege is distinct from a medical diagnosis.

2. "Treating" means selection and performance of those therapeutic measures essential to the effective execution and management of the nursing regimen, and execution of any prescribed medical regimen.

3. "Human Responses" means those signs, symptoms and processes which denote the individual's interaction with an actual or potential health problem.[3]

Two states have adopted the New York definition, together with its subordinate definitions, essentially verbatim. Six other states have adopted the New York definition and seem to have incorporated the same concept as the New York definition of the nurse's medical role. Analysis of the New York definition and those based on it reveals a clear dichotomy between "medical" and "nursing" functions. Although the classic medical terms "diagnosing" and "treating" are used, they are carefully defined as distinct from their medical counterparts. What, in fact, they are intended to consist of in the nursing context is somewhat less than clear. In addition, where the term "medical regimen" appears, the nurse's role is confined to "execution," in a phrase strikingly reminiscent of the phrase "administration of medications and treatments prescribed by a licensed physician" which appears in the older ANA definition. *It is therefore questionable at best whether the New York definition and its progeny have relaxed at all the traditional prohibitions against any independent functioning by a nurse in the medical sphere.*

The second broad type of new definition is that adopted by Maryland[4] and Minnesota.[5] This definition does not include any of the terminology used in the New York definition, but does have much the same effect in restricting the medical role of a nurse to traditional concepts. This effect is achieved by a sentence which describes nursing as consisting of "independent nursing functions...[and] delegated medical functions." Again, the parallelism between this statement and the reference in the traditional definition to "administration of prescribed medications and treatments" is obvious.

The third format has appeared in the California definition and is the only one of the new definitions which not only manages to avoid perpetuating traditional concepts of the nurse's medical role but explicitly adopts the view that a nurse's and a physician's functions are to some extent overlapping and that the two professions work in collaboration in this shared area. The preamble states the legislative intent to recognize "the existence of overlapping functions between physicians and registered nurses" and to permit "additional sharing of functions within organized health care systems which provide for collaboration between physicians and registered nurses."[6] The definition itself is rather lengthy and at least arguably narrower in its description of a nurse's medical role than the preamble. It consists of a detailed description of four nursing functions. The first of these seems clearly nonmedical in nature ("services that insure the safety, comfort, personal hygiene, and protection of patients...."); the second consists of the administration and implementation of medical treatments. The third and fourth consist of limited medical activities ("basic health care, testing, and prevention procedures,.... observation of ... symptoms, implementation of appropriate reporting ... or changes in treatment regimen"), the performance of which in both cases is tied to "standardized procedures." This term is in turn defined as "policies and protocols developed ... through collaboration among administrators and health professionals including physicians and nurses." The question raised, therefore, is how all-inclusive must the required "standardized procedures" be—how wide a range of acts must they cover and how much room may they leave for the exercise by a nurse of her own judgment.

In summary, the preamble to the California definition indicates clearly that the Legislature recognized what the expanded role of the nurse consists of with respect to the performance of medical acts and intended to legitimize it, without any overriding blanket requirement of physician delegation or supervision. However, the actual definition shows the pitfalls which will almost inevitably stem from any attempt to express substantively and to itemize the functions of the nurse at any given time. It is that much more difficult, *a fortiori*, to formulate a substantive redefinition of the practice which will also be appropriate in future years, as the role of the nurse continues to evolve.

PROHIBITIONS OF PRACTICE OF MEDICINE

Eight states share a provision in their nurse practice act, usually found in a section other than the definition, which has a powerful effect on the meaning which might otherwise be given the definition standing alone. This provision is a statement to the effect that nothing in the act shall be construed as conferring the authority to practice medicine.* With such a

*Of interest in this connection is that California had such a provision prior to its 1974 amendment of the definition of nursing, at which time it amended it to read as follows: "Except as otherwise provided herein this chapter confers no authority to practice medicine or surgery."[7]

provision it becomes virtually impossible to argue that nurses may legally perform medical acts, except as delegated by a physician, inasmuch as performance of them in any other capacity would constitute the illegal practice of medicine.

PROHIBITIONS OF PRACTICE OF MEDICINE BY NONPHYSICIANS IN MEDICAL PRACTICE ACTS

The prohibitions against the practice of medicine discussed above parallel comparable prohibitions aimed at all nonphysicians—not just at nurses—which are found in the medical practice acts of all the states. Almost half the states, however, exempt nurses from this prohibition. Seven others exempt persons legally practicing another profession under another law of the state, which exception could, depending on the terms of the nurse practice act, extend to nursing. Of the remaining states about half have some form of a limited exemption (often referred to as a "delegation provision") for nurses or nonspecified persons acting under the direction and supervision of a physician, and the rest have no exemption for nurses at all. Some of these latter states have a delegation provision which applies only to physician's assistants, not to nurses. It should be noted also that a few of the states which specifically exempt nurses, without any requirement of delegation, also include nurses in a delegation provision, thereby raising the question whether delegation is intended as a limitation on exemption. In any case, the lack of any exemption is in fact no more restrictive than an exemption for delegated acts only.

MEDICAL AND NURSE PRACTICE ACTS CONSIDERED TOGETHER

In determining the legal scope of nursing practice in any given state it is imperative, therefore, to look not just at the nurse practice act, but also at the medical practice act. The two are not separate entities; for the meaning of one can affect the meaning of the other. Where the two acts are inconsistent, as where one grants (or at least does not preclude) a latitude which the other specifically prohibits, one cannot with absolute confidence ignore the latter and rely exclusively on the former to supply legal authority for the medical aspect of the expanded nursing role. Ideally, the two acts should speak consistently on the subject of nurse practice, but few do.

In conclusion, the flurry of legislative activity in the last few years attests to the widespread realization that nursing as a profession has undergone a significant change. It is in the interests of optimal health care to provide clear legal sanction for this change. However, the new definitions of the practice of nursing largely have been counterproductive since they have failed to acknowledge the role which a nurse practitioner plays in the medical area. Rather, they have perpetuated the traditional view that in the overlap between medicine and nursing the nurse acts in a dependent capacity. The only state which to some extent has avoided this pitfall—California—has nonetheless come up with a wordy, detailed definition which raises semantic questions of its own. Indeed, any new definition would raise some such questions. The most fruitful approach, therefore, would be the simple additional acts amendment which does not attempt to deal substantively with the content of nursing practice, but incorporates a criterion of legality, such as professional opinion, which can be counted on to delimit the scope of nursing practice in a meaningful, responsible manner.

Anyone contemplating a statutory amendment would be well advised to focus on the following areas of concern:

- Does the proposed amendment restrict nursing to something other than medicine?
- Does it assume or explicitly provide for a dependent role in the performance of medical acts?
- Does it contain terms which create ambiguities?
- Does it rely on implementation by rules and regulations or on a meaningful, self-executing criterion?
- Is it consistent with medical practice acts?

Whatever form of statutory change is chosen, all these concerns must be satisfactorily resolved before one can fully achieve the desideratum of a law which is at once flexible in permitting new professional developments and at the same time responsible to the public. Only then, in turn, can nursing feel free to devote its full attention to what should and must be its primary concern: determining what role it can best fill in the delivery of health care now and in the future.

Notes

1. This chapter is based on a survey prepared by the author in 1974 for the National Joint Practice Commission entitled "Statutory Regulation of The Scope of Nursing Practice—A Critical Survey." Omissions in the original survey have been corrected, to the extent discovered, and the survey has been updated to include new developments which have come to the author's attention. However, the author can give no assurance

that the article is fully current. In addition, the author does not purport to speak authoritatively as to the law of any state other than Massachusetts.

2. New York Educ. Law § 6902 (1)(McKinney Supp. 1973) (Amended 1972).

3. Ibid.

4. Maryland Ann. Code art. 43, § 291(b)(1)(ii) (Supp. 1974) (Amended 1974).

5. Minnesota Stat. Ann. § 148.171(3) (Supp. 1975) (Amended 1974).

6. California Business and Professional Code § 2725d (West Supp. 1975) (Amended 1974).

7. Ibid.

Chapter 8

Physician's Assistant and Nurse Practitioner Laws for Expanded Medical Delegation

Philip C. Kissam

This chapter reviews a new development in state medical practice laws: the attempt to provide a permanent legal structure to authorize and regulate innovative delegations of medical acts by physicians which will be referred to as expanded medical delegation.[1] This attempt to reform the basic structure of medical practice laws has resulted in two types of new laws: One is the so-called "physician's assistant" (PA) statute that authorizes expanded medical delegation to any qualified nonphysician. The other, which may be referred to as the "nurse practitioner" (NP) statute, authorizes expanded delegation only to qualified professional nurses and, in a few cases, to qualified practical nurses as well.

THE NATURE OF EXPANDED MEDICAL DELEGATION

The nature of expanded medical delegation suggests the potential medical and economic feasibility of delegating a wide range of medical acts to a variety of nonphysicians, delegation that transcends the scope of traditional medical responsibilities of allied health personnel. Medical practice may be defined as all acts of patient care that physicians are trained to perform. It will help to think of these acts as forming a spectrum that consists of three distinct, albeit overlapping, categories. At one end of the spectrum are *diagnostic and treatment judgments*, which include initial determinations of disease based upon an evaluation of symptoms and the development of an appropriate treatment plan for the diagnosed condition. The middle category consists of *treatment modifications*, which include judgments about the severity of symptoms and the need to continue or modify the prescribed treatment. (These first two categories have sometimes been referred to as a "doctor's diagnosis" and a "nursing diagnosis" respectively.) The third category of medical acts consists of *medical procedures*, which include all remaining acts necessary to implement diagnostic and treatment judgments or treatment modifications. Medical procedures include diagnostic procedures such as physical examination, medical history, laboratory tests and therapeutic procedures such as administering medication by injection and suturing wounds. These categories cannot be defined in a precise way because many medical acts will not be classified easily in one or another category. For example, should the interpretation of X-rays be classified as a diagnostic judgment or a data-gathering procedure? It also will be difficult in some cases to draw a line between the administration of a prescribed treatment and a treatment modification, or between a treatment modification and the diagnosis and treatment of a new condition. Notwithstanding this lack of precision, these three categories will be helpful in describing the possibilities for expanded medical delegation and in analyzing many of the new legislative rules that make use of these terms.

Traditionally, some delegation of medical acts has been utilized. For example, physical therapists prescribe and carry out treatments upon referral from physicians; and nurses administer physician-prescribed medications and treatments. But traditional medical delegation has not included even the most relatively simple, routine medical acts. Physical examination, medical history, diagnosis and treatment of common illnesses, minor surgery, and decisions to continue or modify prescribed treatment for convalescing or chronically ill patients generally have not been delegated. Furthermore, medical acts that have been delegated have been entrusted only to limited groups of licensed allied health personnel, notwithstanding other nonphysicians' ability to perform the same acts. For example, a practical nurse qualified by on-the-job training to give inoculations may not have legal authority to do so because only professional nurses have been licensed to give inoculations.

Diagnostic and treatment judgments, treatment modifications, and medical procedures vary from relatively simple, routine acts to highly complex ones. It would seem *a priori* that many simple, routine acts in all three categories might be performed as competently by nonphysicians as by physicians.[2] For example, compare the decision whether an upper-respiratory tract complaint is a symptom of a common cold, a streptococcal throat infection for which penicillin should be prescribed, or some more complex disorder. Recent medical studies suggest that such limited medical acts which include diagnostic judgments and treatment modifications, may be performed competently by nonphysicians with limited and varied medical training.[3] The nonphysicians studied ranged from PAs with one or two years of training in diagnosing certain types of medical complaints under supervision or written protocols, to professional nurses with additional medical training who conducted a general medical practice on an independent basis, referring more difficult problems to physicians.

The usefulness of expanded medical delegation will depend on its economic as well as its medical feasibility. Economic feasibility requires that the value of the services delegated exceed the costs of such delegation. The high cost of physicians' services relative to the cost of nonphysicians' services suggests that a much expanded delegation may be economically feasible. Physicians' incomes today appear to be in excess of four times those of professional nurses, the allied health professionals whose functions most closely approximate those of PAs and NPs. For 1973, as an example, the American Medical Association's estimates for average net incomes of physicians by specialty ranged from $40,000 for pediatricians and general practitioners to more than $58,000 for surgeons. For the same year, the Department of Labor's statistics show that the average annual salaries of general duty registered nurses in public hospitals of 21 major cities ranged from $8,000 to $11,000, with salaries over $9,800 only in two of the 21 cities. It will be necessary to pay PAs and NPs something more than professional nurses. In view of relatively low PA and NP training costs it may not be necessary to pay PAs and NPs much more than professional nurses. Thus, for example, if PAs and NPs earn a salary equal to one-third of physicians' incomes, and if their use increases physicians' productivity by more than a third, it will pay physicians to employ them. Recent economic evaluations of PAs and NPs indicate that gains in physician productivity from effective use of full-time PAs and NPs are likely to be far in excess of 33 percent.[4]

Finally, feasible medical delegations are likely to vary substantially in the manner in which they are implemented. The different types of nonphysicians and the nature of the physician-nonphysician relationship also may vary. Depending upon the nature of the delegated acts and the skills of the nonphysician, these acts might be performed on a limited, independent basis, with referral of more difficult problems to physicians; upon referral from a physician after an initial diagnosis has been made; or under a physician's supervision, which may vary from personal observation to periodic communication with and review of the nonphysician's work. The medical acts considered delegable and the necessary qualifications of any nonphysician to perform them also will vary over time, as physicians and nonphysicians obtain new knowledge and skills from experience and as medical technology and economic conditions change.

LEGAL BARRIERS TO EXPANDED DELEGATION: THE NEED FOR STATUTORY AUTHORIZATION

Traditionally, state statutes governing medical and allied health practices have limited the legal rights of physicians to delegate medical acts in an innovative manner. Thus, some form of statutory amendment is necessary to obtain clear legal authorization for expanded medical delegation.

The medical practice acts of all states require that the practice of medicine be conducted only by licensed physicians or persons specifically exempted by the acts. These acts typically define the practice of medicine in broad although imprecise terms. For example, New York defines medical practice as the "diagnosing, treating, operating or prescribing for any human disease, pain, injury, deformity or physical condition."[5] These acts provide criminal, civil and administrative sanctions (fines, imprisonment, injunctions and revocation of physician license) for the unlicensed practice of medicine and for aiding and abetting another in such practice. In the few relevant court decisions testing the legality of delegation of medical acts to unlicensed persons, courts have tended to give a broad reading to the practice of medicine and thereby to find the delegation illegal. They also have rejected the defense that unlicensed persons working under physician supervision were not themselves practicing medicine but acting as mere agents of the delegating physician.

Any unlicensed person to whom medical acts are delegated, any physician who supervises such a person, and any employer also may risk imposition of additional liability in malpractice cases because of the delegation. This additional liability may result from judicially created rules that disfavor the unlicensed practice of medicine such as a presumption of negligence, conclusive or rebuttable, from the fact of unlicensed practice despite the custom's relevance to the unlicensed person's ability to perform the delegated act with reasonable care. These disfavoring rules, like broad interpretations of medical practice and rejection of the agency defense in criminal and administrative proceedings concerning the unlicensed practice of medicine, have been based upon the policy underlying medical practice acts of protecting the public by licensure.

State statutory law does recognize two types of medical practice by nonphysicians. The first type is authorized by specific exemptions from the medical practice acts. These exemptions are limited to well-identified groups such as consulting physicians from out of state, good samaritans, and medical students and interns. Generally, however, these exemptions have not provided legal authority for expanded medical delegation.

Allied health personnel licensure laws authorize a second type of medical practice by nonphysicians. These laws generally are not appropriate for authorizing expanded medical delegation because they authorize only limited medical practice by specific allied health personnel, who qualify by showing competence to perform an entire range of medical and nonmedical acts. In terms of expanded medical delegation, professional nursing practice acts are probably the most important of these laws, as they reveal the legal problem for expanded medical delegation that is common to all such statutes. Nursing practice acts typically require that the practice of professional nursing be conducted only by licensed, registered professional nurses (RNs). The practice of professional nursing is also defined in broad and imprecise terms except that specific authority is usually provided for RNs to perform limited types of medical acts, typically, "the administration of medications and treatments as prescribed by a licensed physician." Frequently these acts also provide that professional nursing practice shall *not* include "acts of diagnosis or prescription of therapeutic or corrective measures." Thus, traditional professional nursing practice acts appear to preclude the delegation to RNs of medical diagnostic and treatment judgments. Moreover, the ambiguous definition of nursing practice, which includes specific authority for quite limited medical acts, creates substantial uncertainty about the legality of other new medical delegations to RNs. To establish legal authority for such delegations, it is necessary to rely upon case-by-case interpretations of the statutes by state Attorney Generals, state licensing boards and occasionally the courts, with the possibility of subsequent reinterpretations as well. This procees is likely to inhibit even those innovative medical delegations that might be authorized by the new statutes.

In summary, traditional state law substantially limits the legal rights of physicians to delegate medical acts, both as to whom they may delegate and as to the nature of delegated acts. Delegations to unlicensed personnel are authorized only if the acts are deemed not to constitute "the practice of medicine." Statutory change is necessary to provide clear legal authority for any expanded delegation.

THE NEW LEGISLATION

The feature common to PA and NP legislation is the use of broad terms to authorize expanded medical delegation to nonphysicians. The statutes differ as to the nonphysicians covered, the nature of administrative controls imposed over expanded medical delegation, and the manner in which a number of important rule-making issues have been resolved.

This part of the chapter will describe four basic types of new statutes—two types of PA statutes and two kinds of NP statutes. The following part will discuss several important rule-making issues that have been resolved in different ways by the statutes and regulations promulgated thereunder.

The PA Statutes: Regulation and Delegation

At least 37 states had enacted PA statutes by the summer of 1975. These statutes authorize varied groups of nonphysicians to qualify as PAs and they authorize supervising physicians to delegate a broad range of medical acts to qualified PAs. PA statutes generally recognize that any allied health professional with appropriate medical training may qualify as a PA. The determination of appropriate training by and large has been left to administrative agencies and, in some cases, supervising physicians.

These statutes typically authorize PAs to perform "medical services" or "patient's services" under the "supervision" of a licensed physician. For example, in California PAs may "perform medical service . . . under the supervision of a licensed physician,"[6] and in Georgia PAs may "provide patients' services not necessarily within the physical presence but under the personal direction or supervision of a physician."[7] Generally the statutes do not limit the nature of medical acts that may be delegated, except for the frequent requirement that PAs not function as or compete with certain other health professionals, usually optometrists, podiatrists, chiropractors and dentists. A few statutes, however, do prohibit diagnostic and treatment judgments and drug prescription. For example, Oregon has prohibited PAs from exercising "independent judgment in determining and prescribing treatment except in life-threatening emergencies,"[8] and Virginia has prohibited PAs from "the establishment of a final diagnosis or treatment plan for the patient . . . [and] the prescribing or dispensing of drugs."[9] In contrast, Colorado's Child Health Associate Law authorizes child health associates to "practice pediatrics"[10] and to prescribe certain nonnarcotic drugs approved by the state medical board.

PA Regulatory Statutes

The great majority of PA statutes provide explicitly for some form of administrative control over expanded medical delegation and are referred to as PA Regulatory Statutes. These statutes delegate broad regulatory authority to an administrative agency or agencies to determine the competence of all nonphysicians who perform delegated medical acts under the authority of such statutes. Most PA Regulatory Statutes also authorize an administrative agency to regulate PAs' scope of practice. In at least 17 states, a primary form of such regulation is the requirement that an individual job description be approved by the administrative agency before a PA may practice. Most PA Regulatory Statutes delegate all responsibility for administrative control to state medical licensing boards.

PA Simple Authorization Statutes

A very few PA statutes recognize expanded medical delegation without explicitly authorizing administrative regulation of expanded delegation and are referred to as PA Simple Authorization Statutes. These statutes consist merely of specific exemptions to state medical practice acts for services rendered by nonphysicians who work under a physician's "supervision" or "direction and control." Three of these statutes (Arkansas, Connecticut, Tennessee) define qualified nonphysicians as "a physician's trained assistant, a registered professional nurse or licensed practical nurse;"[11] Michigan refers to "a person qualified by education, training and experience;" and one simply refers to any person.[12] These PA Simple Authorization Statutes define expanded medical delegation simply as "services" or "selected acts, tasks or functions." None of these statutes provides further terms or procedures that otherwise define or limit PA practice, and it would appear that a physician has relatively broad discretion to select nonphysicians to perform medical acts.

The general statutory authority of medical licensing boards to ensure competent practice by physicians arguably might be sufficient authority for a board to promulgate specific PA regulations. These boards generally are also authorized to promulgate rules and regulations necessary or convenient to carry out their duties. Under such authority and the more general implied authority to ensure competent medical practice, it could be argued that a medical board is empowered to issue regulations defining the qualifications and scope of practice of PAs authorized by PA Simple Authorization Statutes. One medical board (Michigan) that has tried to do so, however, has been effectively restrained by an unfavorable opinion from the State Attorney General as to the scope of the board's general regulatory authority. In view of medical boards' traditional reluctance to regulate how physicians practice and the more general reluctance of state administrative agencies to promulgate regulations without explicit statutory authority, the promulgation of administrative regulations under PA Simple Authorization Statutes seems unlikely.

The NP Statutes—Regulation and Delegation

At least 28 states had enacted NP statutes by the summer of 1975. Typically, NP statutes consist of simple amendments to the statutory definition of the practice of professional nursing, expanding the definition to include additional acts that are authorized by administrative regulations or are performed "under the supervision" or "in collaboration with" a licensed physician.

NP Regulatory Statutes

A substantial majority of NP statutes require that expanded medical delegation to RNs be authorized by some form of administrative regulation and are referred to as NP Regulatory Statutes. At least nine NP Regulatory Statutes use "acts of medical diagnosis" and "prescription of therapeutic measures" or similar terms to define expanded delegation.[13] Typically, other NP Regulatory Statutes define expanded delegation as "additional acts" authorized by regulatory action.[14] In both adopted and proposed regulations under NP Regulatory Statutes, the marked tendency is to require prior certification of an NP's competency by the responsible licensing board. Such regulations also usually establish a job description for NPs or require approval of an individual job description by the responsible board before an NP may practice. NP Regulatory Statutes typically authorize state nurse licensing boards to administer regulations for expanded medical delegation, often promulgated jointly with the state medical licensing board or in accord with expanded nursing functions recognized "by the medical and nursing professions."

NP Simple Authorization Statutes

At least ten states[15] have enacted NP statutes that authorize expanded medical delegations to RNs and, in three cases, to licensed practical nurses as well, without explictly authorizing an administrative agency or professional society to regulate the process. It should be noted, however, that the nurse licensing board in at least one state (South Dakota) is in the process of developing NP regulations notwithstanding the absence of explicit statutory authority. NP Simple Authorization Statutes define qualified NPs simply as RNs or as RNs "with appropriate training to perform special acts ... delegated by a physician," and three of these statutes include licensed practical nurses as well. These statutes define the new medical acts that are delegable to NPs in varying ways, ranging from California's "standardized procedures, or changes in treatment regimen in accordance with standardized procedures," to Florida's and

Oklahoma's "services," to Colorado's, New Jersey's, and New York's "executing medical regimen[s] as prescribed by a ...physician." [16]

California's NP Simple Authorization Statute deserves special mention because of the unique way in which it authorizes and regulates expanded medical delegation to RNs who work within licensed health care facilities. The California legislature added the following language to the statutory definition of the practice of nursing:

> Observation of signs and symptoms of illness, reactions of treatment, general behavior, or general physical condition, and (1) *determination* of whether such signs, symptoms, reactions, behavior, or general appearance exhibit *abnormal characteristics*; and (2) *implementation, based on observed abnormalities,* of appropriate reporting, or referral, or *standardized procedures or changes in treatment regimen in accordance with standardized procedures,* or the initiation of emergency procedures.
>
> "Standardized procedures" as used in this section means ... policies and protocols developed ...through collaboration among administrators and health professionals including physicians and nurses. (Cal. Business & Professions Code, §2725d) [italics added].

The California NP statute classifies policies and protocols into two categories: those developed for use in licensed health care facilities, including hospitals and nursing homes; and those developed for use outside such facilities, primarily physicians' offices. California's medical and nursing boards are authorized to promulgate joint "guidelines" to which the latter category of policies and protocols will be subject, but these guidelines may not require approval of standardized procedures by either of the two boards. It is unclear whether such guidelines are intended to be advisory or to have some binding effect, but in any event they apply only to expanded delegation in a noninstitutional setting. California's NP statute appears to grant broad legal authority to physicians and RNs for expanded medical delegation in institutional settings, including the making of diagnostic and treatment judgments by RNs, provided only that the RNs work in accordance with policies and protocols—presumably written ones—developed by decentralized decision-makers. This approach avoids prior administrative controls over expanded medical delegation but attempts to ensure quality of medical care by requiring that the decentralized decision-makers think through and presumably write out precisely what RNs will be doing in the medical field.

Many NP statutes have been enacted by states that previously or concurrently had enacted PA Regulatory Statutes. Since the latter provide authority for expanded medical delegation to qualified RNs as well as other PAs, the enactment of these NP statutes might seem to be a wasteful duplication of effort, undertaken merely because of organized nursing's desire that NPs be recognized and controlled as members of the nursing profession rather than as adjuncts of the medical profession. NP statutes, however, may be more effective than existing PA Regulatory Statutes in promoting expanded medical delegation to RNs, who constitute the largest source of readily available personnel for expanded medical delegation. NP statutes contain fewer restrictions on expanded medical delegation than PA Regulatory Statutes. In addition, many NP statutes, particularly NP Regulatory Statutes, authorize the making of diagnostic and treatment judgments by nonphysicians more clearly than do PA statutes.

MAJOR LEGISLATIVE ISSUES

In establishing the PA and NP legislation, legislatures and administrative agencies face a number of important choices among different approaches to expanded medical delegation. This part of the chapter analyzes the choice between Regulatory and Simple Authorization Statutes, examines PA and NP qualifications under these statutes and looks at issues underlying scope of practice rules.

The dominant theme of this part is that unnecessary prior controls over expanded medical delegation have been established by the new legislation. Expanded delegation is innovative and in some cases experimental. It is tempting to conclude that an appropriate legislative policy should provide for strict prior legal controls over expanded medical delegation until it has been shown to be medically feasible.[17] The danger is that strict prior controls may become rigid, thus unduly limiting expanded medical delegation. This approach also ignores a fundamental characteristic of government regulation of medicine. With the exception of new drugs, medical innovations and experiments generally are not subject to prior legal controls to ensure the quality of patient care. The basic legal control in these situations is the law of malpractice, which imposes liability for personal injuries resulting from incidents that have already occurred. Because of these considerations, policy makers should question carefully any claim for prior legal controls over expanded medical delegation. If prior controls are adopted, careful consideration also should be given to ensure against overly rigid administration of the controls. Judgments about the value of different legislative rules can only be tentative at this time because of limited experience with the new legislation governing expanded medical delegation. It seems important, nonetheless, that such judgments be made. Present decisions will help determine and perhaps limit future patterns of expanded delegation because political inertia and the development of vested interests in existing regulatory patterns may hinder rule changes in the future. If current decisions remain unexamined on the grounds that additional empirical data are needed before passing judgment, maximum benefits from expanded medical delegation may never be realized.

Finally, a number of issues are closely related to each other. For example, a fundamental choice facing legislatures has been whether to adopt a Regulatory or Simple Authorization Statute. But this choice affects and is affected by several other legislative issues that may and indeed should influence it. The choice of a Simple Authorization Statute will largely determine who qualifies as a PA or NP and what a PA or NP may do, because these statutes appear to authorize any person to perform any delegated medical act if the supervising physician determines he or she is qualified. On the other hand, the difficulty of establishing rules about PA and NP qualifications and practice may influence legislatures to adopt a Regulatory Statute in order to delegate these decisions to administrative agencies believed to have the necessary expertise.

Another issue is the relationship between PA and NP qualifications and scopes of practice. If extensive training is required for qualification, relatively liberal rules on scope of practice seem more easily justified. Conversely, if extensive training requirements are not established, one may believe that more restrictive rules on scope of practice are necessary. This phenomenon may be seen by a comparison of the language of NP Regulatory Statutes with corresponding language in NP Simple Authorization Statutes. Many NP Regulatory Statutes, which provide for administrative determination of NP qualifications, expressly authorize the performance of "acts of medical diagnosis" and "prescription of treatment." On the other hand, NP Simple Authorization Statutes, which do not provide for administrative determination of NP qualifications, typically authorize only the performance of "services" or "medical regimens prescribed by the physician," language that appears to be more limiting.

The Choice of Regulatory or Simple Authorization Statute

The great majority of PA and NP statutes are Regulatory Statutes that authorize professional licensing boards to regulate expanded delegation through one or more forms of prior control. Prior controls may be any of three types: (1) a requirement that PAs or NPs must graduate from a training program approved by an administrative agency; (2) a requirement that PA or NP competency must be certified by an administrative agency; or (3) a requirement that PA or NP job descriptions must be approved by an administrative agency. Three factors appear to explain this pattern: the ostensible concern of legislators with the quality of care to be provided in expanded medical delegation; the interests of organized medicine in controlling expanded delegation through the use of state medical licensing boards; and the interests of organized nursing in limiting expanded delegation to RNs and in controlling the process through state nurse licensing boards.

The official position of the AMA on this issue has been clear and significant. In December 1970, when political interest in the use of PAs was just beginning, the AMA's House of Delegates recommended that state medical practice acts be amended "to remove any barriers to increased delegation of tasks to allied health personnel by physicians." [18] This recommendation defined allied health personnel to include unlicensed but trained PAs, RNs, and licensed practical nurses; and, importantly, it suggested that the amendment be in the form of a Simple Authorization Statute. In June 1972 the AMA's House of Delegates recommended that PA legislation empower state medical licensing boards to approve on an individual basis the supervising physician, the PA, and a job description of the proposed functions of the PA. The Delegates endorsed this form of PA Regulatory Statute because prior controls were deemed necessary to ensure the quality of PA services and thereby to assure third-party payors, insurance companies and government health service programs, that reimbursements could appropriately be made to physicians for PA services rendered under physician supervision. Although the AMA's resolution indicated that such reimbursement questions had arisen only as to PAs working in "a location physically remote from an employing physician," [19] the AMA recommended that all proposed PA functions be given individual approval by a state medical licensing board, no matter where the PA might be located. The resolution also recommended that reimbursement for PA services be limited to services that had individual licensing board approval, thereby inviting the cooperation of third-party payors in implementing the AMA's recommended form of legislation. One may ask whether the AMA's 1972 recommendation was not prompted more by an interest in establishing organized medicine's control over expanded medical delegation than in solving a particular reimbursement problem. [20]

Two related social benefit arguments have been made to justify adoption of Regulatory Statutes instead of Simple Authorization Statutes:

(1) That some form of prior legal control over expanded medical delegation is necessary to protect the public from incompetent performance by unqualified nonphysicians, and

(2) Prior controls are necessary to promote expanded delegation by helping assure consumers, physicians, and other potential employers that PAs and NPs are competent to perform particular medical acts.

Analysis suggests that these arguments are not persuasive and that the choice of a Regulatory Statute instead of a Simple Authorization Statute may diminish social gains from expanded medical delegation. The claim that prior controls over expanded delegation are necessary to protect the public will be persuasive only if potential benefits of preventing harm caused by unqualified PAs and NPs seem likely to outweigh potential costs to society from using prior controls. Unfortunately, these future benefits and costs cannot be measured and weighed against each other in a precise way. However, analysis of several underlying factors suggests that the likelihood of substantial harm from unqualified PAs and NPs is not great and that the potential costs of a prior control system may be significant. The social benefits from a prior control system will consist of the harm prevented by excluding from expanded delegation those nonphysicians for whom a reasonable showing of competency could not be made before a panel of disinterested medical experts. Claims that the amount of such harm would be substantial seem to rest upon an implicit analogy between the practice of medicine by physicians and expanded medical delegation. One searches in vain among writings that propose prior controls over expanded medical delegation for justifications beyond the assertion that protection of the public requires them. The analogy between expanded delegation and the practice of medicine by physicians is a natural one, however, and might provide a powerful argument for prior controls.

Licensure of physicians may be justified on social welfare grounds since without licensure the relatively high incomes and social status of physicians might attract many unqualified persons into the occupation. The variability in the quality of physicians' services, the importance of that variability to patients' treatment, and the relative inability of consumers to evaluate the quality of physicians' services suggest that substantial harm may be caused to consumers by the practice of unqualified physicians. It does not follow, however, that prior controls over expanded medical delegation are similarly justified. Physician status and income will not accrue to PAs and NPs. Rather, nonphysicians will be attracted into PA and NP occupations largely to the extent that physicians choose to employ them. Expanded medical delegation will consist of simpler, more routine medical acts, indicating that variability in quality of nonphysicians' services and the importance of that variability in the outcome of patients' treatment will be much less than in the case of physicians' services. Most significantly, expanded delegation, with the exception of limited independent practice,[21] will interpose a licensed physician between the individual consumer and nonphysician. The physician will be legally responsible for his or her negligence in selecting the nonphysician, in selecting the acts to be delegated and in supervising the nonphysician's performance. The physician also will be responsible under the master-servant doctrine for negligent performance by PA and NP employees and arguably should be similarly responsible for PAs and NPs supervised by the physician but employed by another person. In effect, physicians will be buying PA and NP services for consumers, thereby substituting physicians' abilities to evaluate the quality of nonphysicians' services for the relative inability of consumers to do so.[22] These characteristics of expanded medical delegation suggest that the frequency with which unqualified PAs and NPs will be employed is low and that little harm will result from their performing medical acts in the absence of a system of prior controls.

A prior control system over expanded medical delegation will result in greater economic costs because the imposition of quality standards will tend to diminish the amount of expanded medical delegation and the price of medical services will be higher than without such controls. In this situation it is likely that some consumers will forego necessary medical services, thereby suffering harm, and that other consumers will be forced to pay higher prices for higher quality medical services than they desire to purchase.

It has been argued that the inherent nature of expanded delegation and malpractice constraints upon physicians make it unlikely that many unqualified PAs and NPs would be employed in the absence of prior controls. One might conclude that prior controls will not diminish substantially the amount of expanded medical delegation and that the entire issue is *de minimis*. This assumption, however, ignores an important distinction between the theory and practice of administrative regulation over medicine in general and expanded delegation in particular. In theory, an administrative agency operating under a Regulatory Statute would preclude by prior controls only those medical delegations for which a reasonable showing of competent performance cannot be made. In practice, administrative agencies with the power to preclude are likely to preclude too much. These agencies are likely to make overly restrictive judgments about competence because of a lack of techniques and resources to determine competence and because of the vested interests of organized medicine and nursing in limiting the supply and types of non-physicians participating in expanded medical delegation. Much of the following discussion is devoted to demonstrating how this gap between theory and practice can develop and that in fact such a gap does exist under PA and NP Regulatory Statutes.

The foregoing analysis of potential benefits and costs of prior controls over expanded medical delegation suggests that the harm from allowing unqualified PAs and NPs to practice without prior controls does not seem likely to be substantial or outweigh the benefits from allowing individual physicians to decide what to delegate to whom. At the very least, the analysis suggests that distinctions might be made among different types of expanded medical delegation, imposing prior controls only over delegations closely analogous to the medical practices that justify prior controls over physicians. For example, prior controls might be limited to expanded delegation involving (1) limited, independent practice by non-physicians; (2) nonphysician practice in locations physically remote from the supervising physician; or (3) issuance of drug prescriptions by non-physicians. Similar distinctions have been recognized to a limited extent under some PA and NP Regulatory Statutes. Under a few PA Regulatory Statutes, an administrative agency's approval of a specific job description is required only for acts to be performed in a setting physically remote from the supervising physician. The NP Regulatory Statutes of Alaska and New Hampshire, cited elsewhere in this chapter, have been interpreted by the nurse licensing boards of those states to authorize expanded medical delegation to two distinct categories of RNs—those working under the relatively close supervision of a physician in a hospital setting, without prior controls, and those required to exercise greater medical judgment who are subject to prior controls.

The second social benefit claim for Regulatory Statutes is that prior controls are necessary to promote expanded medical delegation in several ways. It has been argued that such controls will reassure both consumers and potential employers about the competence of PAs and NPs, thereby promoting their acceptance and effective use by physicians. A closely related argument is that administrative regulation can help resolve physicians' uncertainties about the legality of particular medical delegations by providing detailed answers to specific questions. Physicians' uncertainties might be a significant obstacle to expanded medical delegation, particularly in view of the generally broad but ambiguous statutory provisions authorizing delegations and the resulting physician concern about disciplinary, civil and criminal liability. Regulatory

Statutes also have been supported on the ground that they will ensure a better flow of information to health planners and funding agencies about the employment of PAs and NPs, thereby facilitating the evaluation and expansion of medical delegation.

These secondary claims for Regulatory Statutes seem largely misplaced because there are less restrictive alternatives that would accomplish the same purposes. First, voluntary certification of PA and NP qualifications by state or professional agencies, and a legislative or judicial requirement of patients' informed consent before performance of services by a PA or NP would provide the same information to consumers and physicians about PA and NP qualifications as prior controls, without excluding from practice noncertified PAs and NPs whom physicians might want to employ. Consumers desiring to purchase only qualified PA and NP services might pay higher prices for services of certified PAs and NPs, but other consumers would be free to pay lower prices for services of noncertified PAs and NPs. Second, voluntary certification also would provide a procedure by which uncertain physicians and other employers could establish a presumption of legality for delegation of specific acts without binding more confident employers to decisions by administrative agencies. To ensure that voluntary certification does not have a dampening effect upon physicians who desire to use noncertified PAs and NPs, a statute might provide that the failure to obtain voluntary certification shall not be used as evidence in any subsequent legal proceedings. Otherwise courts and medical licensing boards in subsequent civil, criminal and administrative proceedings involving use of noncertified PAs or NPs might employ the traditional presumptions against the unlicensed practice of medicine. Third, simple registration of all PAs and NPs, without qualifying conditions, would provide accurate information for the evaluation, planning and policing of expanded medical delegation. All this could be done without incurring the potential losses that seem likely to accompany imposition of prior controls.

PA and NP Simple Authorization Statutes thus seem more likely than comparable Regulatory Statutes to promote social good. One would be better assured of the validity of this conclusion if two relatively simple provisions were added to the typical Simple Authorization Statute. First, a Simple Authorization Statute might require physicians to specify protocols to be followed in the course of any expanded medical delegation. This proviso would help ensure that both physicians and nonphysicians think carefully about their respective responsibilities before engaging in them. These protocols, if reduced to writing, also might make malpractice litigation and physician disciplinary proceedings more effective mechanisms for preventing incompetent delegations. Second, voluntary certification by a state agency of PA or NP qualifications to perform any particular medical act might promote expanded medical delegation in the face of potential consumer and physician uncertainty. Consumers and physicians then would have the opportunity to use nonphysicians whose qualifications have been state approved.

PA and NP Qualifications

The legal standards and procedures that define who may qualify as a PA or NP differ substantially between Regulatory and Simple Authorization Statutes. Regulatory Statutes contain specificity. They reflect a marked tendency to limit PAs and NPs to persons who have undergone successful completion of a formal training program. Such rules seem likely to preclude expanded delegation to persons with limited medical skills or to persons who acquire their medical skills through informal on-the-job training. Under Simple Authorization Statutes, on the other hand, supervising physicians appear to have been granted a great deal of discretion in selecting nonphysicians to whom they may delegate medical acts.

Qualifications under Regulatory Statutes

Under a Regulatory Statute, the most important qualification issue is whether any nonphysician who can demonstrate the skill to perform a particular medical act may qualify or whether only nonphysicians with relatively comprehensive skills may qualify. PAs and NPs may be limited to persons with comprehensive skills by two related rules: (1) a requirement that the PA or NP successfully have completed a training program approved by the administrative agency, or have demonstrated training and experience equivalent to such a program, and (2) a requirement that approved training programs provide relatively comprehensive training.

The first requirement is in effect under most PA and NP Regulatory Statutes. The second requirement, that training be relatively comprehensive, is specified under several PA and NP Regulatory Statutes. In addition, standards for PA and NP training programs developed by the AMA and other professional organizations are at least the minimum training requirements for qualification under several other Regulatory Statutes. These standards seem to require relatively comprehensive training of PAs and NPs within given medical specialities. In view of this pattern and the traditional emphasis in medical licensure on formal education, it would be surprising if most other medical and nurse licensing boards do not follow such standards in making individual determinations of competency, even if they do not establish the training standards as formal rules.

Two factors appear to explain the decision to limit PAs and NPs to persons with comprehensive medical training. The first is medical licensors' tradition of assessing a person's competency by evaluating the quality of the candidate's formal education rather than the quality of his or her patient care. Medical and nurse licensing boards will certainly find it administratively easier and less expensive to measure PA and NP qualifications by traditional methods that rely on accreditation of relatively comprehensive formal educational programs. The national standards and accrediting mechanism for formal PA training programs already established by organized medicine also encourage the use of comprehensive qualification standards. A second reason for requiring broad training may be that the quality of a given medical act will be better to the extent that the provider has relatively comprehensive training in related medical acts. For example, the quality of diagnostic procedures may be better if the person performing the procedure also is trained in treatment. This argument overlooks two features of expanded medical delegation—that medical studies already have shown that narrowly limited medical acts may be performed competently by persons with training limited to those acts and that expanded delegation often involves a supervising physician who can supply the comprehensive medical knowledge and clinical judgment that the nonphysician lacks.

National certification examinations to assess the competency of PAs or NPs can help promote medical delegation. First, national certification can help provide consumers and physicians with information about the quality of those PAs or NPs who obtain certification. Second, nationally certified PAs and NPs will have greater job mobility across state lines, particularly if national certification entitles them to automatic qualification under Regulatory Statutes. Such mobility may serve both private and public interests as it increases career attractiveness and allows PAs and NPs to be employed where they are needed most. Where passage of a national certification examination is made a condition of qualification, however, the quality control imposed thereby might be unduly restrictive to many informally trained PAs and NPs.

Qualification under Simple Authorization Statutes

Under Simple Authorization Statutes, the statutory language designating who may perform delegated medical acts and decisions of supervising physicians will determine in the first instance who may function as PAs or NPs. One possible statutory limitation on physicians' discretion to choose PAs and NPs is the reference in some statutes to "trained assistant" or "training," which might be interpreted narrowly to mean medical training in a formal educational program. To support this interpretation, it might be argued that a particular legislature enacting a Simple Authorization Statute intended to restrict qualified PAs or NPs to graduates of formal training programs in view of the importance such programs have played in the development of expanded medical delegation. This interpretation again would have the unfortunate effect of precluding expanded delegation to persons trained in particular medical acts and to persons who have obtained medical skills on an informal basis. A broader interpretation of "trained" and "training" seems preferable as a matter of policy so that expanded delegation could be made to nonphysicians who meet the malpractice law standard of competency.

Scope of Practice Rules

Scope of practice rules define medical acts that may or may not be delegated to PAs and NPs, as well as the nature of physician supervision over those acts. With certain major exceptions noted below, legislation generally leaves scope of practice questions to a case-by-case resolution. On the whole such resolution seems desirable, but an analysis of the major exceptions together with legislative silence on certain important issues suggests that legislatures and administrative agencies may be implementing an overly conservative policy toward PA and NP scope of practice.

All Simple Authorization Statutes and some Regulatory Statutes provide for scope of practice questions to be resolved initially by supervising physicians. Approximately half of the Regulatory Statutes leave scope of practice questions to be resolved initially by administrative agency approval of job descriptions on a case-by-case basis, but job descriptions are not likely to answer all questions and may leave some discretion to supervising physicians. Ultimately, of course, particular scope of practice questions may be decided by disciplinary, civil and criminal proceedings.

The general absence of scope of practice rules seems desirable because the diversity of potential delegations makes it difficult to legislate effectively PAs and NPs with widely varying skills who might work under quite different degrees of physician supervision. The absence of rules or standards governing the outer boundaries of expanded medical delegation, however, may create certain obstacles to the full realization of benefits from expanded delegation. There are three related scope of practice questions which help define the outer boundaries of expanded medical delegation: (1) May PAs and NPs make diagnostic and treatment judgments? (2) May PAs and NPs practice in locations remote from their supervising physician? and (3) May PAs and NPs prescribe or dispense drugs? Studies suggest that under certain conditions PAs and NPs competently do any of these. The following discussion analyzes the problems created by legislative silence on these questions and the few legislative choices that have been made to date.

The absence of statutory standards governing outer boundary delegations may create substantial legal uncertainty that will retard the development of maximum feasible delegation in several ways. First, under the Regulatory Statutes, administrative agencies may prohibit or hesitate to authorize these delegations. Second, without explicit authorization by statute or regulatory action, physicians may hesitate to make the most effective use of PAs and NPs because of the possibility of subsequent legal proceedings. Finally, with legislative silence on outer boundary delegations, the seemingly conservative policies of organized medicine about PA and NP scope of practice are likely to carry greater weight with administrative agencies, physicians and tribunals involved in legal proceedings concerning expanded delegation. The written policies of organized medicine on PA and NP scope of practice described below would seem to constitute some evidence of customary practice. The importance of medical custom in malpractice cases and in criminal and administrative proceedings involving the interpretation of medical practice acts has been well documented.

In December 1971, the AMA's House of Delegates approved the *Essentials of an Approved Educational Program for the Assistant to the Primary Care Physician* (see Appendix A), a set of standards for training primary care PAs and NPs. To establish such standards, it was necessary to define the scope of practice for which primary care assistants should be trained. The AMA Essentials begin by noting that the primary care assistant "will not supplant the doctor in the sphere of decision making required to establish a diagnosis and plan therapy." No justification was given for this recommendation, either in the Essentials or in a task force report that preceded it. A mere assertion by organized medicine that licensed physicians must "make diagnoses" and "plan therapy" is apparently enough. If established by law, this prohibition would help ensure that PAs and NPs merely supplement rather than substitute for physicians' services. A possible explanation for the AMA's position is that supplemental services by PAs and NPs are likely to generate new demand for medical services, thereby protecting physicians' fees and incomes.[23] The AMA Essentials define PA and NP services to include "executing [a physician's] standing orders." Although this term is not defined further, its customary use by health professionals indicates that it includes treatment modifications by nonphysicians working under a physician's written directions. In other words, a nonphysician working under standing orders may determine the severity of symptoms of an already diagnosed disease or other abnormal condition and choose to modify treatment, perhaps by the dispensation of drugs. PA and NP services are also defined to include the "independent performance of evaluative and treatment procedures essential to provide an appropriate response to life-threatening, emergency situations." This provision establishes that in case of dire need a PA or NP may make a diagnosis and initiate treatment until a physician is contacted. The AMA Essentials do not mention remote practice or drug prescriptions by PAs and NPs, although a general reference is made to the variations in practice that may result from "geographic, economic and sociologic factors." The recognition of standing orders for PAs and NPs also implies authority to engage in limited, independent decision-making with respect to drugs. In sum the AMA Essentials seem to be conservative on the question of diagnostic and treatment judgments, and they are unclear on outer boundary questions of standing orders and emergency care.

If any generalization can be made about scope of practice rules under the new legislation, it is that they tend to be at least as conservative as the AMA Essentials. The typical provisions in PA statutes that allow PAs to perform medical services under a physician's supervision do not resolve the outer boundary questions. Medical services are not further defined by statute, and their ambiguous nature easily allows interpretations that prohibit PA practice along the outer boundaries of expanded medical delegation. The language of NP Simple Authorization Statutes is similar, authorizing "delegated medical acts," "standardized procedures," "services," or merely the "execution of medical regimens." In contrast, approximately half of the NP Regulatory Statutes authorize NPs to perform "acts of medical diagnosis" and "prescription of medical therapeutic or corrective measures" to the extent authorized by regulation. This language provides clearly that state regulatory agencies may authorize NPs to make diagnostic and treatment judgments and to prescribe or dispense drugs.

Rules under a few PA Regulatory Statutes provide or imply that PAs may make diagnostic and treatment judgments that they are competent to perform. The Colorado Child Health Associate Law authorizes child health associates to practice pediatrics under physician supervision, and the South Dakota PA statute authorizes PAs to "make tentative medical diagnosis and institute therapy or referral ... [and] to treat common childhood diseases."[24] By administrative opinion, Nebraska has authorized PAs to prescribe certain drugs, without limiting this authority to follow-up treatment after an initial diagnosis by a physician.[25] The absence of such a limitation suggests that the Nebraska medical licensing board is willing to recognize diagnostic and treatment judgments by PAs through individual approval of job descriptions. Nevada and Washington by regulation recognize remote practice by PAs.[26] Because this authority would be ineffectual without concomitant authority for PAs to make diagnostic and treatment judgments about more common medical disorders, these regulations also suggest that the medical boards in these states are authorizing such judgments on the basis of approved job descriptions.

As noted, many NP Regulatory Statutes appear to allow diagnostic and treatment judgments by NPs to the extent authorized by regulatory agencies. Among the few available regulations addressing this issue, Nevada and Washington clearly have authorized NPs to perform diagnostic and treatment judgments. In addition, New Hampshire and Vermont have authorized nurse-midwives to "manage" or "assume responsibility" for normal or low-risk obstetrical patients, authorization that includes the initial judgment that the patient is low-risk.[27] New Hampshire has authorized psychiatric NPs to "identify and interpret problems related to the mental health of the patient . . . and provide appropriate therapy or referral." In contrast, New Hampshire has limited NPs other than nurse-midwives and psychiatric NPs to making an initial judgment of normal or abnormal condition, with referral of abnormal conditions to physicians required. Virginia has limited NPs to recommending diagnoses and treatment plans to physicians.

PAs and NPs are precluded from practicing in remote locations, that is outside of the supervising physician's office, a hospital in which the physician has patients or patients' homes, under at least ten PA regulatory Statutes and one NP Regulatory Statute. To the contrary, Nevada, South Dakota, Washington, and Wisconsin have authorized remote practice by PAs, and Alaska, Nevada, and New Hampshire have recognized self-employed NPs who may work "in collaboration with" or "upon referrals" from physicians, an apparent authorization of remote practice by NPs.

The authority of PAs and NPs to make independent decisions regarding the use of drugs, either by prescribing drugs to patients or by dispensing drugs directly to patients in hospitals, nursing homes and physicians' offices, depends not only on the relevant PA or NP statute and regulations but also on federal and state drug control laws that place certain limitations on who may prescribe and dispense drugs. Federal law relies generally on state law to determine practitioners' qualifications to prescribe or dispense drugs, but it does establish two significant conditions. The Food, Drug, and Cosmetic Act requires that retail sales of prescription drugs be made only upon the written or oral "prescription of a practitioner licensed by law to administer such a drug."[28] It seems clear that a PA or NP whose qualifications have been individually approved by an administrative agency and who has been granted explicit authority to administer drugs by legislative rule or approved job description would satisfy this requirement, because the determination of "those licensed by law to administer drugs" is a matter of state law. Clear answers are not similarly available for two other cases: (1) prescriptions by PAs and NPs whose qualifications have received state approval by a form of license but who have been neither granted nor denied explicit authority to administer drugs, and (2) prescriptions by PAs and NPs who have not been licensed to administer drugs but who complete prescription order forms previously signed in blank by their supervising physician. Resolution of the first case will depend on whether the nonphysician's general authority to perform medical acts is interpreted to include the authority to administer drugs. An interpretation recognizing such authority seems reasonable in view of the general lack of statutory limitations on PAs' and NPs' authority to perform medical acts and the obvious importance of drug prescriptions to modern medicine, but such an approach is uncertain because of the typically ambiguous scope of practice provisions mentioned above. Determination of the second issue will depend on whether PAs and NPs who prescribe drugs on forms signed in blank by their supervising physicians are recognized as agents who are merely carrying out a physician's prescription or whether they are considered independent practitioners. The former view is supported by the policy underlying the Food, Drug, and Cosmetic Act, which relies on state law to govern the medical aspect of drug prescriptions, and by the authority of physicians under the new state laws to employ PAs and NPs generally as agents who perform medical acts. The ambiguous nature of statutory scope of practice provisions, however, renders uncertain the resolution of this issue.

The second condition imposed by federal law is that narcotics, barbiturates, amphetamines and other dangerous drugs deemed "controlled substances" under the Drug Abuse Prevention and Control Act may be prescribed or dispensed only by a person "licensed . . . or otherwise permitted by . . . the jurisdiction in which he practices . . . to distribute or dispense . . . a controlled substance in the course of professional practice. . . ."[29] Regulations make it clear that physicians' agents who prescribe controlled substances must be "licensed . . . or otherwise permitted" by the jurisdiction in which they practice to so prescribe and must be registered with the federal government. Agents who merely dispense controlled substances directly to patients need not be registered but must be "licensed . . . or otherwise permitted" by state law to dispense controlled substances. Under these provisions, state licensure is not necessary to grant permission to PAs and NPs to prescribe or dispense controlled substances, but the exact nature of the required permission is unclear. Thus questions may arise that are similar to the scope of practice issues under the Food, Drug and Cosmetic Act.

State pharmacy and narcotics control acts regulate the flow of drugs in the same manner as the federal drug control laws, relying mainly on state licensure laws to determine practitioners' qualifications to prescribe or dispense drugs. A survey of these laws is beyond the scope of this chapter, but it should be noted that these laws may add additional restrictions to those imposed by federal law. For example, a state pharmacy act may provide that only "licensed practitioners" can prescribe drugs, rather than "authorized persons," and it may regulate the dispensing of all prescription drugs, not merely controlled substances. To the extent that additional restrictions are imposed by these laws, they create added uncertainties about the legal authority of PAs and NPs to prescribe or dispense drugs.

Explicit authority for PAs to prescribe or dispense drugs has been granted under at least four PA Regulatory Statutes. Colorado's statute provides that child health associates may prescribe specified prescription drugs that have been approved by the state medical board.[30] South Dakota's statute is less clear in providing authority for PAs to "prescribe medication for symptoms and temporary pain relief" and in authorizing the medical board to approve "such other tasks" for PAs "for which adequate training and proficiency can be demonstrated."[31] By administrative opinion, Nebraska has recognized a physician's right to delegate his "prescribing authority" to PAs for drugs other than controlled substances.[32] New York by regulation has authorized PAs to dispense drugs including controlled substances to hospital inpatients if the order is countersigned by the supervising physician within 24 hours.[33] To the contrary, PAs appear to be precluded from prescribing or dispensing prescription drugs under at least ten PA Regulatory Statutes, explicitly in four cases and implicitly in the others by prohibitions against the exercise of diagnostic and treatment judgments and treatment modifications.

Only a few available regulations under NP Regulatory Statutes address the drug prescription issue. Washington has authorized NPs to use drug therapy "persuant to protocols jointly recognized by the medical and nursing professions."[34] New Hampshire and Vermont have authorized nurse-midwives to dispense "medications" to normal or low-risk obstetrical patients. New Hampshire's regulations, however, limit NPs other than nurse-midwives to "recommending non-prescription drugs," to "regulating and adjusting" physician-prescribed medications and to dispensing certain prescription medications in emergency situations only.[35]

In summary, outer boundary delegation most effectively allows PAs and NPs to substitute their services for those of physicians, rather than merely to supplement physicians' ministrations. Not coincidentally, such outer boundary delegations most threaten physicians' fees and incomes. Most PA and NP statutes and available regulations thereunder do not clearly resolve the three important scope of practice issues that define the outer boundaries of expanded medical delegation: diagnostic and treatment judgments, remote practice and prescription of drugs. When legislative rules have been promulgated, they have tended to preclude PAs from making diagnostic and treatment judgments or prescribing drugs. Too few NP regulations are available to indicate a trend one way or the other on these issues. Under a majority of Regulatory Statutes, it is possible for authority for outer boundary delegations to be awarded on a case-by-case basis through administrative approval of job descriptions. In view, however, of the general absence of statutory standards on these questions, organized medicine's conservative position, and the control of the confirmation process by state medical boards and state medical societies, authorization for outer boundary delegations through approved job descriptions may be quite limited. Empirical studies of what is happening under the mechanism of approved job descriptions is clearly a next step in the study of PA and NP statutes. The consequence of this legal structure will be uncertainty about or denial of the rights of PAs and NPs to make diagnostic and treatment judgments for more common illnesses, to prescribe drugs for such disorders, and to practice in locations remote from their supervising physicians, despite the fact that such practices seem medically feasible in many instances. In scope of practice regulation, as with other issues under the new legislation, organized medicine seems to be protecting successfully the economic interests of physicians.

RECOMMENDATIONS

Recommendations for legislative rules to improve the prospects for maximum feasible expanded delegation are presented in summary form in order to pull together the various analyses in preceding parts of this chapter. The recommendations are presented in the form of a "Model Simple Authorization Statute" and a "Model Regulatory Statute" because statutory change is necessary to authorize expanded delegation in some states. Nonetheless, many of these recommendations may be implemented under existing Regulatory Statutes by administrative action in view of the broad authority generally delegated to administrative agencies by these statutes.

The author recommends the Model Simple Authorization Statute. The arguments for regulatory alternatives seem insupportable on the grounds of social good. As previously pointed out, prior legal controls over the independent practice of medicine by physicians may be justified, but the analogy between such practice and expanded medical delegation seems weak if for no other reason than the ethical and legal responsibility of physicians for acts performed under their supervision. Prior controls over expanded delegation may well limit the social benefits from expanded delegation if administrative agencies implement prior controls in an unduly conservative manner, as seems likely. This prediction is strengthened by the observation that administrative agencies under Regulatory Statutes in fact seem to be implementing unnecessarily conservative policies.

There are nonetheless several reasons why a Simple Authorization Statute might be rejected and some form of Regulatory Statute adopted. First, a great number of Regulatory Statutes are in effect, and reform may be limited to improving the existing legal structure. Second, legislators reasonably may disagree with the conclusion that social costs of a prior control system over expanded delegation are likely to outweigh social benefits; this conclusion, after all, is not more than a prediction of future probabilities. Third, imposition of prior controls over nonphysicians authorized to prescribe or dispense drugs is justified if uncertainty about the authority of unlicensed physicians' agents to prescribe or dispense drugs under the federal drug control laws effectively prohibits such practice. Unlike legal uncertainty about other forms of expanded delegation, this uncertainty is created by federal law and cannot be resolved by state legislation alone.

A Model Simple Authorization Statute

A Simple Authorization Statute designed to promote expanded medical delegation in the public interest would contain the following provisions:

1. An exemption from the medical practice act for any act of medical diagnosis or prescription of therapeutic or corrective measures performed by any person under a physician's supervision; provided that such performance is in accordance with written policies and protocols established by the physician and nonphysician.

2. Explicit recognition that the authority to prescribe therapeutic measures includes authority for the nonphysician to prescribe and dis-

pense prescription drugs to the extent authorized by the supervising physician.

3. Explicit recognition that the nonphysician may practice in locations remote from his supervising physician to the extent authorized by the physician.

4. A voluntary certification system administered by a state agency to determine the competence of nonphysicians to perform any medical act or acts; in order to ensure that this system is truly voluntary, the statute should also provide that failure to obtain or denial of voluntary certification shall be excluded from evidence in any subsequent legal proceedings.

5. Express provisions that patients shall be informed clearly that direct care services are to be provided by a nonphysician; that evidence of the nonphysician's training, formal or informal, shall be readily available to patients; and that, for purposes of malpractice liability, any supervising physician shall be presumed conclusively to be a principal, master, or employer of any nonphysician performing medical acts under the physician's supervision.

This Model Simple Authorization Statute has four basic advantages over the Simple Authorization Statutes enacted to date. First, the voluntary certification system and the explicit authorization for diagnostic and treatment judgments, drug prescriptions, and remote practice would promote maximum feasible delegations by establishing standards and procedures to provide presumptive legal validity for more innovative delegations—delegations that physicians otherwise may avoid because of uncertainty about potential liability. Second, the requirement of the provision that written policies and protocols be established, which follows California's NP Simple Authorization Statute, would help ensure that physicians and nonphysicians alike focus scrupulously on the quality of care to be provided by the nonphysician. Third, the voluntary certification system, together with the notice requirements, would help provide information to consumers about the relative competencies of nonphysicians, allowing patients the choice of obtaining services from physicians only, state-certified PAs or uncertified PAs. Finally, the conclusive presumption of a master-servant relationship between any supervising physician and supervised nonphysician performing medical acts would remove doubt about the full application of the borrowed servant doctrine to hospital employed nonphysicians.[36]

In lieu of a state-administered voluntary certification program, whose costs would be borne by the state, decision-makers might choose to rely on national PA and NP certification programs operated by professional groups for the dual purposes of promoting expanded delegation and providing consumers with information about relative competencies of nonphysicians. This reliance would seem unwise, however, since these programs apply only to nonphysicians trained to perform relatively comprehensive medical functions and are controlled by organizations with an apparent interest in restricting expanded delegation.

A Model Regulatory Statute

A Regulatory Statute best designed to promote expanded medical delegation would contain the following provisions:

1. Delegation of regulatory authority to the state health agency or, in the alternative, division of regulatory authority between the state health agency for services that are offered within a licensed health care institution and the state medical licensing board for other delegations.

2. An express provision that nonphysicians may qualify to perform any particular medical act and that qualification need not be based on completion of a formal, approved training program; prior administrative determination of PAs' qualifications should be limited to those PAs granted authority to prescribe or dispense drugs if the only justification for a Regulatory Statute is the need to authorize and control drug prescriptions by PAs.

3. Explicit authorization of outer boundary medical delegations to qualified PAs in the same manner as provisions (1), (2), and (3) of the Model Simple Authorization Statute.

4. Explicit recognition that hospitals and other licensed health care institutions may employ PAs and that PAs may be supervised at different times by different physicians.

5. A provision that any general limitation on the number of PAs that may be supervised by a physician shall be waived by the regulatory agency on a showing that supervision of a larger number is reasonable.

The purpose of these recommendations is to implement prior controls in a manner that would avoid the significantly restrictive aspects of the new legislation. Delegation of regulatory authority to the state health agency or division of such authority between the state health agency and professional licensing boards would avoid organized medicine's effective control over expanded delegation through regulation by medical licensing boards. If permitted by law, hospitals and other licensed health care institutions probably will be the centers of much useful expanded medical delegation. State health agencies appear more likely than medical boards to be free from influence of medical professionals who have interests that are threatened by expanded medical delegation; thus health agencies seem more likely to recognize innovative delegations and maximize benefits from the new legislation.

It may be argued that a division of regulatory responsibility would cause jurisdictional confusion and an increase in administrative costs. California's NP Simple Authorization Statute, which appears to provide for a similar division of responsibility, and New York's PA Statute, which divides responsibility along different lines, are precedents that suggest that this is not an insurmountable problem. Moreover, the state health agency might choose to regulate expanded medical delegation largely as part of its overall institutional review, thus modifying any burden of increased cost. Such regulation in effect would delegate most or all prior controls over expanded delegation to the governing bodies of licensed health care institutions. This form of regulation has been labelled "institutional licensure," and it is most closely associated with proposals made by Professor Nathan Hershey of the University of Pittsburgh School of Public Health. The practical effect of the proposed Model Simple Authorization Statute would be similar to institutional licensure. Under Simple Authorization Statutes, health care institutions presumably will establish internal regulations for governing expanded medical delegation.

Provision (2), that nonphysicians may qualify to perform any particular medical acts based on limited and informal training, is designed to avoid the traditional, restrictive practice of relying on comprehensive formal academic training as the standard for competence to perform medical acts. This provision would require use of approved job descriptions to take account of the many different types of possible authorizations. It may be argued that alternative means of determining competency are not available or that the provision would be administratively unworkable, but competency assessments and administrative burdens have not been deemed insurmountable by the large number of states that already approve job descriptions for PAs or NPs. Moreover, as state health agencies gain experience, they will develop categories of approvable job descriptions, thereby easing the administrative burden. This provision also would limit prior legal controls over qualifications to nonphysicians authorized to prescribe or dispense drugs if licensure of drug-prescribing agents of physicians is deemed to be the only justification for prior controls. Because drug prescription is such an important part of medical practice, this requirement would effectively establish prior controls over most or all nonphysicians who engage in diagnostic and treatment judgments and in remote practice. Such a limitation would be similar to the regulation of NPs under the NP Regulatory Statutes of Alaska and New

Hampshire, which provide for certification only of those NPs who engage in outer boundary delegations.

Provision (3) authorizes outer boundary delegations in order to provide clear statutory authority for administrative agencies to recognize such delegations by regulation or approved job descriptions. This would help promote expanded delegation in the same manner as the corresponding provisions of the Model Simple Authorization Statute.

Provisions (4) and (5) are designed to preclude administrative agencies from prohibiting hospital employment of PAs by requiring that only one physician may supervise a PA, or restricting the number of PAs or NPs that a physician may supervise without exception. These kinds of restrictions seem designed to accomplish nothing more than protection of physicians' and nurses' economic interests.

A Final Option: Limited Independent Practice

States suffering from substantial physician shortages in certain locales may discover that expanded delegation by physicians will not provide sufficient expansion of medical services if too few physicians are willing to employ PAs and NPs. These states should have a particular interest in authorizing special categories of PAs or NPs to practice independently, referring more difficult medical problems to appropriate physicians or specialists. A Canadian study by Dr. Walter Spitzer suggests that such practice by NPs at least is medically feasible.[37]

Regulation of independent practice by nonphysicians is beyond the scope of this chapter, but it may be noted that effective authorization and regulation of such practice might best be achieved by a modified form of the Model Regulatory Statute discussed above. First, individual state approval of nonphysicians' qualifications would be necessary because authority to prescribe drugs would be essential to this practice, and Federal law requires that such prescriptions be made by practitioners licensed by the state to administer such drugs. Second, authorization in broad terms for nonphysicians to practice medicine, together with an administrative procedure for defining scope of practice limits on a case-by-case basis, would seem preferable to the traditional approach of attempting to define statutorily the scope of limited independent medical practice. As previously discussed, the latter approach creates substantial uncertainty about the legality of particular medical acts.

Alaska, Nevada and New Hampshire have authorized certain forms of limited, independent medical practice by NPs under their NP Regulatory Statutes.[38] New Hampshire's statute provides that NPs may practice "either in private practice or in a collaborative relationship with physicians." By regulatory action, Alaska and Nevada have recognized "private" or "independent" practice by NPs. Available regulations, however, provide little further guidance or information as to the scope of practice authorized for independent NPs. Nevada and New Hampshire both require some evidence of a "collaborative relationship" between the NP and a physician or physicians, an apparent attempt to ensure that medical problems beyond the NP's competence are appropriately referred. Nevada's regulations do not authorize clearly either diagnostic and treatment judgments or drug prescriptions by independent NPs. Finally, New Hampshire's regulations limit most categories of NPs to making an initial judgment of normal or abnormal condition, while requiring referral of abnormal conditions to physicians, and to modifying drug treatments prescribed by physicians. These regulations do not appear to have been designed to obtain maximum social benefits from limited, independent practice by NPs.

SUMMARY

The foregoing analysis suggests that much of the new state legislation governing expanded medical delegation is unduly restrictive and incomplete in several respects. First, a substantial majority of the statutes have established a regulatory structure that seems wholly or largely unnecessary. These statutes also have delegated most administrative authority to state medical licensing boards, which appear to have a significant interest in restricting the performance of medical acts by nonphysicians. Second, nonphysicians performing medical acts have been limited in many cases to persons trained in formal educational programs to perform a relatively comprehensive set of medical functions. This limitation precludes from expanded delegation persons with less formal training or with training to perform only specific medical acts, an exclusion that seems unjustified and costly. Third, the scope of practice of qualified nonphysicians has in many cases been unduly restricted and has not been defined to promote maximum feasible expanded delegation.

Notes

1. This chapter is a shortened version of the author's article "Physician's Assistant and Nurse Practitioner Laws: A Study of Health Law Reform," which appeared in the KAN. L. REV. 24 (1975) 1-65. The study was supported in part by a grant from the University of Kansas General Research Fund. For discussion of some additional issues pertaining to PA and NP laws, the reader is referred to the original article.

2. The standard for competent performance of medical acts by PAs and NPs will be assumed throughout this chapter to be the level of competence that is expected of physicians. This conservative assumption is made for practical reasons. It relies on an

existing standard of competence and is in accord with both the standard employed in medical evaluations of PAs and NPs and the standard apparently assumed by legislators in enacting new statutes. This assumption begs the important but currently unanswerable question of what the appropriate standard should be. Should it be physician equivalence or some lower standard that is still acceptable in the sense that total social value of services performed exceeds total social cost? The availability of any such lower standard can only be ascertained by further experience with PAs and NPs.

3. At least three recent studies found that initial, limited diagnostic and treatment judgments by trained nonphysicians is performed as competently as by physicians. *See* Chappell and Drogos, "Evaluation of Infant Health Care by a Nurse Practitioner," *Pediatrics* 49 (1972), 871. (A professional nurse with five years' experience in a pediatric emergency room and who had short-term medical training was responsible for all well-baby care and also diagnosed acute illnesses, treating some and referring others); Greenfield, Bragg, McGraith & Blackburn, "Upper-Respiratory Tract Complaint/Protocol for Physician-Extenders," *Arch. Intern. Med.* 133 (1974), 294. (An initial, limited diagnostic and treatment judgment of upper-respiratory tract complaints was performed as competently by trained nonphysicians, working under written protocols, as it was performed by physicians); Spitzer, Sackett, Sibley, Roberts, Gent, Kergin, Hackett & Olynich, "The Burlington Randomized Trial of the Nurse Practitioner, *N.Eng.J.Med.*, 290 (1974), 251. (Professional nurses with three months' additional medical training treated patients in a family practice on an independent basis, referring more difficult problems [approximately one-third of all visits] to appropriate physicians); *see also* Silver, Ford & Day, "The Pediatric Nurse Practitioner Program," *J.A.M.A.*, 204 (1968), 296. (Pediatric nurse practitioners were able to give total care to more than 75 percent of all children who came to pediatric clinics, including almost all well children and approximately half of the sick or injured children.) A larger number of studies have found that various types of nonphysicians can perform as competently as physicians certain treatment modifications and medical procedures not traditionally delegated. Bessman, "Comparison of Medical Care in Nurse Clinician and Physician Clinics in Medical School Affiliated Hospitals," *J. Chron. Dis.* 27 (1974), 115; Charles Stimson, Maurier & Good, "Physician's Assistants and Clinical Algorithms in Health Care Delivery," *Ann. Intern. Med.* 81 (1974), 733; Charney & Kitzman, "The Child-Health Nurse (Pediatric Nurse Practitioner) in Private Practice," *N.Eng.J.Med.*, 285 (1971), 1353; Komaroff, Black, Flately, Knopp, Reiffen and Sherman, "Protocols for Physician Assistants—Management of Diabetes and Hypertension," *N.Eng.J.Med.*, 290 (1974), 307; Lewis, Resnik, Schmidt and Waxman, "Activities, Events and Outcomes in Ambulatory Patient Care," *N. Eng. J. Med.* 280 (1969), 645; Runyan, "The Memphis Chronic Disease Program: Comparisons in Outcome and the Nurse's Extended Role," *J.A.M.A.*, 231 (1975), 264. Cf. Dellaportas, Swords and Ball, "Diagnostic Efficiency of Paraprofessionals," *Am. J. Pub. Health* 64 (1974), 993. (This study of physicians and nonphysicians diagnosing gonorrhea patients found that physicians exhibited diagnostic superiority, but that the diagnostic competence of the nonphysicians was sufficient to be useful in treating male but not female patients.)

4. One economic study has found that current use of PAs in physicians' offices may increase physician productivity from 49 percent to 74 percent, depending upon the extent of delegation by the physician. (Smith, Miller and Golladay, "An Analysis of the Optimal Use of Inputs in the Production of Medical Services," *J. Hum. Res.* 7 (1972), 208, 218-23.) A less rigorous economic evaluation of NPs found some economic benefit

for physicians employing NPs instead of professional nurses in their office practices, although this study did not take into account the possibility of increased physician time spent supervising and consulting with NPs or the likely need to adjust assignments and salaries of other personnel in the physicians' offices. (Yankauer, Tripp, Andrews and Connelly, "The Costs of Training and the Income Generation Potential of Pediatric Nurse Practitioners," *Pediatrics* 49 (1972), 878, 882-84.)

5. New York Educ. Laws §6521 (McKinney 1972).

6. California Business and Professional Code §2510-22 (1974) (Enacted 1970).

7. Georgia Code Ann. §84-6203(c) (Supp. 1974).

8. Ore. Rev. Stat. §677.065(3) (1974).

9. Virginia Code Ann. §54-281.4(a) (1974).

10. Colorado Rev. Stat. Ann. §§ 12-31-102(2), -103(2) (1974).

11. Ark. Stat. Ann. §72-604(2)(p) (Supp. 1973); Conn. Gen. Stat. Ann. §20-9 (Supp. 1975); Tenn. Code Ann. §63-608 (Supp. 1974).

12. Mich. Comp. Laws Ann. §338.1816(1)(f) (Supp. 1975); Colo. Rev. Stat. Ann. §§ 12-31-101-115 (1973) (Enacted 1963).

13. Alaska Stat. §§ 08.68.410(5), (9) (1974); Idaho Code §54-1413(e) (Supp. 1974); Me. Rev. Stat. Ann. tit. 32, §2102(2)(3) (Supp. 1973) and Ch. 354, §1, (1974); Miss. Gen. Laws 405, amending Miss. Code Ann. §73-15-5(2) (1972); Nev. Rev. Stat. §632.010(7) (1973); N.H. Rev. Stat. Ann. §326-A:2 (I) (Supp. 1973); N.C. Gen. Stat. §90-158(3)(a) (Supp. 1974); Pa. Stat. Ann. tit. 63, §212(1) (Supp. 1974); Wyo. Stat. Ann. §33-279.7(a)(i)(o) (Supp. 1975).

14. See e.g. Ariz. Rev. Stat. Ann. §32-1601(5) (Supp. 1974).

15. Cal. Bus. and Prof. Code §2725(d) (West Supp. 1975); Colo. Rev. Stat. Ann. §§ 12.38-202(7), (9)(c) (1973); Minn. Stat. Ann. §148.171(3) (Supp. 1975); N.Y. Stat. Ann. §45:11-23(1)(b) (Supp. 1975); N.Y. Educ. Law §6902(1) (McKinney Supp. 1973); Tenn. Code Ann. §63-740 (Supp. 1974); Fla. Stat. Ann. §458.13(4) (Supp. 1975); Kansas Stat. Ann. §65-2872(g) (1972); Okla. Stat. Ann. tit. 59, §492 (Supp. 1974); S.D. Compiled Laws Ann. §36-9-3(1) (1972).

16. Cal. Bus. and Prof. Code §2725(d) (West Supp. 1975); Fla. Stat. Ann. §458.13(4) (Supp. 1975); Okla. Stat. Ann. tit. 59, §492 (Supp. 1974); Colo. Rev. Stat. Ann. §§ 12-38-202(7), (9)(c) (1974); N.J. Stat. Ann. §45:11-23(1)(b) (Supp. 1975); N.Y. Educ. Law §6902(1) (McKinney Supp. 1973).

17. As suggested in footnote 2, medically feasible delegations may be considered those delegations that can be performed by nonphysicians as competently as by physicians.

18. Licensure of Health Occupations, recommendation (a) prepared by the AMA Council on Health Manpower: adopted by the AMA House of Delegates, Dec. 1970.

19. AMA Board of Trustees, Report 2, Guidelines for Compensating Physicians for Services of Physician's Assistants 2, Recommendation 1 (Approved by AMA House of Delegates, June 1972).

20. The essential reason for organized medicine's desire to control expanded medical delegation is that substantial expanded delegation of medical services might threaten the collective economic interests of physicians. This argument is developed in detail in the author's article, "Physician's Assistant and Nurse Practitioner Laws: A Study of Health Law Reform, KAN. L. REV. 24 (1975), 1, 13-20.

21. Limited, independent practice by PAs and NPs is generally outside the scope of this chapter. Regulatory statutes would appear to be the appropriate statutory form for

authorization and regulation of such practice, because the analogy with licensure of physicians is stronger and federal drug laws require state licensure for independent practitioners who prescribe drugs.

22. Of course, the ability of individual physicians to evaluate and supervise the quality of nonphysicians' services may vary substantially. One may ask, however, whether the significance of this variability with respect to patient harm is likely to be greater than the significance of physician variability in many other types of medical acts that are not subject to prior legal controls, e.g., intricate surgical operations, combining drugs to treat a specific patient for a specific disease, or the use of medical equipment as a physician-substitute in various diagnostic and treatment procedures.

23. It seems likely that *quality* in addition to the *quantity* of medical services will be expanded and that physicians will be able to generate new demand for such higher quality services.

24. Colo. Rev. Stat. Ann. §§12-31-101(2), -103(2). (1974); S.D. Compiled Laws Ann. §§36-4A-1 to -42. (Supp. 1974) (Enacted 1973).

25. Memorandum from Rex Higley, Director of the Bureau of Examining Boards, Nebraska Department of Health, Aug. 12, 1974.

26. Regulations for the Certification of Physician's Assistants, Board of Medical Examiners of the State of Nevada §I.(4); Wash. Ad. Code §308-52-130, §5(b)(i).

27. Rules and Regulations—Advanced Registered Nurse Practitioner (New Hampshire Board of Registration in Medicine and Board of Nursing Education and Nurse Registration, adopted Dec. 3, 1973), Part B, §§3.1(B)(d), (e) Statement of Policy on Nurse-Midwives, Vermont State Nurses Association, Vermont State Medical Society, Vermont Hospital Association, adopted March 1974, §III.

28. 21 U.S.C. §353(b)(1) (1970).

29. 21 U.S.C. §§802(20), 829(a), (b) (1970).

30. Colo. Rev. Stat. §12-31-103(2)(b) (1973).

31. S.D. Compiled Laws Ann. §36-4A-23.

32. Memorandum, Rex Higley, op. cit.

33. Regulations of the New York Commissioner of Health, §94.2(e).

34. Wash. Ad. Code §§308-120-190 to -250 (effective Feb. 1975).

35. N.H. NP Regs, see note 27, Part B, §§3.2(B)(g), (h), 3.3(B)(j), (K), Part C.

36. Hospitals have been prohibited from employing PAs as PAs under a number of PA regulatory statutes. The justification for this exclusion is unclear. However, one argument that might support exclusion is that under the existing borrowed servant doctrine of malpractice law, physicians supervising hospital employed PAs may not be fully liable for all medical acts of the PA. The conclusive presumption of a master-servant relationship is intended to answer this claim.

37. W.O. Spitzer et al., "The Burlington Randomized Trial of the Nurse Practitioner," *N.Eng.J.Med.* 94 (1974) 251-256.

38. Alaska, Nev. and N.H. Stat., see note 13.

Chapter 9

Third Party Payment for the Services of the Assistant to the Primary Care Physician

Stephen B. Morris*

Third party payment plays a major role in meeting the costs of health care in the United States. Third party payment policies for medical services provided by physician assistants will, therefore, influence the economic viability of physician assistants. Current third party policies vary with regard to medical services provided by physician assistants, but the prevailing attitude appears to be that physician assistants are not a well identified or uniform class of medical provider. The major unresolved issues include legal and professional definitions, quality of care, and the cost implications of payment for physician assistant services. The Social Security Administration's Physician Extender Reimbursement Study will address most of these issues and should make useful information available for developing sensible and fair third party payment policies.

ROLE OF THIRD PARTY PAYMENT IN MEETING PERSONAL HEALTH CARE COSTS

Third party payment plays a major role in the United States in determining economic demand for certain health services, especially hospital and physician's care. About 87 percent of persons under 65 years of age were covered by some type of health insurance as of 1973. Of these, 78 percent were enrolled in private insurance plans while 17 percent participated in public health programs. Of those in private programs, 78 percent had some hospitalization and surgical coverage (61 percent of the total population). Only 35 percent, however, had some coverage for physician office and home visits and even fewer (11 percent) for dental care.[1]

*The views expressed in this article are the author's and do not necessarily reflect the view of the Social Security Administration.

Reprinted with permission from the *P.A. Journal*, Vol. 6, no. 2 (Summer 1976): 72-78.

Almost all persons 65 and older are eligible to participate in the Medicare program. This program provides hospitalization insurance and, for a monthly premium, supplementary medical insurance to meet physician and other charges, both in and out of the hospital.

The impact of health insurance coverage on sources of payment for health care services is significant. For fiscal 1974, third party payers met 65 percent of these costs while 35 percent were met directly by individuals. In comparing source of expenditure for health care services in fiscal 1966 (the year immediately preceding the start of the Medicare program) and 1974, a shift away from direct payment can be seen in both the under 65 and over 65 population.[2] While both public and private insurance assumed larger roles in payment of health care costs in the under 65 groups, it was government, primarily Medicare, whose responsibility grew from 30 to 60 percent of the health care costs for the 65 and older group. Private insurance shrank from 16 to 5 percent in this age group.

For all insured persons, 89 percent of hospital costs and 61 percent of physician's charges are met by third parties, with only 11 percent and 39 percent respectively being paid directly. Dental services and drugs remain largely direct payment items while other care is split about evenly between direct and third party payers.[3]

CURRENT THIRD PARTY PAYMENT POLICIES FOR PHYSICIAN ASSISTANT SERVICES

Given the significant role of third party payment in meeting personal health care expenses, it is clear that third party reimbursement policy on services provided by physician assistants (PAs) could influence consumer demand for these services and employer demand for these providers. Yet few public or private health insurance programs recognize a PA (or a nurse practitioner) as a bona fide provider of medical care. It is equally true that few have established procedures for looking beyond a physician's claim for reimbursement as to whether the physician or a PA provided a particular service.

The Social Security Administration does not recognize PAs or nurse practitioners as independent providers of medical care or other covered services under the Supplementary Medical Insurance provisions of Medicare.[4] Presently, Medicare reimbursement for services performed by PAs is limited to those provided incident to a physician's professional service. "Incident to" services must be of the kind commonly furnished in physicians' offices as an adjunct to a physician's personal service and must be provided under the direct supervision of the physician. Also, "incident to" services are commonly rendered without charge or are included in the physician's bills. If a PA provides a service typically and characteristically rendered only by a physician, such as examining a patient or prescribing medication, the service cannot be reimbursed. A physician may provide a personal identifiable "physician's service" in conjunction with a PA (such as during a physical exam) but under no circumstances can a PA service itself be reimbursed if it does not meet all of the "incident to" criteria.

Medicaid is a state-federal cooperative health insurance program for the poor and medically indigent. Medicaid policy on reimbursing for PA services varies from state to state. In some states, only PA services are reimbursable, while in others only nurse practitioner services may be paid. There are 25 states with some type of reimbursement policy for PA services. In all of them, claims for PA services must come from the supervising physician or employing clinic. No reimbursement is permitted for PA services in 25 other Medicaid programs except as may inadvertently be made as part of a physician's service and claims. Many of the Medicaid programs which will reimburse for PA services require the immediate availability of a physician as a condition of reimbursement. Physicians must be on the premises with, although not necessarily in the same room as, a PA. This requirement would appear to preclude Medicaid reimbursement for PA services in satellite facilities, hospital, home or nursing home visits unless the physician also makes the trip.

At the present time, there are 37 states in which the PA is recognized by statute as a dependent provider of medical services under the supervision of a licensed physician. It is interesting to note, however, that legal recognition of PAs is neither a necessary nor a sufficient condition for Medicaid reimbursement. The Medicaid programs in 15 of these 37 states will not reimburse for their services. On the other hand, four Medicaid programs in states without PA laws *will* reimburse for their services.[5]

A number of private third party payers were contacted by the author for information on their current reimbursement policies for PA services. The National Association of Blue Shield Plans reported that it generally supports the concept of Blue Shield reimbursement for PA services which are provided under the supervision of a licensed physician. In canvassing its member plans, it has found that some have been reimbursing for these services for four to five years, while others do not yet reimburse for PA services. The National Blue Shield Association also supports the concept of reimbursement at a lower rate for PA services than for physician's services.

In 1972, the Health Insurance Council of the Health Insurance Association of America conducted a survey of commercial health insurance companies to determine their reaction to reimbursement guidelines for

PA services prepared by the American Medical Association. The Council received responses from 35 companies. Of these, the Council reported that 27 did not exclude benefits for services performed by PAs under coverage then available. It is not clear, however, that these companies are reimbursing PAs or physicians for PA services. Six of the country's largest commercial health insurance companies reported that they do not recognize PAs as independent providers of medical services and that they have had little experience with claims for reimbursement filed by PAs or by physicians for medical services where a PA was specified as the provider.

In general, the companies' comments on the rate of reimbursement reflected an overriding concern that broadening the definitions of eligible providers of services to include PAs would further escalate the inflation of health care expenditures by increasing service charges or number of services or both. Several companies said that if reimbursement was to be made separately for PA services, either to the PA or the PA's employer, then the rate of reimbursement should be lower than that for a physician providing the same service. Other companies expressed an interest in seeing whether PAs would have a stabilizing effect on physician charges for health care services.

Commercial insurance companies find differing state laws and regulations with regard to PAs an impediment to substantial change in their current definitions of eligible providers of care. These companies often write large contracts covering groups of employees spread across several states. It would be difficult to guarantee, as some groups insist, the same range of benefits for all those covered under these contracts when one benefit—PA services—may be legal in one state but not another.

ISSUES OF REIMBURSEMENT FOR PA SERVICES

At the present time, the numbers of PAs in primary care practices is relatively small but growing rapidly.[6] Whether they continue to do so depends in part upon whether public and private third party payment is available for their services. The issue of whether public third party reimbursement is made available for PA services will be resolved only after a number of other issues are dealt with first. These include the legal and professional ambiguities in defining what a PA is and does, the nature and quality of the services PAs provide, and the effects of reimbursement on the cost inflation in health care programs such as Medicare.

Will PAs be recognized by the medical and legal fields according to some generally accepted system of certification or licensure? In 1971, the Secretary of Health, Education, and Welfare in conjunction with the

American Medical Association and the American Hospital Association called for a two-year moratorium on state licensing of new types of health manpower. This request was extended into 1974 and 1975. The purpose of the moratorium was to give the Federal Government and the professional societies an opportunity to assess how best to address a rapidly expanding list of new health providers. During the moratorium the American Medical Association, with Department of Health, Education, and Welfare support, developed an accreditation plan for PA training programs. Also, the Department of Health, Education and Welfare (HEW) and the National Board of Medical Examiners began developing a certification examination for the assistant to the primary care physician, given first in December 1973. In 1975, an HEW sponsored evaluation of the examination's ability to predict performance of a PA in actual practice was undertaken and is scheduled to be completed in 1977.

These activities will, hopefully, serve to establish universally accepted standards of training and tests of competence for primary care PAs. Until they do, it will remain difficult for states to define, certify, or license PAs, and for third party payers to develop appropriate reimbursement policy for physician assistant services.

Universally accepted standards of preparation and tests of competence may serve as one means of measuring the quality of PA care. Almost all studies conducted to date indicate that the quality of physician assistant services is at least as good as that provided by primary care physicians. Unfortunately, the measures used in many of these studies have been patient and physician attitudes about PAs and the care they provide. More objective quality measures are included in only a few small scale studies which most often observed nurse practitioners rather than PAs.[7] Duncan, et al. obtained independent assessments of the conditions of 182 children by pediatric nurse practitioners and their supervising pediatricians. The results showed complete concurrence in 82 percent of the assessments and insignificant differences in 17 percent. In only two cases or one percent was there significant disagreement in the assessments.[8] Spitzer, Sackett, et al. conducted a randomized control trial in two suburban Ontario practices which consisted of a physician and a family nurse practitioner. Patients' health status, as measured by changes in quantitative indicator conditions as well as by patient satisfaction, showed no significant difference between those seen by physicians and family nurse practitioners.[9]

Much remains to be learned about the quality of physician assistant care. The problem is whether or not the services being reimbursed are of satisfactory quality. If the existing evidence can be reinforced by more objective quality studies, the question could be more satisfactorily resolved.

The costs and benefits of employing PAs is another crucial issue both to potential employers and third party payers. Does it pay to employ a physician assistant as opposed to additional physicians or other personnel; does it pay to set up a satellite facility staffed by a PA rather than circuit-riding or not serving another community? One MEDEX program reported that employers were either breaking even or experiencing small profits from the employment of their PAs. A more recent study of 12 primary care practices employing Medex showed substantial excess revenues from the PAs after their costs had been met.[10]

From an economic perspective, high potential profits could serve as an incentive to hire PAs. To the extent that employer demand exceeds physician assistant supply, physicians or clinics would bid up the salaries for available PAs. This, in turn, would increase the demand for PA training programs. However, this process would not necessarily provide any relief from the inflation in medical care expenditures. In fact, a major question which remains to be answered is the extent to which third party payment would intensify inflation in expenditures by increasing both the price of services and the number of services delivered.

The dilemma for public policy on third party reimbursement is how to encourage the productive use of PA resources while containing the inflationary trend in medical care expenditures. The growth of third party payment has been attended by a rise in health care expenditures.[11] How can utilization of PAs reduce the rate of inflation in these expenditures and increase access to needed primary care for those who would not otherwise receive it? Certainly, the Congress and the Social Security Administration do not wish to see third party payment for PA services result in additional inflationary pressure on Medicare expenditures or the addition of unnecessary care for the adequately served portions of the population. These concerns led to the decision by the Congress to conduct research on the impact of third party payments for PA services before establishing a reimbursement policy for PA services. The question to be answered is what sort of reimbursement policy would make sense from the point of view of the employer, third party payer, and the consumer, who ultimately absorbs the costs.

SSA PHYSICIAN EXTENDER REIMBURSEMENT STUDY

Under congressional authority provided in the Social Security Amendments of 1972,[12] the Social Security Administration is conducting a nationwide study which addresses most of these issues. This effort, referred to as the Physician Extender Reimbursement Study, will make Medicare Part B reimbursement available on an experimental basis to participating noninstitutional primary care practices for services provided to beneficiaries by physician extenders. Physician extender, or "PE," is the generic term used in SSA to refer to primary care physician assistants including Medex and nurse practitioners who have received formal training in diagnostic and therapeutic skills necessary to provide primary health care services under the general supervision of a physician.

The purpose of the study is to determine under what circumstances payment for services provided by PEs would be appropriate and the most appropriate, equitable, and noninflationary alternatives which, if accepted for general use, would not impede continuing efforts to expand the supply of qualified physician extenders. Also, physician extenders are to be "clearly" trained and legally authorized to perform the specific services for which reimbursement is claimed. Further, reimbursement is to be made only to employers of physician extenders and only for services which are delivered independent of an employing physician's direct involvement. The results of the study are to provide a basis for economical and noninflationary reimbursement for physician extender services, at a rate which may be less than a physician's reimbursement. The recommendations, if implemented, should enhance the PE's ability to extend the physician's productivity and bring necessary care to those who would otherwise not receive it.[13]

The Physician Extender Reimbursement Study will attempt to answer the following questions: (1) Does the value of services provided by a PE exceed the costs of his or her employment? (2) Do PEs make a greater contribution to practice productivity when working independently of physicians or when working under the close supervision of physicians? (3) Do practices employing PEs deliver more services than other practices? (4) Is the quality of services delivered by a PE as good as that delivered by a physician? (5) Does utilization of PEs result in a shift in locations where services are delivered by the practice (e.g., more home visits)? (6) Does Medicare reimbursement for PE services result in a shift in PE utilization towards serving Medicare beneficiaries? (7) Do Medicare total program expenditures increase with reimbursement for PE services. If so, why? (8) Does reimbursement for PE services at a rate less than that allowed for physician services nevertheless stimulate the utilization of PEs? If so, how?

The study consists of two major phases, the baseline data collection activity and the reimbursement experiment. It is anticipated that about 800 practices which employ PEs will agree to participate in the baseline effort. These practices will be identified through a survey of PE graduates whose names and addresses were obtained from their training programs.* Also included in the baseline activity will be a group of comparison practices which do not employ PEs, but which are matched on the basis of practice location, practice arrangement, specialty, and size of staff. The matching data and eligibility information will be collected through a brief questionnaire mailed to both PE and comparison practices.

The baseline activity will be conducted through the use of a log-diary and questionnaire to be completed by PEs, their supervising physicians, and physicians in the comparison practices. This information will be used to describe differences between PE and comparison practice organization and productivity. Specific information which will be collected includes professional characteristics of physicians and PEs, types and volume of services delivered by them, charges for services, and patient characteristics.

The baseline activity began in December 1975 with the mailing of log-diary and questionnaire booklets to approximately 100 practices employing PEs. Subsequent mailings will be made monthly to groups of 100 practices until all practices have participated in the baseline activity. Practices which satisfactorily complete the baseline activity will be contacted by the appropriate Medicare carrier about 30 days after returning the booklets, and after claims processing procedures are explained, should be submitting Medicare claims for PE services within the following month.

Reimbursement to participating practices for PE services will be made at the lower of the actual charge or a maximum allowable charge (less deductible and coinsurance payments). The maximum allowable charge will be calculated according to one of three possible methods: a rate equal to the Medicare allowable charge now being applied to the supervising physician's services, 80 percent of the supervising physician's allowable charges, or an average cost-related rate. In authorizing this study, the Congress expressed the opinion that the rate of experimental reimbursement should be lower than the rate for physicians. This rate was, according to the Congress, to contain costs while not impeding the training (and thereby employment) of PAs. The rate chosen by SSA for experimentation—80 percent of the physician's maximum allowable charge—is considered to meet these goals.

---

*The baseline phase is being conducted by the Division of Research in Medical Education, University of Southern California School of Medicine under contract to the SSA. Invaluable assistance was provided by PA program directors, program graduates, supervising physicians, the American Academy of Physicians' Assistants, and the APAP-AAPA National Office staff.

Experimental reimbursement will continue for two years. At intervals throughout this period, data similar to those collected in the baseline activity will be collected in the participating PE practices. For a subsample of PE and comparison practices, more detailed studies of productivity, costs, and quality of care will be conducted. Also, summary information on Medicare claims for PE services will be used to measure the impact of experimental reimbursement on program costs and costs to beneficiaries.

Preliminary results should be available early in 1977 of: (a) the baseline activity—assessing the impact of physician extenders on primary care practices and (b) the reimbursement experiment—assessing the impact of Medicare reimbursement for PE services on program costs and practice activity.

CONCLUSION

There are those who believe that the issues of defining the physician assistant and proper PA roles and functions are resolved, and that third party payment should be made for PA services. Others, including the Congress, SSA, and many private third party payers have taken a "wait and see" position, recognizing that much remains to be learned and understood about PAs and their impact upon the provision of primary care. The Social Security Administration hopes that, through its study, some light will be shed in this important area for use in developing sensible and fair reimbursement policies.

EXHIBIT 9-1

Below is an excerpt of the U.S. Finance Committee Report which authorized the S.S.A. Physician Extender Reimbursement Study.

PHYSICIANS' ASSISTANTS

Under present law, part B of medicare pays for physicians' services. Within the scope of paying for physicians' services, the program pays for services commonly rendered in a physician's office by para-medical personnel. For example, if a nurse administers an injection in the office, medicare will recognize a small charge by the physician for that service.

Medicare will not pay where a physician submits a charge for a professional service, performed by a para-medical person, in cases where the service is traditionally performed by a physician. For example, the program would not recognize a charge for a complete physical exam conducted by a nurse.

Additionally, medicare will not recognize a physician's charge for a service performed by a para-medical person outside of the physician's office. In other words, he would not be reimbursed for an injection administered by a para-medical employee in a nursing home.

Over the past few years, a number of programs have been developed to train physicians' assistants. These assistants are seen as a way to extend the physician's productivity and to bring necessary care to many who would otherwise not receive it. HEW is currently supporting the training of these physicians' assistants. There are some 100 experimental training programs for physician assistants and nurse practitioners. Each of these, however, is structured differently, reflecting the lack of agreement among professionals on the experience and education that should be required of training program applicants, the content of the programs, or the responsibilities and supervision that are appropriate for their graduates. These unresolved issues have prompted the American Medical Association, the American Hospital Association, the American Public Health Association, as well as the Department (in its "Report on Licensure and Related Health Personnel Credentialing") and other organizations to ask for a moratorium on State licensure of the new categories of health personnel.

Some feel that it is inconsistent for HEW to support the training of these personnel, while medicare does not, in some instances, recognize all their services as reimbursable items.

Others argue that medicare does reimburse physicians for services provided by these new physicians' assistants, so long as they are services commonly provided by para-professional personnel in a physician's office. They contend that, until the training and licensure of physicians' assistants becomes more uniform, it would be inappropriate for medicare to take the lead in encouraging doctors—by generous reimbursement—to use physicians' assistants to work independently or to expand their responsibilities.

The committee has included a provision authorizing demonstration projects to determine the most appropriate equitable methods of compensating for the services of physicians' assistants. The objectives are development of non-inflationary alternatives which, if accepted for general use, would not impede the continuing efforts to expand the supply of qualified physicians' assistants.

Reimbursement under these demonstration projects would not be made to physicians for services performed by physicians' assistants unless such services are of kinds performed independent of the employing physician's immediate supervision and unless such assistants are clearly trained and legally authorized to specifically perform those independent services.

In addition it would seem inappropriate to reimburse a physician his regular fee-for-service rate if the service was performed wholly by the physician's assistant. This would merely serve to vastly increase and inflate medical care costs in large part by increasing physicians' incomes.

Medicare would be given demonstration authority to study, develop, and make such types of reimbursement on a demonstration basis as might serve to provide bases for equitable, economical and non-inflationary compensation for the independently rendered services of physicians' assistants.

U.S. Senate
Senate Finance Committee Print 92-1230

Notes

1. Mueller MS: Private Health Insurance in 1973: A Review of Coverage, Enrollment, and Financial Experience. Social Security Bulletin, DHEW Publication No. (SSA) 74-11700, February 1975.

2. Mueller MS, Gibson RM: Age Differences in Health Care Spending, Fiscal Year 1974. Social Security Bulletin, DHEW Publication No. (SSA) 75-11700, June 1975.

3. Worthington NL: National Health Expenditures, 1929-1974. Social Security Bulletin, DHEW Publication No. (SSA) 74-11700, February 1975.

4. United States Senate, Committee on Finance. The Social Security Act (As Amended Through January 4, 1975) and Related Laws. Washington, D.C., U.S. Government Printing Office, Sec. 1861 (r), 455-456, 1975.

5. Simpson J: Reimbursement to Physician's Assistants and Nurse Practitioners Under Medicaid. National Health Law Project Staff Paper. November 25, 1974.

6. Appel GL, Lowin A: Physician Extender. An Evaluation of Policy Related Research. Minneapolis, Interstudy, January 1975.

7. Social Security Administration, Office of Research and Statistics. Impact of Physician Extenders on the Delivery of Medical Care—A Review of the Literature Including an Annotated Bibliography and References. Division of Health Insurance Studies Staff Paper. 32-36, July 1974.

8. Duncan B. Smith, AN, Silver HK, Comparison of the physical assessment of children by pediatric nurse practitioners and pediatricians. Am. J. Pub. Health 61:1170-1176, 1971.

9. Spitzer WO, Sackett DL, et al.: The Burlington randomized trial of the nurse practitioner, N Engl J Med 290:251-256, 1974.

10. Nelson EC, et al: Financial impact of physician assistants on medical practice. N Engl J Med 293:527-530, 1975.

11. Social Security Administration, Office of Research and Statistics. Monthly Statistical Report Summary of Selected Price, Cost, and Utilization Data for the Health Care Market in the United States. Division of Health Insurance Studies, January 1975.

12. Public Law 92-603, Sec. 222(b)(1)(G).

13. United States Senate, Committee on Finance, Social Security Amendments of 1972. Washington, D.C., U.S. Government Printing Office, 1972.

Chapter 10

Economic Effectiveness of Family Nurse Practitioner Practice in Primary Care in California

Mary O'Hara-Devereaux, John V. Dervin, Len Hughes Andrus
and Leona Judson

The economic factors associated with the utilization of family nurse practitioners (FNP) and physician assistants (PA) is a critical consideration of primary care. The University of California at Davis Family Nurse Practitioner Program[1] has implemented several studies to analyze the impact of their graduates on primary care practices throughout California. If FNPs and PAs are to be appropriately utilized within the health care system, their economic feasibility in a variety of primary care settings needs to be established. If rational decisions are to be made about type and level of reimbursement for these new health practitioners, appropriate data must be gathered to support those policy decisions. This chapter will summarize the results of two of these studies. In addition, it includes a study of the integration of the FNP Program into the Sonoma County Family Practice Residency (FPR) Program.

PILOT STUDY OF NINE PRIVATE PRACTICES IN CALIFORNIA

In an effort to gain a frontline look at the economic factors of FNP practice in the private sector, nine private practices througout California were selected where an FNP/MD team had been working together for at least one year. Of the nine study sites, five were predominantly rural settings and the other four in urban areas. Evaluation staff visited each site and interviewed the FNP/MD team, collected productivity data, and reviewed actual billings and financial reports.

Practice Description

The FNPs spent about 38 to 40 hours a week in professional activities, and the physicians tended to devote 50 to 60 hours (not including after-hours call time) to their practice. While in the office, these MDs and

161

FNPs saw similar kinds of patients in the broad diagnostic categories. None of the practices screened patients for the FNPs. All the practices reported that the FNP was able to see from 75 to 80 percent of the patients without direct physician consultation. In general, the FNPs spent more time in preventive activities, such as physical examinations and prenatal and well baby care, than the physician members of the team. The physicians tended to do more procedures such as biopsies, fracture reductions, and laceration repair.

Productivity

Table 10:1 summarizes the office practice load and charges for an office visit of the nine practices. Each site was requested to monitor the actual number of patient visits and charges to each FNP or MD provider for a two-week period. Gross annual income was projected from these data and cross-checked with the former year's gross receipts. Number of patients seen per day by the FNP averaged about 17 (range 9-25). Physician visits averaged 25 (range 15-32) patients per day in the office setting. FNPs had a mean charge per patient of $10.30 (range $10-$13). The physician's mean charge per patient among the nine practices was $17.30 (range $11-$21).

Physican Income

A summary of the source of physician income is detailed in Table 10:2. The nine physicians derived 69 percent of their income from their office practice. The range of office-based services among the nine practices varied from 52 percent to 100 percent with one physician having no out-of-office-based activities. The average salary for the physician in the practice was $58,000. Twenty-eight percent of physician income came from hospital activities and other sources, such as lab and X-ray consultations, and 12 percent of the physician's net income came from the FNP practice. The average dollar amount accrued to the physician's net

TABLE 10:1

Pilot Study Summary of Nine Practices' Office Practice Load and Charges

	FNP	MD
Patients per day	17.1	25
Patients per annum	4,104	6,000
Charge per patient	$11.30	$17.30
Gross annual income	$46,375	$103,800

TABLE 10:2

Pilot Study of Nine Practices

	Physician Income
Net Physician Income	
From office practice (69%)	$34,935
From hospital and other sources	$16,238
From FNP practice	$ 6,904
Total Physician Income	$58,077

income from the FNP practice was $6,904 (range $1,178 to $12,000). The nine practices reported an average overhead of about 50 percent, with a range from 46 to 58 percent.

The FNPs had an average salary of $17,151 (range $9,363 to $21,000). All their income was generated from office-based activities. All practices reported that the FNP salary reflected productivity factors, with some having a periodic review of salary based on productivity and some receiving a straight percentage of income.

All the FNP/MD teams were satisfied with the arrangement of their practice style. All felt that FNP practice should be office-based. However, many were interested in expanding the FNPs' activities to the hospital and nursing home as soon as California hospital regulations and reimbursement issues were settled. The FNP/MD teams also felt that FNPs would take more after-hour calls as soon as the FNPs were more widely known and accepted by other physicians in the community.

All agreed that the graduate FNP was paying her own way and was able to reach the break-even point a month or two after entering the practice. The result of this pilot study of nine private practices of FNP/MD teams in California supports the premise that FNPs are economically feasible.

SURVEY OF 93 PRIMARY CARE PRACTICES

In August of 1976 a confidential survey was mailed to FNP/MD and PA/MD teams who were graduates of two FNP programs and one PA program in California. Ninety-three primary care practices responded, which represents 215 FNPs and 44 PAs, a response rate of 84 percent. Table 10:3 summarizes the type and location of the practices responding. The practices were asked to detail specific productivity and income data of these three primary care providers. The PAs and FNPs in the practices in Table 10:2 have been in their roles for an average of two and a half years with a range of eight months to six years. The vast majority of the primary care practices reported that the addition of an FNP/PA increased the income of that service unit. Only two percent of the practices in the private sector reported a decrease in income for the practice with the addition of the FNP/PA.

Although there are few reports of nationwide salaries of FNPs and PAs in the literature, most of them suggest a lower salary than the respondents in these California primary care settings. With a range of $11,000 to $27,000, these 259 FNPs and PAs made a mean salary of $17,420. The average salaries of the FNP and the PA were about the same; however, FNP salaries are higher by two percent. The highest salaries were paid by group practices, followed by solo practice settings, and last, hospital and public community clinics. Thirty-eight percent of salaries were determined in specific relationship to productivity, and these were usually in the private sector. Other salaries were determined by institutions or practice settings through the usual administrative process used to determine all other health care worker salaries.

Productivity

In August 1976 practices were asked to indicate their average daily patient load and average charge per patient visit during the week they received the survey. Table 10:4 details the responses. The FNP-PA/MD in solo practice saw an average of 15.2 and 28.2 patients per day, respectively. The physician in group practice saw 27.9 patients per day, and his team member FNP/PA saw 18 patients. In both the community and hospital clinics the physician saw about 21 patients per day; the FNP/PA saw 15.6 in the community clinic and 17.7 in the hospital clinic. Within the sample, physicians working with FNPs tended to see fewer patients (21 per day) than physicians working with PAs (30 per day). Likewise, the

TABLE 10:3

Type and Practice Location of 93[1] Sites Responding to Economic Survey

Type of Practice	Number	Percent (%)	Location[2]	Number	Percent (%)
Solo	25	27	Urban	34	37
Group	17	19	Suburban	29	31
Public Community Clinic	19	20	Rural	26	28
Hospital Clinic	16	17	No response	4	4
Other	16	17	—		
TOTAL	93	100%	TOTAL	93	100%

[1]Represents 93 MDs, 214 FNPs, 44 PAs
[2]Sites classified themselves

TABLE 10:4

Productivity and Charges Per Patient Visit

Type of Practice	Numbers of Patients Seen Per Day		Average Fee Per Patient Visit — Office	
	MD	FNP/PA	MD	FNP/PA
Solo	28.2	15.5	$15.80	$15.07
Group	27.9	18.0	14.09	10.65
Public Community Clinic	21.9	15.6	9.20	8.84
Hospital Clinic	21.6	17.7	15.54	15.54

TABLE 10:5

Factors Contributing to Physician Gross Income (By Percent)

Income Source:	Mean Percent	
	MD	FNP/PA
Office visits	72.5%	91.2%
Hospital	14.3%	1.9%
Nursing home	1.7%	2.6%
Emergency room	6.83%	—
Home visits	.66%	2.0%
Lab and X-ray charges	6.5%	4.2%
Other	1.6%	—

PAs saw an average of 19 patients per day, and the FNP saw 15. The physicians working with PAs had a higher average charge per patient visit ($18.53) than the physicians working with FNPs ($15.74). There was also a difference between PAs and FNPs; the FNPs had a higher charge per patient ($15.18) than the PA ($13.48).

The solo and group practices in the private sector reported an average of 52.8 percent overhead with a range of 48 to 66 percent. These practices reported that the addition of an FNP or PA increased overhead by about 17.63 percent, which includes the salary of this new health professional. Overhead costs of these practices categorically showed that about 46 percent of the cost was attributable to personnel, 14 percent to general supplies, 10 percent to rent and utilities and about 6 percent to malpractice insurance. The rest of the overhead (24 percent) is distributed among equipment, maintenance, and other miscellaneous categories.

Table 10:5 details the percent income of physicians and the FNP/PA by category of service. These data indicate that the FNP and the PA produce income mainly from the office setting in contrast to the physician who receives a substantial proportion of his salary from hospital-based activities. Currently, California hospital regulations are somewhat prohibitive concerning the utilization of the FNP/PA in hospitals. A change in this area will provide an increase of activity in the hospitals and, in particular, nursing homes.

The results of this survey of 93 practices and their reported economic data support the thesis that the addition of an FNP/PA to a variety of primary care settings is economically feasible. Projecting the FNP/PA patient volume per day with the average charge per patient indicates that the FNP/PA's potential gross income is over $40,000 per year. This amount more than covers the cost of their salary and overhead.

FNPs IN A COUNTY HOSPITAL-BASED FAMILY PRACTICE PROGRAM

Community Hospital of Sonoma County is a 140-bed hospital located in Santa Rosa, California. The hospital conducts an approved residency program in Family Practice with 27 residents in training.* Outpatient services are concentrated in the Model Family Practice Unit (MFPU), an 11,000-square-foot structure. There were 35,000 patient visits at the MFPU in 1976.

FNPs were introduced into the MFPU in 1973. There was interest in utilizing FNPs to provide residents with an education experience in team care with FNPs, to lower the cost of primary care county service obligations by replacing some physicians with FNPs, and to improve the cost-effectiveness of the MFPU through better space utilization, reorganization of support personnel, and increased general primary care services provided by FNPs.

FNPs are utilized in a number of activities. Approximately two-thirds of FNP time is allocated to Family Practice clinics. In these three- to four-hour clinic sessions, FNPs are teamed with second and third year residents, and together they see their patients. FNPs also spend a small amount of time working with the faculty physicians in their clinics.

FNPs perform a number of county services previously reserved for physicians. The FNPs are responsible for various health requirements of Sonoma County employees such as pre-employment examinations, periodic health testing for management level personnel, and other routine health maintenance. In addition, various special county contracts have been developed for performance of medical tasks by FNPs in areas previously served by physicians. Specifically, FNPs provide health maintenance and acute care services to county agencies such as the jail, juvenile hall, and the drug dependence unit.

---

*In affiliation with the University of California, San Francisco Medical Center.

To assure continued utilization of the FNP in the MFPU, it was necessary to demonstrate their economic viability to the county administration. Data acquired since 1973 indicate the economic success of the FNP concept in MFPU. Productivity of practices of Family Practice Residents (FPR) has increased with the addition of FNPs. From a sample of patients visits in 1974 and again in 1976, it was determined that in FNP/FPR team practices, FPRs were responsible for 53 percent of visits, and FNPs 47 percent of visits in both years.

In 1975, a controlled study was implemented to compare the productivity of FNP/FPR teams to that of FPR practices without FNPs. Practices with FNPs averaged 83.2 visits per month. Practices with FNPs were 31 percent more productive than those without FNPs. A follow-up study in 1976 showed that practices with FNPs were 38 percent more productive than those without FNPs.

Economic viability of any endeavor ultimately comes down to a comparison of cost versus income. Before looking at these aspects of the FNP project, however, two considerations are essential: salary savings as a result of change in the support personnel mix in the MFPU and ancillary income from FNP services.

Upon initiating this project, support personnel in the MFPU included a number of registered nurses (RN). A task analysis of RN functions showed that RNs spent a considerable amount of time in licensed vocational nurse (LVN)/aide functions. By replacing RN support personnel with aides and LVNs, and by shifting those duties from the RN to the FNP, a salary savings of $24,250 resulted, in 1976. RNs replaced in this changeover were encouraged to complete an FNP training program, and the majority chose this alternative. These savings must be considered when studying the economics of the FNP Program in the MFPU.

When the FNP sees a patient, charges other than the actual visit charges are generated as a result of that visit (e.g., X-ray, pharmacy, lab charges). In the Sonoma County system, all of these charges are grouped in the single category of ancillary income. An understanding of ancillary income allows a more realistic evaluation of the total financial benefit of FNP activities to the county. The cost of FNPs in 1976 was essentially that of their salaries and benefits, with no appreciable increase in overhead costs. There were several reasons for this: architecture of the MFPU was relatively spacious, personnel were underutilized, and no increase in support personnel or space was necessary with introduction of the FNPs. Cost for five full-time FNPs was $96,000 in 1976. Income attributable to the FNP Program in 1976 is summarized in Table 10:6. The sum of income and economic benefits attributable to FNP activities for 1976 was $221,450. The summary of economic value to the hospital versus cost for

TABLE 10:6

Income for FNPs in Model Family Practice Unit 1976

Income Categories:	
Resident/FNP clinics	$49,100
Faculty physician/FNP clinics	$13,000
Employee health activities	$28,000
Special contracts	$10,500
Total Income Attributable to FNP's	$100,600
Other Economic Benefits:	
Ancillary income	$96,600
Savings by change in personnel mix	$24,250
Total Economic Benefits Attributable to FNPs	$120,850

the MFPU as a whole, and specifically for the FNP Program, is included in Table 10:7. The FNP activities were responsible for about 20 percent of the total income of the MFPU. The economic success of the FNP in the MFPU at Community Hospital of Sonoma County has been demonstrated.

DISCUSSION

The results of these three studies show that family nurse practitioners and primary care physician assistants are economically feasible in a wide variety of primary care settings. Economic evaluation of the FNP has not received as much attention in the literature as evaluation in areas such as productivity, attitudes, and quality of care. Some literature does exist on the economic feasibility of the FNP and PA concept and the results of these studies generally support the data reported in this chapter.

Schiff et al.,[2] as early as 1969, demonstrated that PNPs could generate sufficient income to cover their expenses. In this situation, there was a minimal increase in practice overhead. Yankauer et al.,[3] in a 1972 study of pediatric nurse practitioners (PNPs), demonstrated that the PNPs could cover the costs of their salary and overhead. Their findings were based on a standard $5.00 charge and a 40 percent overhead figure.

In a study from private practices of general practitioners and internists utilizing Medex, Nelson et al.[4] demonstrated income gains for 10 of the 12 practices studied. In that study, a method was developed to proportion costs of shared visits (in which both physician and Medex saw the patient) between Medex and physician. A similar method was utilized to allocate income from shared visits.

At the Everett Clinic, 30 miles north of Seattle, a nurse practitioner generated between $28,000 to $31,000 inpatient services over a 10.5-month period in 1974, against her salary of $10,085.[5] She saw an average of 10 to 12 patients daily, but occasionally saw as many as 20 patients.

A dissenting study from a large teaching hospital outpatient clinic challenges the economic feasibility of the FNP concept. Spector et al.[6] studied patient charges for the three months before and three months after NPs and showed average patient costs of $53.94 and $66.76 for each phase. Conclusions drawn were that quality of care delivered by NPs seemed good, but increased cost could not justify the program. It should be noted that cost to the patient was the only basis for determining economic viability.

PROBLEMS AND ISSUES

Productivity—The overall productivity of an office family practice was increased by the addition of an FNP/PA for all the settings studied. The determining factors seem to be adequate patient volume, access by the FNP/PA to a broad spectrum of patients, adequate space, positive physician attitude towards maximum utilization and a well-trained FNP/PA with a broad clinical base who knows the economic factors involved in office practice. Productivity as measured by patient visits alone cannot be utilized as a criterion for the success of team practice. Addition of an FNP/PA to a practice can decrease the burdensome workload of a physician, can add needed comprehensive services to an episodic illness-focused practice, and can provide time away for the physician for educational and personal pursuits. It has also been our experience that the ad-

TABLE 10:7

Economic Benefits of Family Nurse Practitioners in a Model Family Practice Unit[1]

	Revenue Generated In MFPU	Portion Generated By FNPs[2]
Direct income	$486,000	$100,600
Ancillary income	457,705	96,600
Personnel savings	24,250	24,250
Total Income	$967,955	$221,450
Total Cost	$495,000	$ 96,000

[1] Data for year 1976
[2] These income and cost figures are included in the revenue generated by the MFPU.

dition of an FNP/PA to a practice allows extension of services to Medicaid patients, who are definitely an underserved group.

Finally, a different view of both the health care team's economic producitivity and its impact on health status needs to be advanced. The team concept of family practice challenges the belief that patients benefit from only a single provider each visit. The issue of who should see the patient provides a focus of attention counterproductive to good team relationships. Although the patient may see only one of the providers on a given visit, he actually benefits from the availability of the total services of the team. When looking at patient care over a time, the shared responsibility of the team for total care is demonstrated.

Salaries—Issues related to salaries of the FNP/PA are complex. It is essential that physicians be appropriately renumerated for supervising and consulting with the FNP/PA. In this study the $6,000 per annum increase in income for the physician seems a fair return for medical supervision of the FNP/PA and legal responsibility for all patients in the practice. In isolated cases financial returns to the physician for such supervision may be excessive. This issue needs to be addressed openly and some reasonable guidelines developed.

Trends in team practice indicate that straight salary arrangements will be replaced by increased risk and profit-sharing by the team members. Employer/employee relationships between the physician and the FNP/PA will probably be replaced by legal and administrative partnership agreements.

Overhead—It appears that an addition of an FNP/PA to existing practice results in little increase in practice overhead above their salaries and benefits. Most practices are not efficiently using their space and personnel and find the FNP/PA a cost-effective approach to better resource utilization.

Reimbursement—Physicians are reimbursed at the same rate for services rendered in the practice regardless of whether or not an FNP/PA participates in rendering those services. In other words, current practice is fee-for-service rather than fee-for-physician-service. In the practices studied the cost of rendering services was similar regardless of whether the FNP/PA or the physician rendered the actual care. The comparison of costs includes reasonable compensation for physician supervision and consultation of the patient's care. The argument for lower reimbursement for the FNP/PA based on salary differentials with physicians is inaccurate. Physician salaries reflect more broad complex medical care activities and longer hours. Secondary and tertiary care constitute the bulk of health care costs; therefore, establishing lower reimbursement rates to physicians for FNP/PA services will not result in significant cost savings and may result in decreased utilization of these new primary care providers who have proven to be competent and cost-effective.

Architecture—Existing medical care facilities were built around the physician provider concept. The need to increase examining space per provider is essential to the success of the FNP/PA office practice. Contrary to the success of the FNPs in the Sonoma program where space is abundant, progress is slow in other county systems, residency programs, and educational networks which lack such space.

NATIONAL IMPLICATIONS

There are implications from studies such as these that should influence national education and health care policies. It is clear that FNPs and PAs can be economically feasible in a broad spectrum of primary care settings. The specific discussion of economic factors of office practice with students and preceptors is essential if successful practice relationships are to be developed. The unsuccessful economic ventures in FNP/PA practice stem in a large part from poor planning and lack of information by the employers. Educational programs should clearly take responsibility to insure the appropriate utilization of their graduates, or all their training investment will be in vain. Funding for such activities should be included in training grants.

A national policy decision is necessary to increase the training and employment opportunities for cost-effective new primary care providers. The spiraling costs of health care are due mainly to secondary and tertiary care. The development of a system focused on primary care will be the most important step in curtailing these costs. The full utilization of the FNP/PA in teams with family physicians may have the greatest and most immediate impact.

Notes

1. L.H. Andrus and M.D. Fenley (O'Hara-Devereaux), "Educational Evolution of a Family Nurse Practitioner Program to Improve Primary Care Distribution," *J. Med. Educ.* 51 (1976): 317-324.

2. D.W. Schiff, C.H. Fraser, and H.L. Walters, "The Pediatric Nurse Practitioner in the Office of Pediatricians in Private Practice," *Pediatrics* 44 (1969): 62-68.

3. A. Yankauer et al., "The Costs of Training and the Income Generation Potential of Pediatric Nurse Practitioners," *Pediatrics* 49 (1972): 878-887.

4. E.C. Nelson et al., "Financial Impact of Physicians Assistants on Medical Practice," *N.E.J.M.* 293 (September 11, 1975): 527-530.

5. M.A. Draye and L.A. Stetson, "The Nurse Practitioner as an Economic Reality," *Med. Group Management* 22 (July/August 1975): 24-27.

6. R. Spector et al., "Medical Care by Nurses in an Internal Medicine Clinic," *J.A.M.A.* 232 (1975): 1234-1237.

Chapter 11

Cost Effectiveness of FNP Versus MD-Staffed Rural Practice

Barbara Seigal, David A. Jensen and Earl M. Coffee

Cooperative Health Services (CHS), a joint venture of presbyterian Hospital Center and St. Joseph Hospital in Albuquerque, was formed in 1971 to pursue solutions to the broad problem of cost and availability of health care in both urban and rural New Mexico and to encourage application of resources from the private sector. During the past several years, CHS has developed five primary care practices, three of which served rural communities with no other source of medical care. Two practices are staffed by a physician; three practices are staffed by family nurse practitioners (FNPs). The FNPs care for patients in solo practice settings at a distance of 20-85 miles from physicians in private practice and the hospitals which provide medical supervision and backup.

This chapter addresses the outreach activities of Cooperative Health Services in providing primary care in rural communities and analyzes comparative data collected during a 12-month period in 1974-1975 on the costs of operating MD and FNP staffed rural practices. One of the two physician practices was established in Bernalillo when a Spanish-speaking, general surgeon with a strong interest in general practice was recruited to staff a clinic serving a population of approximately 5,000 persons. The costs of operating this clinic are compared with those of two family nurse practitioner clinics, at Estancia 65 miles east and at Pecos 85 miles northeast of Albuquerque. All three rural communities and patients are different; the professional backgrounds of the primary care providers are different; the range of services available at each site varies; and overhead expenses vary depending on local economic conditions. In evaluating each of the rural areas in which CHS has assumed provision of services, serious consideration has been given to: (1) need for medical service (Is there no other provider?); (2) distance from the nearest medical community (at least 20 miles); (3) population base to be served (at least 2,500 to 4,000); (4) central management capability (within 100 miles); (5) availability of physicians to assume supervisory responsibility; (6) CHS recruitment of primary care providers for the site; (7)

history of the community in recruiting or retaining a provider; (8) commitment of the community to assist with funds to equip, fund or remodel a site; (9) the community's understanding of the role of the family nurse practitioner in providing care; and (10) community commitment to use and pay for services provided.

At the three sites, a local community health committee serves as an advisory council to the clinic and reviews future plans, fees, financial reports, helps raise funds to pay for special equipment and so forth, and meets with staff several times per year. However, management of each clinic rests with CHS which has assumed the financial risk for providing care. Although operating deficits have occurred at several sites, they have decreased over the years. These deficits, along with start-up costs, have been assumed by the sponsoring hospitals in Albuquerque.

VARIATIONS IN VISITS AND REVENUE AMONG THE PRACTICES

In 1974, an encounter form (see Exhibit 11:1) was instituted at each primary care clinic in order to facilitate collection of uniform cost and clinical data for comparative studies of the practices at each location. New providers and clerical staff were taught to use similar definitions in coding the forms. The encounter form is used by the receptionist to bill for services and procedures. The age and sex of the populations seen at the three respective clinics are shown in Tables 11:1 and the types of visit in Table 11:2.

TABLE 11:1

Patient Visits by Age and Sex, July 1974-July 1975

TOTAL VISITS	5,000 BERNALILLO MD		3,000 HOPE-ESTANCIA FNP		2,800 PECOS FNP	
AGE	FEMALE	MALE	FEMALE	MALE	FEMALE	MALE
0-4	5%	5%	7%	5%	9%	11%
5-12	6%	6%	8%	6%	6%	10%
13-19	6%	6%	8%	7%	7%	9%
20-64	27%	17%	30%	16%	20%	18%
65+	6%	7%	4%	4%	5%	4%
Not Recorded	5%	4%	3%	2%	—	1%
TOTALS	55%	45%	60%	40%	47%	53%

TABLE 11:2

Patient Visits by Type of Encounter, July 1974-July 1975

TOTAL VISITS	5,000 BERNALILLO MD	3,000 HOPE-ESTANCIA FNP	2,800 PECOS FNP
Episodic Illness	71%	46%	57%
System Initiated Follow-up Care	5%	6%	16%
Emergency	2%	3%	7%
Chronic Disease Management	18%	17%	4%
Specialty Consultation	—	—	—
Other Medical	—	2%	—
Prenatal	—	2%	1%
Well Baby	—	2%	1%
Immunizations Only	—	2%	1%
Family Planning	—	1%	—
Mental Health Care	—	1%	—
Physical Examinations	1%	4%	4%
Other Preventive	2%	9%	6%
Health Guidance	—	2%	—
All Other Care	1%	3%	3%
TOTALS	100%	100%	100%

The Bernalillo clinic served an older population group with chronic and acute disease conditions, and care at Bernalillo was provided by a general surgeon for two years and subsequently by an internist. It is possible that the physician's specialist status attracted the older patients. Also, because both a public health department (providing well child services and family planning) and a satellite clinic of the Albuquerque Maternal and Infant Care Project operate in Bernalillo, the CHS clinic sees little obstetrics. Bernalillo, 20 miles north of Albuquerque, is also close enough to Albuquerque so that many patients continue some relationship with medical specialists there. Care is largely episodic, with patients and families seeking care for acute illnesses from several sources.

The well-established Hope-Estancia Center, 65 miles from Albuquerque, provides care to a representative cross section of families. It provides more preventive services and family-centered care than the other sites. The FNP at Hope continues to follow a large number of patients with chronic disease, many of whom have been coming to the FNP for years. They are periodically referred for consultation to Albuquerque specialists, who review their medical status and send the patients back to Hope for followup by the FNP.

At Pecos, 85 miles from Albuquerque, the FNP, although experienced, had to face the problem of building a practice; there, the practice included more pediatrics than at other sites. The Pecos site was backed up by Santa Fe, where primary care providers also are in short supply. The Pecos Clinic which opened in August 1974, was staffed by a family nurse practitioner whose first visits were for school and athletic physicals, for immunizations for children and TB tests for teachers, and subsequently became involved with the throat culture program and treatment for strep. The practice has always served both children and adults. A larger number of emergency patients seek care at the Pecos Clinic, located in a heavily traveled tourist area at the edge of the Pecos Wilderness. Because the clinic was in its first year, the volume of chronic disease patients was relatively small; most of the patients were new patients with acute illnesses.

The distribution of patient revenue by procedure is described in Table 11:3. The MD clinic at Bernalillo derives most of its revenue from office visits for episodic treatment of illness. Although the clinic has X-ray and laboratory equipment, these facilities are used less than at the other two sites. Either the MD does not request their use or the nurse at the clinic does not feel comfortable performing the tests and has them sent out. Another possibility is that because Bernalillo is relatively close to Albuquerque, it is frequently more convenient to ask patients to go directly to the hospital or laboratory for diagnostic X-rays or studies. New laboratory equipment was added recently and the use of this additional equipment will be studied.

TABLE 11:3

Distribution of Patient Revenue by Procedure, July 1974-July 1975

	BERNALILLO MD	HOPE-ESTANCIA FNP	PECOS FNP
TOTAL REVENUE	**$55,000**	**$39,600**	**$25,200**
Procedure			
Office visits	77%	56%	53%
Emergency room	2%	3%	4%
Medical supplies	1%	2%	1%
Medications	7%	12%	23%
Laboratory	8%	18%	13%
X-ray	4%	8%	—
Clinical procedures	1%	1%	2%
Other medical services	—	—	4%
TOTALS	100%	100%	100%

The Estancia clinic, because of its large volume of chronic disease patients, performs many laboratory studies relevant to patient management. Many tests are sent to one of the backup hospital laboratories by bus, as are the X-rays to be interpreted. The office fee for the FNP ($6.00) is less than the physician fee ($8.00); hence, the percentage of office revenue related to total revenue is smaller. The Hope Medical Center bills efficiently as a result of the emphasis on charging for services rendered.

The Pecos Clinic, unlike Bernalillo and Hope, is located in a community with no pharmacy. Through a relationship with a community pharmacy in Santa Fe, the clinic dispenses prepackaged medications. The Pecos facility, which derives more income from walk-in visits, is crowded, comprising only 800 square feet, and has no X-ray equipment on site.

The revenue by source of payment for each site is compared in Table 11:4. New Mexico is a poor state and Medicaid reimburses on a fee-for-service basis for public assistance beneficiaries. None of the sites has any publicly funded, health care centers for poor people. To further aggravate the situation, Medicare does not reimburse for services rendered by an FNP.

Both Hope and Pecos are participating in the Social Security Administration study on experimental reimbursement under Medicare, Part B, as authorized in the 1972 Social Security Administration Amendments. The CHS has sought Medicare reimbursement for FNP services since 1969. At

TABLE 11:4

Clinic Revenue by Source of Payment, July 1974-July 1975

	BERNALILLO MD	HOPE-ESTANCIA FNP	PECOS FNP
TOTAL REVENUE	$55,000	$39,600	$25,200
Medicaid	18%	12%	12%
Medicare	11%	3%*	7%*
Medicare/Medicaid	2%	3%	2%
Mastercare	—	—	—
Insurance	14%	17%	3%
Insurance/Self-Pay	3%	8%	—
Self-pay	51%	55%	75%
Charity	—	—	—
Other	1%	2%	1%
TOTALS	100%	100%	100%

*Self-Pay—Medicare does not reimburse FNP services.

Pecos, 75 percent of the patients are self-pay, and the bill collections are good in spite of the poor patient population. Medicaid beneficiaries comprise from 12 to 18 percent of the visits.

At Bernalillo, which is closer to the Albuquerque labor market, some families have good insurance for outpatient care. Bernalillo also serves an older patient population which qualifies for Medicare benefits; but Pecos and Hope lose Medicare patients to specialists because Medicare does not cover FNP services. Even though Hope is located 65 miles from Albuquerque, some area residents commute to Albuquerque to work. They carry group insurance, as do local employees of adjacent school districts. Hope serves a broad socioeconomic cross-section—from local ranchers and businessmen to migrants. However, at all sites, at least 50 percent of the patients pay out-of-pocket. New Mexico is a state with a high proportion of families who are working poor with no insurance (or, at best, some hospital insurance) and no access or income to afford a group insurance policy. The working poor in rural areas, however, still pay their medical bills; the closer to Albuquerque, the more difficult is the collection of overdue bills and the more transient the patient. In rural areas, the clinic staff know the patients, and the patients know that the continued availability of services is dependent on payment. Many small hospitals in New Mexico have closed; most people live a long distance from medical care; and access to primary care has become an important community concern.

COSTS OF OPERATING A RURAL CARE PRACTICE

The CHS clinics in these rural areas are small operations staffed by three people—the primary care practitioner (MD or FNP), a clinical assistant and a clerical assistant. Accounts receivable are managed on site under central supervision. A clinic coordinator manages all sites from Albuquerque. Payroll, accounts payable, accounting, legal, personnel, and other business and administrative functions are provided centrally. The allocation of central support expense amounts to $6,000 per year per clinic.

Table 11:5 shows that the operating expenses, in the period studied, for an MD clinic were about $68,000, and for an FNP clinic, under $50,000 per year, with variations in overhead expense. Hope pays little rent, as the facility is owned by a local board and leased to CHS at a nominal yearly rental. However, Hope has an expensive but essential telephone line to Albuquerque, since it permits the site to call physician supervisors, backup hospitals and central staff.

Bernalillo's modern medical facility is relatively expensive, as is insurance for physician professional liability; at Pecos the cramped 8,000 square feet space is inexpensive to rent. The CHS philosophy has been to put resources into services rather than buildings. Maintaining a large

TABLE 11:5

Operating Expenses—Rural Solo Practice Primary Care Clinics, July 1974-July 1975

	BERNALILLO MD	HOPE-ESTANCIA FNP	PECOS FNP
Salaries			
Primary Care Provider	30,000	14,000	13,500
Clinical Assistant	8,400	6,000	5,000
Clerical Assistant	4,800	6,000	5,000
Janitor	1,000	1,000	1,000
Payroll taxes and employee benefits	2,756	1,618	2,052
Staff development and training	—	31	165
Medication supplies	671	284	3,402
Medical supplies	2,608	2,153	2,103
Laboratory supplies	247	300	713
X-ray supplies	965	300	—
Office supples	2,638	1,970	2,239
Janitorial supplies	97	141	85
Minor equipment and supplies	167	121	235
Professional fees—doctors	1,120	900	5,055
Legal	780	775	772
Outside Laboratory	—	—	1,145
Equipment rental	—	—	42
Freight out	—	540	22
Books and health education materials	157	915	633
Repairs and maintenance	320	46	258
Utilities	1,023	1,031	665
Telephone	1,189	2,397	788
Insurance	1,268	466	643
Public Relations	—	—	—
Travel	20	1,004	511
Dues, fees and registration	163	248	193
Miscellaneous expense	450	170	194
Rent expense	5,700	100	1,200
Start-up costs	—	—	—
Depreciation	1,300	1,512	892
Total direct expenses	$67,839	$44,022	$48,507
Central Supportive Expenses			
Administration			
Accounting			
Personnel and Payroll	6,000	6,000	6,000
Total expenses	$73,839	$50,022	$54,507

pharmacy inventory is expensive, however. Also, at Pecos, the nurse practitioner, in his first year in a rural solo practice setting, felt strongly that part-time on-site physician services were required, and $5,000 was spent for physicians to go to the clinic and work with the FNP and review medical charts, among other activities. The amount of physician involvement that would be required by the FNPs in the new Pecos clinic was badly underestimated and should have been budgeted. The FNP at Hope required little on-site physician involvement in her sixth year of practice, but she did have large amounts of MD involvement on-site in the early years. Also, the MD supervisors from Santa Fe and the FNP in Pecos did not have the same degree of mutual understanding of the role of a nurse practitioner or the same level of professional working relationship as existed at Hope. The Pecos Clinic has been reorganized subsequently and in 1975 was staffed by a Primary Care Physician Assistant supervised by one physician.

The first FNP at Pecos experienced a heavy work load, personal problems in adjusting to rural living and dissatisfaction with solo practice because of the lack of leisure time or relief from after-hours calls. He had to train the office staff, set up the records and learn to bill on a fee-for-service basis. It was a difficult and very busy first year. The unanticipated heavy utilization of clinic services swamped operations and several administrative problems never received prompt and early attention.

SUMMARY AND CONCLUSIONS

Can rural practices be operated effectively and efficiently so as to be self-sustaining in sparsely populated areas with less than 5,000 people? As indicated in Table 11:6, a break-even point for the physician clinic

TABLE 11:6

Comparative Costs of Primary Care Clinics, July 1974-July 1975

	BERNALILLO MD	HOPE-ESTANCIA FNP	PECOS FNP
Direct Expenses/Year	$67,839	$44,022	$48,507
Actual Average Revenue/Visit	$11	$11	$9
Patient Visits Required/Year to Cover Direct Expenses	6,167	4,002	5,389
Patient Visits Required/Day (4.5 Days/Week) to Cover Direct Expenses	26	17	23
Actual Patient Visits	5,000	3,600	2,800
Deficit	($12,839)	($4,422)	($23,307)

was 6,167 visits for the period under study. At Hope, 4,000 visits were needed, and at Pecos, 5,400 visits to sustain direct operations. At Pecos, average revenue was lower because of a large volume of brief visits in pediatrics. Revenue at Bernalillo should have been higher, but lack of laboratory and X-ray revenue resulted in a lower average revenue per visit. The physician clinic lost more money than did the FNP clinic. The FNP clinic is close to breaking even, substantiating the assumption that the FNP model is a cost-effective way of providing quality care to rural communities. The loss on the physician operation reinforces the reluctance of private physicians to locate in solo practice and to remain in poor, sparsely populated, low-income areas. It is even difficult to recruit physicians for a site 20 miles outside of Albuquerque.

CHS activities at present are focusing on improved productivity and an increase in fees at each site. Each clinic will be asked to set its own productivity goals and will be monitored for performance. The number of patient visits required to sustain operation is realizable; and fees, even after an increase from $8 to $10 per visit, will still be very reasonable. It has been difficult for FNPs to adjust to a fee-for-service practice and, as nurses, to charge for time spent with patients.

In terms of the future of rural solo practice, several major issues remain to be resolved:

1. Are rural solo practice settings, although financially viable, acceptable professionally to most nurse practitioners, physician's assistants, or physicians?

2. Should rural communities make do with 50 hours per week of patient service? It is virtually impossible to find coverage if the solo practitioner gets sick, goes on vacation or away for continuing education.

3. If small health care teams, such as a full-time nurse practitioner and a full-time physician are required to meet the professional requirements for a practice setting and to provide 24-hour-a-day, 7-day-a-week coverage, without undue provider burden in rural areas, who is to subsidize provision of such care for communities which financially cannot support such teams?

4. How can comprehensive and preventive services be made available in rural areas where the residents barely can afford treatment for acute illness or emergency care?

In order to meet the professional needs of the practitioner, the needs of the community for better 7-day-a-week, 24-hour-a-day coverage, and the growing demand for ambulatory care visits and preventive services in the next few years, placement of a National Health Services Corps physician has been requested at each site, so that each of these three sites will have a team of two providers. The addition of a physician will solve significantly the problem of Medicare reimbursement, and the presence of the physician should enable CHS to raise fees to a more realistic level and to attract those patients seeking physician care elsewhere. The addition of a physician at the FNP sites also will provide continuity of patient care for those patients requiring hospital admission. The physician supervisors will continue to serve as specialty consultants and are encouraging the FNPs to move in new directions. At one time or another, more than 25 private physicians have served as unpaid physician supervisors for the FNP sites. The role of FNPs in both urban and rural areas is well established and accepted in New Mexico. The CHS looks forward to having sites with both physicians and nurse practitioners and will keep a careful accounting of the financial viability of such sites for a later report.

The concept of the need for the nurse practitioner to relate the content of a patient visit to reimbursement for the specific services she renders may be one of the most significant issues highlighted by the CHS experience.

THE THREE SITES REVISITED

An update on the development of these three clinics in August 1976 indicated that several changes had occurred. CHS still is the managing organization for the Hope Medical Center, and a National Health Service Corps physician has been added to the staff. The operation of the Bernalillo clinic was turned over to the Bernalillo Development Corporation, a community agency, in August 1976. A National Health Service Corps physician has also been recruited for this site. The Physician's Assistant who had been practicing in the Pecos clinic left, and a young physician from the area has been recruited. The Pecos Village Council has taken over management of the clinic and is raising funds for a new building.

Patient volume in all three sites has increased, undoubtedly a response to the addition of physicians to all three sites. The gradual take-over of the management of two of the clinics by the respective local communities may result in an increased community commitment in the forms of increased patient volume and a potentially sounder economic base for the clinics.

The evolution of the three clinics, briefly highlighted here, serves as an example of the vicissitudes of establishing optimal staffing patterns in the provision of primary health care in rural areas. The impact of federally sponsored health professionals in these clinics, coupled with anticipated changes in reimbursement policies which can reflect accurately the contribution of nurse practitioners, needs to be examined in order to deal seriously with the financial problems of providing rural health care.

EXHIBIT 11:1

SOUTHWEST HEALTH CARE CORPORATION **PRESBYTERIAN HOSPITAL CENTER/ST. JOSEPH HOSPITAL**

I.
1) CLINIC ENCOUNTER NUMBER B 5269   2) PATIENT S NAME
3) CLINIC: HMC   BMC   PVMC
             TCMC   OTHER   4) TOWN OF RESIDENCE

                                                            PATIENT
5) DATE   6 AGE   7) SEX   8) I D NO

II. 9) SOURCE OF PAYMENT   10) PATIENT STATUS   12 TIME OF DAY
       MEDICAID   NEW   MORNING
       MEDICARE   ESTABLISHED   AFTERNOON
       INSURANCE   NIGHT
       SELF-PAY   11) APPOINTMENT STATUS   13 CLINIC PROVIDER
       CHARITY   APOINTMENT   N P   OTHER
       OTHER   WALK-IN   M D   NONE

14) SITE OF ENCOUNTER   15) TYPE OF ENCOUNTER
       CLINIC   EPISODIC ILLNESS
       HOSPITAL   SYSTEM INITIATED FOLLOW-UP CARE   IMMUNIZATIONS ONLY
       HOME   EMERGENCY   FAMILY PLANNING
                                    CHRONIC DISEASE MANAGEMENT   MENTAL HEALTH CARE
                                    SPECIALTY CONSULTATION   PHYSICAL EXAMINATIONS
                                    OTHER MEDIAL SPEC FY   SCHOOL EMPLOYMENT NsURANCE
                                    PRENATAL   OTHER PREVENTIVE
                                    POST PARTUM   HEALTH GUIDANCE
                                    WELL-BABY   ALL OTHER CARE

III. 16 SERVICES & PROCEDURES PROVIDED

OFFICE VISITS	FEE	LABORATORY	FEE	EMERGENCY ROOM	FEE
		HCT	——		
MINIMAL SERVICE	——	WBC	——	MINIMAL SERVICE	——
BRIEF EXAM	——	UA WHITE	——	BRIEF	——
LIMITED EXAM	——	UA LABST x	——	LIMITED	——
COMPREHENSIVE EXAM	——	URINE CULTURE	——	INTERMEDIATE	——
		THROAT CULTURE	——	EXTENDED	——
		BLOOD SUGAR EXTRUST X	——		
		COLLECTION & HANDLING			
		FOR OUTY H AB			
HOSPITAL VISIT	FEE		——	**X-RAY**	FEE
INPATIENT	——				——
ER	——	**MEDICATION**	FEE		——
HOME VISIT	FEE	THERAPEUTIC INJECTIONS			
		OF MEDICATIONS SEE FY		**ECG**	FEE
	——		——		——
OTHER	FEE	IMMUNIZATIONS			——
	——				
	——	THERAPEUTIC INJECTIONS		**MED/SUR SUPPLIES**	FEE
	——	AN BO CS			——
	——	OTHER DRUGS			——

IV. 17) EXTERNAL REFERRALS/SERVICES ORDERED
       ECG TO
       X-RAY TO
       PHYSICIAN CONSULTATION TO
       HOSPITALIZATION TO
       LAB TESTS TO
       OTHER TO
       HOSPITAL ER TO
       PRESCRIPTION WRITTEN FOR

Chapter 12

Physician Supervision of PAs: How Much is Enough? And What Does it Cost?

Jane Cassels Record, Robert H. Blomquist, Benjamin D. Berger and Joan E. O'Bannon

The Kaiser Health Plan in the metropolitan area of Portland, Oregon has about 200,000 members, more than 18 percent of the area's total population. Comprehensive, prepaid health care is provided in the system's two hospitals and in six outlying clinics, one of which is in Vancouver, Washington. Medical services are under the direction of a physician partnership legally titled The Permanente Clinic. The partnership contracts with the Health Plan to provide services for Health Plan members at a negotiated capitation rate. As of spring 1976 there were 151 partners, plus 37 physician employees of the partnership who will be eligible for membership after two years of employment. The 188 physicians represent most of the medical specialties.

Twelve PAs presently practice in the system—three in surgery, three in orthopedics, one in pathology, and five in medicine. Although physicians determine PA numbers and modes of practice, the PAs are employees of the Health Plan rather than of the partnership. This chapter is concerned only with the five Medical PAs, the first of whom entered the Department of Medicine in September 1970, as the first PA employed anywhere in the system. The last Medical PA was added in 1974. All five are graduates of the Duke University PA program.

The first PA was employed at a salary of $13,000 plus fringe benefits of approximately $2,288—a total of $15,288. The present basic salary range (without fringes) is $16,800 to $21,000 in six annual steps. In 1975, salary and fringe benefits for the five Medical PAs averaged $19,265. The PAs get three weeks of vacation (four weeks after three years tenure) and one week of educational leave. (Physician partners get four and two weeks, respectively, and physician employees three and one.)

Although the PA's productivity, measured per clinic day or hour, compares favorably with that of the MD in handling noncomplex outpatient services, the PA's work week is only 33.5 hours, in contrast to an estimated 52.7 hours for the MD.[1] The PA's work week is shaped by clinic hours, because system policy confines the Medical PA to outpatient services, and the basic clinic day is between six and six-and-a-half hours. About 93.5 percent of the PAs' work week is spent in the regular clinic and another 4 percent in the same kind of primary-care services at the hospital on Sundays. The remaining 2.5 percent of their work hours are taken up by meetings and by travel time between system facilities. The meetings, except for department or general staff conferences, relate largely to PA business rather than to matters of more general system policy.

Adult primary medical care is provided in the Department of Medicine by 49 internists, four general practitioners, the five PAs, and five primary care nurse practitioners, added recently, who do health-appraisal exams. Two family practitioners spend about half time on adult medicine but are now considered a separate administrative unit.

Staff at the Kaiser Foundation Health Services Research Center have collected data on the PA program since its inception.[2] The study from which this chapter issues was begun in July 1974, after the Project was funded by a Health Manpower Education Initiative Award (HMEIA) from the Bureau of Health Resources Development within the Department of Health, Education, and Welfare. Although the primary purpose of the proposed research was to assess the cost effectiveness of PAs,[3] an important secondary purpose was to analyze changes in PA policies and practices during the system's first five years of experience with PAs.

In 1970, PAs were new not only to Kaiser-Permanente but to the rest of the medical-care world as well. Policy had to be developed with respect to the kind of supervision PAs would have, the services PAs would provide, the access of PAs to system resources, the relation of PAs to other staff and the manner of presenting PAs to patients. In this chapter, physician supervision—the most important PA issue at Kaiser-Permanente—is examined with respect to evolving policies and costs.

THE PHYSICIAN'S SUPERVISORY FUNCTION

One of the most elusive goals associated with PA programs is the definition and effectuation of a satisfactory supervisory arrangement—satisfactory in the sense that it adequately guards the consumer and public interests in quality maintenance, protects the employer from an elevated malpractice risk, permits the PA to grow in professional competence and avoids a waste of scarce physician (and PA) resources in over-supervision.

Supervision policy must comprehend many questions:

How many PAs may a physician supervise? Should a PA have a regular supervisor, as opposed to a rotation of physicians? Should the supervisor be physically proximate and immediately available? In a system employing more than one PA, should supervisory policy be centralized or left largely to the individual supervisor?

Should the supervising physician see every PA patient? Should the supervisor review each chart before the patient leaves the clinic? If not, should the charts be reviewed later in that same day? Should every chart be reviewed or is sampling adequate?

Should PAs be permitted to prescribe independently, except for narcotics and other drugs restricted by law to physicians? Or should PAs be permitted to prescribe only within a physician-determined protocol, where prescribing can be routinized? Or should all PA prescriptions require physician countersignature?

Should PAs be permitted to order laboratory tests and X-rays without clearing with the supervisor? Should PAs make referrals to specialists in other departments or to subspecialists within the Department of Medicine without the supervisor's approval?

Should PAs practice within formalized diagnostic and treatment protocols, such as algorithms, or is it sufficient to develop an informal, modal interaction between PA and supervisor? When should a PA consult his supervisor? Should PA initiative govern here or should the consultation decision be more structured?

How much physician time should be allotted for supervision? What compensatory time arrangement should be made?

Answers to some of these questions are dictated by law. The Washington and Oregon PA laws were passed in the second year of the PA program at Kaiser-Permanente. The Washington law and administrative regulations have been somewhat more permissive than their Oregon counterparts, largely on the issue of physician supervision.

Both states allow an MD to supervise only one PA but the states differ with respect to physical proximity of the supervisor. In Washington, PAs can practice in satellite clinics, supervised from another locality. The Oregon bill originally contained a statement that the monitoring physician need not be personally present, but that sentence was deleted by amendment from the floor. Although the resulting law does not stipulate immediate supervision, the State Board of Medical Examiners, which administers the law, has required quick physical access to the supervisor. The K-P system has followed that criterion even in its Vancouver clinic.

In all four clinics (including Vancouver) where PAs practice, each PA has a regularly assigned supervisor, who monitors the PA except when the supervisor is off duty, in which case a substitute MD is designated. In one clinic, where the PA has an essentially walk-in practice, whichever physician is on walk-in duty for the day assists the regular supervisor in prescription signatures and chart review.

Although the Washington law did not require physician chart review until 1974—and then the stipulation was merely that the review be done at least once a week, when the supervisor must be present in the PA's place of practice—the K-P physician supervising the first PA at Vancouver was asked by the system to review and countersign all PA charts by the end of the clinic day. The first PAs in Oregon clinics were much more restricted, largely because of specific legal constraints or uncertainties. Physician monitors were asked to discuss each patient with the PA before the patient left the clinic, to reexamine the patient where necessary or advisable, and to sign patient charts. No patient was to be seen by a PA three times in the same illness episode without being seen also by a physician. About a fifth of all persons seen by a PA were also examined by an MD under these various rules. In the Oregon clinics, the supervisory MDs were asked also to sign all prescriptions; and PAs were not to order lab or X-ray services, or make referrals to specialists, or make a diagnosis, without conferring with the supervisor.

As the system gained confidence in the PAs and as the legal environment was relaxed somewhat, the K-P restrictions were softened. The Oregon supervisors no longer review charts routinely while the patient is still present, although until quite recently the PA or his/her nurse took prescriptions to the supervisor to be signed while the patient waited. Now the Board of Examiners has ruled that an Oregon PA can phone in or write a prescription without physician signature. On the other side of the Columbia River, the Washington Board already had reversed itself from the opposite direction. Until 1974 it had not required a physician signature for drug orders; since that time, countersigning by an MD has been necessary.

After observing the conservative use of lab and X-ray services by PAs during the first years, physicians in all clinics receded from the requirement that PAs secure an MD signature for such orders. The referral policy also changed. Initially, the chart carried a note saying that the supervisor had approved the referral. The first charts that reached some specialists without such a note evoked complaints, particularly from some of the ophthalmologists, urologists, and ear-nose-and-throat physicians, but the resistance soon subsided.

The PAs have not used formalized schemata for diagnosis and treatment; the system has depended, rather, upon close interaction between the PAs and their supervisors. Perhaps the most important kind of knowledge that PAs have—the most important kind of judgment that they exercise—concerns *when to consult the physician.* In the K-P system the consultation decision is primarily the PA's initiative. How does one objectify the decision? Can one objectify the decision?

There is substantial variance among the PAs in frequency of consultation. Data from a 1974-75 clinical observation show that the 5 PAs consult their supervisors, on the average, in about 12 percent of the office visits but the individual rates differ: 5 percent, 6 percent, 12 percent, 15 percent, and 20 percent. The differential might be attributed to many variables: personality, case load, case mix, type of visit (walk-in versus appointment), tenure, regularity of supervision and so on. The only objective factor which seems to correlate reasonably well in the observation data is physical distance between supervisor and supervisee. Adjoining offices appear to promote consultation, different corridors to discourage it. For example, the PA who consults most frequently on the whole has a marked drop in consultations when he and his supervisor, who normally have adjacent offices, occasionally move to separate quarters for the day.

On the assumption that the answer to the consultation question must be less simple than mere physical arrangements, it was decided to go to the medical charts themselves to seek clues. Which morbidities prompt consultation? Unfortunately, the answer is not neat. The observation data showed that for a substantial number of office visits (OVs) with the same presenting morbidity, one PA might consult and another not consult; indeed, the same PA sometimes consulted and sometimes did not.

From the observation printouts, a mixed set of morbidities was selected. An attempt was made to identify variables, other than the morbidity itself, which might affect whether or not to consult. Eight variables were chosen: the particular PA (for interpersonal variation), the number of associated morbidities, the presence or absence of a chronic disease, whether the chart was available at the time of the visit (sometimes for walk-ins there is not enough time to retrieve the chart), the age and sex of the patient, whether the visit was initial or follow-up, and whether it was a walk-in or a scheduled appointment. Information on these variables already was available for each OV observed.

Upper respiratory infection (URI) had the largest absolute number of consultations: after all, it is a very frequent morbidity. For comparison with the nine URI consultations, 23 URI visits for which there was no consultation were selected, to match the nine consultation visits as closely as possible with respect to the eight variables described above.

Seven of the nine charts where consultation had occurred were located. In four cases "the consultation" appeared to be only for an MD signature on a prescription.[4] In the other three, physical conditions—e.g., a heart murmur—discovered by the PA during the examination caused the PA to confer with the supervisor. In none of the three instances was the reason for the consultation "triagable"—that is, identifiable at the triage level as requiring a physician opinion.

With respect to the 23 URI visits handled by a PA alone, without consultation, it was the opinion of the medical review team that the chart revealed no reason for consultation. In 17 cases where MDs handled URI visits alone—with cases chosen to match the consultation and "PA-alone" OVs in regard to the eight variables insofar as matching was possible—the medical team saw nothing in the chart which a PA could not have handled.

A similar approach was made to consultation for six other morbidity categories: synovitis, strep throat, gonorrhea, abdominal pain, bronchitis and physical exam. Here again, all consultation charts, plus matching charts for "PA-alone" and "MD-alone" visits, were reviewed. The numbers were smaller, but the pattern of findings was similar. In the case of synovitis, for example, there were two consultations about the appropriateness of an injection, one about an abnormal physical finding, and one to decide whether the patient should see a surgeon. For two physical exams the PA had to get the MD's signature on a form, and for a third there was an abnormal physical finding. In two cases of gonorrhea the PA was uncertain about the diagnosis, and in a third he wished to consult about a rash. In the one consultation about abdominal pain, the PA wanted an opinion about a hernia. The only consultations about bronchitis had to do with the prescription of antibiotics.

The chart-review results may be summarized as follows: (1) None of the eight variables listed as possible determinants of consultation decisions appears to be particularly useful, alone or in combination, in predicting consultation; so it probably would not be helpful to try to employ those variables as triage guides.[5] (2) Consultation appears to be prompted primarily by factors discovered by the PA during the examination. (3) The PAs seem to practice conservatively in that the medical-team reviewers in some cases found consultations which probably were not necessary for quality assurance. (4) Of the 55 OVs handled by PAs alone, there was only one instance in which the medical team thought the PA probably should have consulted the supervisor. (5) With few exceptions, the cases handled by MDs could have been handled by PAs; but the morbidities under scrutiny here are, of course, within the PA competence range.[6] These findings seem to support, again, a policy of general rather than detailed instructions to triage personnel, with heavy reliance upon selecting adequately trained PAs and assigning them to competent, responsible supervisors.

The foregoing paragraphs describe an attempt to compare consultation and nonconsultation OVs within specific morbidity categories, to try to determine why a PA might consult his supervisor for one OV and not for another OV even though the two OVs were in the same illness category. Eighty-three OVs recorded by the observers but not included in the above analysis also had a specific physician input. Because they were scattered so thinly over so many morbidities it was not practicable to subject them to the kind of analysis described above. Instead, they were grouped without reference to morbidity. Chart analysis showed that 24 of the 83 OVs designated as "consultation visits" in the observation entailed only a physician signature on a form; 7 others required only the counter-signing of a prescription. Of the 52 remaining, 6 consultations resulted from a need for advice about referring the patient to a specialist, 26 from physical findings during the examination, and 3 from lab test findings. In 9 OVs the PA was unsure of the diagnosis, and in 8 the PA sought advice on the best treatment to order. There was some overlap of reasons. Of the 59 OVs, (not counting the 24 form-signature instances) only 7 were identifiable as consultation-requisite visits at the triage level.

COST OF PHYSICIAN SUPERVISION

Yet another aspect of supervision remains to be discussed; namely, the time allotment. What an adequate supervisory arrangement costs the system with respect to how physicians would otherwise use the time spent in supervision is difficult to measure, partly because supervision takes many forms and because supervisory events are dispersed irregularly through the clinic day. The observation of 1974-75 recorded the time spent by the MD in examining the PA's patient, in discussing specific cases with the PA, in signing prescriptions, and even in signing charts where the act was visible; but most of the supervisory activities were not so discretely measurable. Charts typically are reviewed in batches at ad hoc periods during the day. General instruction or education of the PA also occurs irregularly and, here also, mostly out of observable range.

The measurable—timeable—supervisory activities averaged about an hour per week. How much should be allowed for other duties? For the two Vancouver PAs and two of the Oregon PAs who practice similarly, the supervisors have their appointment schedules lightened by one hour per day or five hours per week.[7]

If one hour is spent in consultation on specific OVs, that leaves four hours for general supervision each week. In the cost-effectiveness study it was discovered that in most cases the minutes spent by an MD in consultation with a PA on a specific OV were about the same as the minutes spent by the MD on that kind of OV when the MD handled it alone; in other words, the OV was more costly when handled by the PA and MD jointly than if handled exclusively by the MD, but the *extra* cost is in PA, not MD, minutes spent. Because of this extra cost, it theoretically would be better to triage such cases directly to the physician; hence the significance of the chart-review results which suggest that in most instances the reason for consultation cannot be identified at the triage level.

The other four hours per week, allotted by the system for general supervision of the PA, are properly viewed as "physician costs" of employing a PA. These four hours annualized constitute 7.8 percent of a physician's work year. In other words, it takes 7.8 percent of a physician to provide general supervision for a PA, and 7.8 percent of $53,593— what it cost the system in basic income and fringe benefits for the average MD in the Department in 1975—is nearly $4,200, which may be defined as the monetized general-supervision cost per PA per year.[8]

But is the four-hour estimate of general supervision accurate? Supervising physicians quizzed in 1975 said that it probably was. Does supervisory time affect physician productivity in office visits handled for their own patients? Daily average OVs for supervising and nonsupervising physicians for the first 6 months of 1975 were reviewed, and it was found that the supervisory group was well above the average (Table 12:1).

The five regular PA supervisors are indicated by the letters A through E in the Table. In three cases the PA and supervisor had the same day off and therefore worked together virtually all of the clinic hours. In the fourth case the PA had a substitute physician supervisor one or two days per week. In the fifth case the PA was monitored by rotating walk-in physicians on four days per week, although his designated supervisor was responsible for general supervision. The supervisors are not identified by letter in the above sentences because that information would also reveal individual productivity rates.

The nonsupervisory MDs varied somewhat in number over the months in response to vacation time and educational leave. It should be pointed out that many of them are substitute PA supervisors on occasion, sometimes as often as one day a week. Even with that and other contingencies taken into account, however, the regular supervisors seem clearly to be performing at a relatively high productivity level in daily output of OVs, despite their supervisory duties, which include admission and care of PA

TABLE 12:1

Daily Average Office Visits for Supervisory and Nonsupervisory Physicians

Month in 1975	Average Office Visits Per Day	Nonsupervisory MDs		Supervisors' Distribution
		%	Cum. %	
January	0-14.9	5.4	5.4	
	15-18.9	21.3	26.8	
	19-22.9	46.4	73.2	A, B
	23-26.9	23.2	96.4	C, D
	27 and over	3.6	100.0	E
February	0-14.9	3.6	3.6	
	15-18.9	15.8	19.4	
	19-22.9	31.6	51.0	A, B
	23-26.9	36.8	87.8	D
	27 and over	12.2	100.0	E, C
March	0-14.9	1.8	1.8	
	15-18.9	23.1	24.9	
	19-22.9	44.7	69.6	B
	23-26.9	25.0	94.6	A, D, C
	27 and over	5.4	100.0	E
April	0-14.9	0.0	0.0	
	15-18.9	21.2	21.2	
	19-22.9	48.1	69.3	B
	23-26.9	25.0	94.3	A, D, C
	27 and over	5.7	100.0	E
May	0-14.9	2.0	2.0	
	15-18.9	24.0	26.0	
	19-22.9	56.0	82.0	B, A
	23-26.9	10.0	92.0	D, E
	27 and over	8.0	100.0	C
June	0-14.9	0.0	0.0	
	15-18.9	21.3	21.3	
	19-22.9	63.9	85.2	A, B, C
	23-26.9	10.6	95.8	D, E
	27 and over	4.2	100.0	

patients who have to be hospitalized, because the PAs provide no inpatient services.

Several conjectures are suggested by the comparative figures. First, the time spent in supervision may be less than the estimated five hours. The walk-in load for the clinic is almost always heavy, and MDs when they are free help with walk-ins. Because the supervisor keeps no log, he would not know exactly how much of the allotted supervision time is being filled up with walk-ins. If there were a clear pattern of supervisors' clinic hours protracting beyond those of nonsupervisors, the elongation might suggest that supervisory duties—in toto or in part—are an "add-on" rather than a substitute for nonsupervisory duties, and therefore no physician cost is incurred in employing a PA. There is no evidence, however, of a disparity in clinic hours. Of course, even if there were, one might conjecture that if there were no PA to supervise, that same physician would stay long hours to see patients of his own.

Can it be that there is a nonconspicuous selective factor in the recruitment of supervisors? Are there personality traits—energy, ability to organize time, capacity for making a patient feel fully listened·to and served in less face-to-face time than it takes other physicians—which permit the supervisor to give an hour a day to the PA and still see enough patients to keep his daily OV average relatively high? Data presently available do not permit a confident answer to these questions, but it should be stated that personality traits such as those described above are part of the overall criteria for selecting PA supervisors in the system.

CONCLUSION

In a large organization it would not be feasible, even if it were desirable, to control supervision policy from the administrative center except in terms of general principles. The PA-supervisor relationship is certain to vary from team to team, and the best method to assure quality and legality appears to be to recruit PAs carefully, with respect to competence and attitude, and to place them under competent, responsible physician supervision.

Adequate supervision is perhaps the most challenging aspect of a satisfactory PA policy, and the issue of "when to consult" is probably the key question. The consultation decision in the final analysis must be placed in PA hands. Because that is true, the single most important test of the PA's competence is his ability to judge where his competence ends. Chart review and other probes on this issue produced data which suggest that, with respect to this criterion, PAs in the K-P system tend to err on the side of restraint rather than overconfidence.

A finding from the chart review—that there is no way of identifying in advance which OVs triaged to PAs will result in a consultation with the physician supervisor—has important cost implications because, as cost data from the Health Manpower Education Initiative Awards (HMEIA) study showed, it would be less costly for the physician to handle most of those OVs alone. The clear-cut cost-effectiveness of PAs in OVs where they do not have to consult with their supervisors is thus offset to some extent by expensive consultations which typically are not predictable and therefore preventable at the triage level. The consultation OVs fortunately are only 12 percent or less of the total PA case load.

Consultation has to do with specific, observable physician inputs into PA services. But there is another kind of supervisory cost not related to particular OVs; namely, the consumption of physician time in general supervisory activities such as routine chart review, instruction, taking care of the PA's patients in hospital, and so on. The best way of calculating that cost is as a "physician fraction," a percentage of a doctor year, although it is quite difficult to measure the time cost with precision. The estimate made for the K-P system is about 8 percent, although there is some evidence that that figure overstates the supervisory cost of using PAs.

Notes

1. The HMEIA Report which contains a detailed description of the method of computation with a breakdown of hours spent in various activities is available on request from the authors.

2. The Center staff also has studied nurse practitioners in Obstetrics-Gynecology and Pediatrics. See J. C. Record and H. R. Cohen, "The Introduction of Midwifery in a Prepaid Group Practice," *American Journal of Public Health*, 3 (March 1972), 354-360; P. D. Lairson, J. C. Record, and J. C. James, "Physician Assistants at Kaiser: Distinctive Patterns of Practice," *Inquiry*, 3 (September 1974), 207-219; and J. C. Record, and M. R. Greenlick, "New Health Professionals and Physician Role: An Hypothesis from Kaiser Experience," *Public Health Reports*, 90, 3 (May-June 1975), 241-247.

3. Preliminary findings are contained in J. C. Record, J.E. O'Bannon, P. D. Lairson, and J. P. Mullooly, "Cost Effectiveness of Physician's Assistants: Kaiser-Permanente Experience," a paper presented to the Health Economics Research Organization of the American Economics Association, Dallas, December 1976. A final version is contained in the HMEIA Report.

4. The observers had been told that if a PA or his nurse merely handed the prescription to the MD supervisor without discussion of the case, that event should not be recorded as a consultation because the prescription countersignature is pro forma in most cases. If, however, there was *any* dialogue about the patient, the exchange was to be recorded as a consultation. Apparently many brief exchanges got so recorded, although nothing in the chart indicates the nature of the exchange. To the extent that pro forma countersignatures may have been counted as consultations, the 12% consultation-rate estimate is high.

5. For a statistical analysis of a larger sample, see Appendix F of the HMEIA Report. These eight, plus other variables, proved in some combinations to be predictive of consultation, but translating the predictiveness into triage guides would be difficult.

6. The well-known limitations of the medical chart should be kept in mind here.

7. In the clinic where the supervising MDs typically are on walk-in duty for that day, there is no appointment schedule to lighten. We are assuming that the supervision time—and therefore the foregone medical services of the physicians—are the same for all clinics. (A more intensive study of supervisory time is planned for the early future.)

8. In 1972 it was estimated that the first PA had an OV consultation rate of 20%, and consumed altogether about 300 hours of physician supervision time per year—12-1/2% of an average physician's year calculated at 2400 hours. J.C. Record and P.D. Lairson, "Physician Assistants At Kaiser: The Question of Substitutability," a paper presented at the American Public Health Association's annual meeting, Minneapolis, November, 1972. Incidentally, the PA's supervisor generally takes over the PA's patients who have to be hospitalized, arranging the admission and giving the physical exam required by the system for all new inpatients.

Chapter 13

Problems of PAs and Medex from Their Own Perspective

Elaine S. Bursic

In 1974, the Project on the Economics of Health Manpower initiated a mail survey of 1,792 formally trained Physician's Assistants and Medex across the country to determine their present job status and the factors affecting their employment. The overall response rate for these formally trained practitioners was 75.6 percent or 1,355 respondents of 1,792.[1] Acknowledging that the respondents could provide some interesting and perhaps valuable information, as well as a different perspective on their status, a sheet was attached to the questionnaire, inviting the respondents to comment on the survey or on their profession in general. Of the 1,355 respondents, 11 percent (124) returned their comments. This chapter is based on that very small subsample of 124 responses, which discuss some of the difficulties PAs and Medex reported in securing employment, and problems faced in the execution of their job activities as well as solutions to these problems suggested by the respondents. In summarizing, the author provides her reaction to both the problems and suggested solutions of the respondents in an attempt to determine the crucial issues facing new health practitioners.

PROBLEMS REPORTED BY THE 124 RESPONDENTS TO THE COMMENT SHEET

A large number of PAs and Medex responded to the query with positive, affirmative letters. Nearly 40 (30 percent), although cognizant of the problems of others in their field, seemed genuinely content with their jobs and co-workers. For them, the concept as originally envisioned had succeeded. They held satisfying, well-paying jobs which perfectly suited their training and capabilities. Rapport with colleagues and patients was excellent, cooperation was optimal. Irrespective of their own ideal employment, however, they understood the frustrations of their colleagues and joined them in making suggestions that they hoped would rectify present problems to the benefit of all.

Lack of Knowledge of PA/MEDEX Concept

Most of the 124 respondents commented on what they felt was an "appalling ignorance" of the PA/MEDEX concept among other health professionals, including physicians. In one way or another, almost all the 124 respondents asserted that the implementation of the PA/MEDEX concept could provide more readily available, more efficient and more economical medical care. They regretted that few other than those involved with the training or the study of their professions appreciated the goal or the existence of this new health practitioner.[2]

Twelve (10 percent) of the respondents complained of the reluctance or refusal of nurses, aides and technicians to accept the instructions or suggestions offered by PAs and Medex. They attributed this problem to the fact that their co-workers simply did not know what a PA or Medex was trained to do and wherein his or her authority lay. They also reported similar problems with respect to physicians, especially in hospital or clinic settings where a PA may have contact with several different physicians, some or all of whom may never have worked with PAs before, nor have knowledge of what they can do. One respondent even reported that a physician he encountered was surprised to learn that PAs are trained to give injections and to suture lacerations.

Respondents noted that the general public remains the least informed about PAs and Medex. Most of those who commented on their direct patient experience expressed regret that the public appeared so misinformed, that it conceived of PAs and Medex as a special kind of nurse or a new type of physician, and had little realistic percepton of what their medical role might be. One respondent felt that popular television drama increased the public's confusion with images of the zealous young paramedic who risks life and limb to rescue accident and disaster victims. He contended that this image stays with the patient and does not easily translate to the PA treating a patient in a family physician's office. Educating the public to understand this identity becomes complicated when in fact several component identities are at question. What it is that a "Type A" PA can do that a "Type B" cannot confuses many people including potential employers and co-workers, not to mention the public who generally has less an idea of what specialization entails than does another professional.[3] A possible solution suggested by a half a dozen respondents would involve standardizing training programs with the goal of producing practitioners of equal skill and knowledge who could be more easily absorbed into the existing medical hierarchy and who could be depended upon to execute that role uniformly.

Many PAs and Medex felt legislators, both state and federal, possess considerable influence over the success or failure of their profession. Several comments emphasized the importance of familiarizing legislators at all levels of government with the potential advantage of nationwide utilization of PAs and Medex, and of lobbying for legislation favorable to PAs.

Licensure and Malpractice

Nineteen (15 percent) respondents cited a lack of precise legislation on the status and permissible job activities of PAs and Medex as a deterrent to securing a job in several states. They remarked that potential employers frequently decided against hiring them because of the ambiguous and delicate legal questions of licensure and liability. Two respondents indicated that they had lost their jobs, one in Illinois and the other in South Carolina, due to charges of practicing medicine without a license. Another two in Missouri and one in Montana were severely restricted in their job duties by the statutes of those states. They felt strongly that it was impractical for a private practice, clinic or hospital in these areas to hire a PA or Medex who would be unable to perform the duties for which he or she had the capabilities and training, or whose job might be jeopardized, due to vaguely defined legislation. In reaction to this situation, some respondents unwillingly uprooted themselves and their families to move to areas where favorable legislation permitted them to work in their chosen profession. Others, who preferred not to relocate, worked at jobs they considered stultifying and unfulfilling, with little hope of using all their training. Four chose to leave their profession in favor of another type of employment that would support them. Even the PAs and Medex who told us that they had found reliable, fulfilling jobs realized the problems inherent in restrictive, inadequate, or nonexistent legislation, if for no other reason than the fact that job mobility remains impossible as long as legislation remains inconsistent across the country.

An issue which linked closely with that of licensure and dismayed some practicing PAs and Medex was the lack of malpractice insurance. Eight (6 percent) cited it as an effective deterrent to the employment of PAs and Medex throughout the country, even in those states whose statutes favor the use of a "Physician Extender" and clearly delineate the job activities concurrent with that use. Three respondents reported that some insurance carriers flatly refused to extend coverage to physicians contemplating the addition of a PA or Medex to their practices.

Another alleged that certain carriers penalized physicians by raising the premium cost for coverage or by threatening to discontinue coverage should "anything go wrong." One effect of this action, he suggested, is that hospitals, clinics and particularly physicians, who are already sufficiently alarmed at the rise in malpractice suits, may refrain from hiring PAs, Medex or similar practitioners. Another effect, he warned, could be a rise in prices for medical services resulting from a rise in the price of insurance coverage. The PAs and Medex believed that this problem may be slow to correct itself as it hinges in great part on legislation regarding the liability for medical services delivered by physician extenders.[4] Several others strongly urged quality control as a means of establishing and maintaining a respected reputation in medical and general societies, as well as improving the health care industry. They believed that professional organizations such as the Association of Physician Assistant Programs or the American Academy of Physicians' Assistants could perform this function of quality control through peer evaluation.

Furthermore, eight (6 percent) of the respondents called for the creation of inexpensive, universal malpractice insurance provided by either private or public means. They also strongly urged the establishment of policies amenable to third party reimbursement by both government and private agencies for medical services delivered by PAs and Medex.[5]

Third Party Reimbursement

Third party reimbursers not paying for services rendered by a physician extender seemed to create additional stumbling blocks to the employment of PAs and Medex. Potential employers faced the impractical situation of hiring personnel whom they might be unable to use effectively to expand health care services due to the inability to get reimbursement for some or all of the care delivered by those personnel. Obviously, this hurts not only the employer and the potential employee, but the patient whose only method of payment for services may be third party payment. Five (4 percent) of the respondents lamented the lack of reimbursement which, they asserted, further damaged the notion that the employment of a PA or Medex can increase productivity and/or income of a practice.

Professional Discrimination

Professional discrimination surfaced as an interesting factor which affected the job market. Three respondents discussed it in detail with respect to their personal experiences. One complained of being in situations time and again where a physician would not delegate any sort of medical task to an "assistant" for fear of appearing incompetent to peers. Another cited physicians in New York State who displayed an apparent resentment of PAs and Medex by refusing them hospital privileges. He continued that the situation then arose of physicians who were willing to hire a PA or Medex deciding against it because of peer pressure, or a feeling that an assistant who could not help in the hospital or clinic would not offer much help.[6] Still another respondent lost his job in a small southern community due to harrassment of him and his employer by another physician in the same town who apparently considered the PA/MEDEX concept a threat to his practice and economic security.

Other health professionals, primarily nurses and nurse practitioners, were reported to have displayed similar hostility toward PAs and Medex. Attributable in some cases to uncertainty about the medical role of the PA or Medex, resistance to working with PAs was thought to occur as a conscious effort on the part of some nurses to undermine the PA/MEDEX concept for fear of losing their jobs. The respondents hoped that this type of resentment would not bias physicians and institutions, wishing to avoid unpleasant employee relationships, against employing them. Most who described this situation reported that after a time, the conflict ceased as nurses realized that the PA/Medex and nurse or NP could coexist without threat to one another. Some went on to acknowledge the parallels in training and functions which presently exist between the NP and the PA or Medex.

Possible Surplus of New Health Practitioners

Four (3 percent) respondents, employed and unemployed alike, protested one particular hazard in searching for a job: an apparent surplus of PAs/Medex and NPs in some areas. These four feared that overproduction within these new health professions might be the largest single problem that PAs and Medex will face in the near future. They also feared that mass production might diminish the quality of the graduates and jeopardize the reputation of the profession, making it hard to find employment.[7] They placed the responsibility for this problem on the training programs. (This is less true of MEDEX than of PA programs, due to the MEDEX practice of training only as many practitioners as there are preceptors available.) Many felt the training programs misled them with anecdotes of dedicated PAs working to effect change in remote areas or in inner cities, of bringing the light of medical science to hundreds who had never known it and of helping the weary but devoted family physician cope with an increasing patient load. Some were disillusioned with the PA concept as they understood it, and especially with a lack of the type of jobs that they believed the concept promised. They asserted that qualified graduates were underemployed by large hospitals and clinics and not optimally employed by the private practice physicians they were intended to assist. Several PAs and Medex were unable to accept employment in California, even if certified through the National Board of Medical Examiners, as they had not received their training there.

Misallocation of Job Responsibilities

The confusion surrounding the capabilities and role of the PA/Medex was reported to result in two opposite circumstances: one in which physician extenders were overtaxed, and the other in which they were underutilized. Those who found themselves overtaxed felt that physicians with whom they worked considered them in, or tried to force them into, the role of another physician. One respondent resented this sort of exploitation, stating that he found physicians very quick to ascertain and overuse his strong points. He realized that his assigned tasks increased overwhelmingly in certain areas in which he excelled. At first, the responsibility pleased him and he felt that he could manage it. Eventually he came to realize that he executed these procedures almost totally alone, without supervision. This alarmed him; he found himself thinking and reacting more like a doctor than a PA as a result of being always left to run the show.

This circumstance seemed less frequent, however, than its reverse in which PAs and Medex performed in the capacity of nurses' aides or Licensed Practical Nurses. This frustrated particularly those who previously held jobs of responsibility and challenge. In one case, a PA who crossed state lines in changing jobs discovered that although his salary and benefits improved significantly on the second job, his tasks resembled those performed by a nurse on the first. He resented the loss of responsibility and attributed it to the fact that the staff physicians where he presently worked simply did not know what he could do. Others complained of similar restrictions resulting in unsatisfactory, boring jobs that wasted their knowledge and skills and in no way approached the ideal of better, less expensive medical care for a greater number of people.

Continuing Education

A surprising conflict experienced by a half dozen or so (5 percent) of the respondents concerned the unavailability of continuing education. Reasons for this complaint centered around these issues: the constant work load so occupied the employing physician(s), the physician extender or both that there remained no time for continuing education; the employing physician(s) considered it a minor activity and did not offer their time for teaching nor allowed their employees time for learning elsewhere; the PA or Medex worked in large hospital or clinic settings which minimized extensive contact with physicians; or finally the PA or Medex worked in a remote locale or satellite which, again, diminished the opportunity of extended contact with physicians or other possible sources of ongoing learning. This frustrated those who mentioned it, since they believed that the best medical care they could deliver depended on opportunities to expand and update their medical knowledge. Such updated skills and knowledge, obtainable through continuing education, would perpetuate a high level of competency among practitioners. One could, moreover, ensure this degree of competency through imposition of an occasional but mandatory retraining period overseen by an organization comprised of members of the profession as well as faculty or staff members of the various training programs.[8]

Salary Inequities

About six (4 percent) of the respondents agreed that salary inequities posed a problem. They defined these inequities as salaries not commensurate with training and/or job activities, as well as salaries that varied so much from state to state as to cause what they believed an imbalance in the geographic distribution of PAs and Medex, legislative and malpractice issues notwithstanding. Resentment of the first stemmed from a natural desire for recognition of one's capabilities; resentment of the second from a fear that such an imbalance would prevent medical care from reaching less affluent areas of the country where the need for medical care outstripped the ability to pay for it. Indeed, one respondent admitted leaving a job in a rural area, where the pay was low, for a job in a more urbanized area offering higher wages. He saw this move as essential to his security, but not without regrettable social implications. In fact, he hoped to return to rural general practice when it became more financially practical, as he felt that the need was greatest there.

Those who complained of salary inequities suggested that an equalization of salaries across the country could produce beneficial results. Their contention was that if a physician or hospital in less populated, less affluent areas would or could offer the same wage as one in wealthier, more densely populated regions, chances of attracting competent medical assistants in those areas increased significantly.

Added to these suggestions, nine (7.3 percent) of the respondents stated goals for themselves and the profession which they felt should be pursued if the profession, as originally intended, expected to survive. These were:

making quality medical care accessible to all persons on all levels of society; developing effective, far-reaching preventive health programs within each practice, hospital or clinic; and creating an efficient and highly skilled primary care practitioner.[9]

Acceptance

The topic of acceptance of PAs and Medex received recognition and some elaboration in the previous section as a suggested deterrent to the employment of physician extenders. Reluctance of other health care providers to welcome the PA or Medex into the health professions for reasons of ignorance, jealousy or uncertainty also, as might be expected, created various uncomfortable working situations for eight (6 percent) of the respondents. These practitioners reported, however, that in most cases the problem subsided after a period of time, and a cooperative spirit replaced it. Moreover, those reporting their experience with patients found acceptance high and consequently gratifying.

COMMENTARY AND CONCLUSIONS

The problems and suggested solutions described above evoke speculation about the critical dilemmas facing PAs and Medex at this time. Although some headway has been made in certain areas such as malpractice and continuing education, on the whole the difficulties exposed by a few respondents in this small subsample of a larger survey serve to point out that the road to progress for a few of these new health professionals has been rough. The PAs and Medex who responded to the comment sheet defined predicaments needing change, but could not always propose methods to implement that change. Their dilemma highlighted the issues of publicizing an accurate image of the PA and Medex, standardizing training programs, modifying salaries across the country to eliminate possible imbalance in distribution and correcting inadequate legislation.

An attempt to produce practitioners of equal qualifications could result in numerous problems, not the least of which would be obtaining a consensus on what skills and knowledge these qualifications should entail and how long a period of time is necessary to acquire the desired level of expertise. Moreover, an adjustment would be necessary for those PAs and Medex graduated and practicing before the new criteria became effective. The benefits of this type of standardization seem likely to offset the difficulties of achieving it by creating a unified, identifiable group. Once standardization was established, the PA profession could proceed to educating other professions and the general public on its existence, role and potential value to the health care system and to society as a whole.

This process of public relations seems crucial and should be accomplished soon lest the profession lose the ground it may have gained over the last ten years in establishing itself as a valuable member of the medical community. Just how to attain this goal remains uncertain, even to the PAs and Medex themselves. Their responses emphasized the need for immediate correct publicity, but offered no vehicle for it. Surprisingly, none suggested that individuals and agencies involved in studies such as this one take the responsibility for wide publication of research findings supportive of new health practitioners. Neither did the respondents look to their professional associations as a means of publicity. Ironically, perhaps the best publicity would stem from increased employment of PAs and Medex bringing them in contact with other medical care workers and the public. Such contact would familiarize these groups with the purposes and potential of utilizing these new health professionals, creating the desire for their services. The unfortunate paradox is, of course, that neither physicians nor the public can demand what they do not know exists.

The problem posed by inadequate legislation entails a similar dilemma. It is reasonable to assume that legislative changes regarding the employment of physician extenders will not precede an acknowledged demand for the services provided by PAs and Medex. The demand would arise from a realization that a desirable service exists; but again PAs and Medex face the problem of educating the public. One short cut to this process, described by one respondent as a personal goal, involves actively lobbying among state and federal legislators until laws are written or changed to accommodate PAs for the benefit of society. Legislative modifications could be an effective, albeit not immediate, solution to several problems mentioned by the respondents. For example, successful lobbying resulting in effective, universal statutes would enable those PAs and Medex not currently fulfilling their potential on the job due to inadequate or nonexistent legislation to assume their intended role in health care. Ideally, it would prevent employers from exploiting the training and capabilities of these new health practitioners. A further benefit would be to clear up confusion surrounding the liability coverage for medical services administered by physician extenders. In some cases, legislation where none existed before would allow private physicians and health care institutions to hire PAs and Medex to augment health services. Favorable universal legislation would likely increase the overall employment of PAs and Medex, thus resulting in a greater knowledge and acceptance of the PA/MEDEX concept.[10]

Several respondents expressed concern over a possible unequal distribution of PAs and Medex due to salary inequities. Instead of practicing in poorer areas with low patient-physician ratios and great need for medical services, PAs and Medex, in an effort to support themselves and their families, would choose to work in more affluent regions offering better pay and increased access to goods and services. There appears no simple solution to this problem, although government subsidies to those areas less capable of supporting additional health care workers constitute one solution. Another would be to standardize salaries across the country for the purpose of attracting practitioners to less affluent areas; the salaries need to be equal in terms of purchasing power rather than in nominal dollar figures. In any case, care should be taken that corrective measures not ultimately increase the cost of medical care, further penalizing low-income patient groups.[11]

The potential for a surplus of PAs and Medex on the job market may be in some way linked to a possible maldistribution of physicians. Or, if one can believe four of the respondents, more PAs and Medex seek employment in the affluent areas than in the poorer regions of the country, due to the pecuniary and other benefits of practice in these wealthier locales. If that is the case, then a surplus may exist only in those affluent areas where a majority of graduates look for jobs.[12] It could be that measures taken to resolve any regional salary differences and eliminate maldistribution could also eliminate regional surpluses.[13] However, one must exercise caution in developing such a policy for fear of creating further financial burdens for patients and practitioners alike.

A few clearly defined solutions exist to rectify the problems of the PAs and Medex now practicing across the country. One such is the malpractice insurance offered by the AAPA, which should minimize the difficulties encountered by these new health practitioners.

For all that the profession itself can achieve, given that the burden of achievement rests upon the shoulders of its members and supporters, most of what it wants remains controlled by diverse and often uninformed persons and organizations. The information gathered here on this small subsample of 124 out of 1,355 PAs and Medex will, it is hoped, stimulate reflection about possible solutions to their problems which could make their employment more productive and enjoyable.

Notes

1. Names and addresses of respondents were provided by the Association of Physician Assistant Programs, in cooperation with its member programs across the country. Nonmember programs were contacted directly by the investigator and asked to provide mailing lists of their graduates. The survey population included graduates of forty-five training programs, PAs and Medex alike, trained in primary care and nonprimary care specialties. Response rates for individual programs varied; in most cases, at least 50 percent of all graduates in each program responded. A formal statistical test for a response bias was performed for the survey and no bias was detected.

2. Other individuals inquired as to their counterparts in different parts of the country, or wrote to complain about the number of such surveys currently circulating, asserting that they all required the same information and seemed to duplicate information in a wasteful manner. A minority wrote not to complain, but to express satisfaction with their employers and gratitude for being asked to express their own sentiments through the comment sheet.

3. The nomenclature "Type A" and "Type B" PA refers to the definition that the National Academy of Sciences applied to the three types of PAs, as listed in its publication "New Members of the Physician's Health Team: Physicians' Assistants," 1970. Type A refers to a highly skilled general practitioner, while Type B indicates a more specialized, less independent one.

4. The American Academy of Physicians' Assistants has responded to the needs of its membership by offering as of June 1975, a National Malpractice Insurance program which provides each member desiring it, coverage at a very reasonable annual rate under a group plan.

5. Progress is being made toward the establishment of such policies. Under the auspices of the Social Security Administration researchers at the University of Southern California are studying the feasibility of third party reimbursement under Section B of Medicare to physician extenders.

6. An interesting note to this is that the same physicians allowed such privileges to Nurse Practitioners. Unfortunately, the respondent did not elaborate on the kind of tasks the NPs performed in hospitals or clinics. He did say, however, that the community favored the use of PAs and Medex; and through community pressure, the situation could change.

7. Such a surplus, if it exists, could result from maldistribution of PAs/Medex and NPs, rather than from overproduction. In the next phase of the current study, efforts will be made to identify the employment demand for PAs and Medex by physicians, hospitals and nursing homes; and to ascertain if that demand can be met by the existing number of these health practitioners, or if more of them should be trained for that purpose.

8. In fact, mandatory continuing education is now in effect under the auspices of the American Academy of Physicians' Assistants. To maintain active membership, current members must complete 90 hours of credit in continuing education before the anniversary date of payment of dues in 1977. Senior membership requires 150 hours acquired over three years.

9. It is interesting to note that primary care was repeatedly offered as the best situation for the PA and Medex, as our study indicates that slightly over half of all PAs and just

over two-thirds of all Medex responding to our questionnaire work with primary care physicians.

10. The second phase of this study dealing with the demand for the services of physician extenders is expected to address the effect of legislation on the hiring practices of physicians and health care institutions.

11. These same groups may suffer similar hardships if the experimental project in third party reimbursement by the federal government of PAs and Medex fails to produce beneficial and satisfactory results. If successful, this model could lay the groundwork for other plans by both private and government agencies to allow reimbursement for services rendered by a physician extender.

12. Although the analysis of location choices of physician extenders is still incomplete, preliminary results indicate that Physician's Assistants tend to locate in the large metropolitan areas of the country. Moreover, although many Medex presently work in less populated, rural areas, they also locate in the more populated urban and suburban areas.

13. This discussion is somewhat simplified. Certainly factors besides salary are considered in a choice of location decision. The suggestion is only that salary is an important consideration and could be an effective tool in alleviating regional health manpower shortages.

Part III

NHP Clinical Impact

One major objective of this book is to provide a collection of evaluative research on the clinical impact of new health practitioners. Data are presented on experimental and innovative use of new health practitioners to provide care. These chapters have been selected to cover the wide range of preventive, acute, and chronic care needed by individuals throughout the life cycle. These studies attest to the capabilities of new health practitioners and may stimulate physicians and health care administrators to examine their patterns of practice and to consider the potential role of a new health practitioner in improving the clinical status of their patients.

Sackett and his colleagues conducted a series of studies on a small sample of nurse practitioners in primary care practices and found them to have a positive impact on patient outcomes.

The role of pediatric nurse practitioners in an early discharge program for obstetric patients is reported by Yanover and his co-workers at Kaiser-Permanente. The health status of infants and mothers during hospitalization and subsequent follow-up was examined and the conclusion reached that the PNPs achieved clinical outcomes comparable to physician care.

The chapter by Spector and his colleagues on care by nurses in an internal medicine clinic presents findings on patient health outcomes which were similar to the health status of patients cared for in a traditional physician clinic. Two subsequent chapters discuss chronic disease care in which nurse practitioners played the major role. In one of the few controlled studies of the use of NPs, Runyan found that 1,006 patients with either diabetes, hypertension or cardiac disease—maintained over a two-year period by nurse practitioners in health department ambulatory clinics near their homes—achieved significant reductions in diastolic blood pressure and blood glucose, and used 50 percent fewer hospital days than a control group of 498 followed in hospital out-patient clinics who showed an increase in hospital days for each disease category. Similarly, Gordon and Isaac's study of diabetics cared for by nurses at

Frontier Nursing Service demonstrated significant improvement of patient clinical outcomes including reduction by half of hospitalization.

Record and her co-workers present the research results on PA practice at the Kaiser-Permanente prepaid health plan, and their chapter compares PA and MD care through an examination of the process of care, patient outcome and patient satisfaction.

These chapters in combination are intended to provide a variety of approaches to evaluating the clinical impact of new health practitioners.

Chapter 14

The Burlington Randomized Trial of the Nurse Practitioner: Health Outcomes of Patients

David L. Sackett, Walter O. Spitzer, Michael Gent,
and Robin S. Roberts*

In collaboration with: W. Ian Hay, Georgie M. Lefroy, G. Patrick
Sweeny, Isabel Vandervlist, John C. Sibley, Larry W. Chambers, Charles
H. Goldsmith, Alexander S. Macpherson and Ronald G. McAuley

In a randomized trial of nurse practitioners as providers of primary clinical services, attention was devoted to the "outcomes" of clinical effectiveness and safety. These outcomes—expressed in physical, emotional, and social function—were assessed with newly developed methods that could be applied easily and objectively by nonclinicians to the two groups of patients under study: patients receiving conventional care and patients receiving care from nurse practitioners. Besides showing the comparability of these groups at the start of this study, these measurements showed similar levels of physical, emotional, and social function in the two groups after 1 year of receiving either nurse practitioner or conventional care. Since the numbers of patients were large enough for a statistical detection of even small differences, the results indicate that the nurse practitioners were effective and safe. This study provides a base from which to explore the "process" of delivering primary clinical services by nurse practitioners.

The availability and distribution of clinical manpower in Ontario, the increasing demand for primary clinical services, and the projected economic implications of this demand indicate the need for determining the feasibility of using the nurse practitioner as a source of primary clinical care.** This feasibility could be determined by measurements of the

*From the Faculty of Health Sciences, McMaster University, Hamilton, Ontario, Canada.

**Spitzer WO, Sackett DL, Sibley JC, et al: The Burlington randomized trial of the nurse practitioner. Methods and principal results. *N Engl J Med*. In press.

Reprinted with permission from the *Annals of Internal Medicine*, Vol. 90, no. 2 (February 1974): 137-142.

"process" of providing clinical services (for example, patients seen, procedures performed, money spent, attitudes of patients and clinicians) or by measurements of "outcomes" among patients receiving these services (end-results measures such as mortality and physical, emotional, and social function), or by some combination of both.

We believe that "process" measurements are meaningful only after proper "outcome" studies have shown that the clinical services under scrutiny are effective and safe. Accordingly, we have applied the strategy of the controlled clinical trial to the health care delivery setting, and we have adapted or developed a series of health outcome measures and applied them to the patients in the trial.

Using the World Health Organization definition of health as a starting point, we have sought indexes of positive physical, emotional, and social health for use as "outcome" measurements. For the purposes of this trial, these outcome measurements had to be objective, positive in orientation, and capable of application to several hundred patients by nonclinical interviewers. Satisfactory measures of physical function that had been developed elsewhere (1-3) were incorporated into a household survey. However, we were unable to find satisfactory positive measures of emotional and social function that were reasonably objective and could be employed and scored by nonclinicians. As a result, our research group had to develop and validate, in an independent investigation, the emotional and social function measurements used in this study.

METHODS

The basic design of the Burlington Randomized Trial is described in detail elsewhere*. In summary, 1598 families receiving clinical services from two family physicians in a middle-class suburb were randomly allocated, in a ratio of 2:1, to a conventional group (designated RC), in which they continued to receive their primary clinical services from a family physician working with a conventional nurse, or to a nurse practitioner group (designated RNP). Patients in the RNP group received their first contact, primary clinical services from one of two nurses who had successfully completed an educational program that stressed clinical judgment in the evaluation and management of conditions arising in primary care (4). Accordingly, the nurse practitioner either totally managed each patient's office visit by providing reassurance or specific therapy, or requested consultation from the associated physician.

---

*Spitzer WO, Sackett DL, Sibley JC, et al: The Burlington randomized trial of the nurse practitioner. Methods and principal results. *N Engl J Med.* In press.

Outcome Measures

Four "outcome" measures were applied to members of the RC and RNP groups.

Mortality: A surveillance system identified deaths of RC and RNP patients during the 1-year experimental period. Decedents were categorized by age, sex, cause of death, and group assignment, and crude mortality rates were generated. On two separate occasions, the clinical records for each decedent were assembled, purged of any notation that would indicate the experimental group to which they had been randomized, and submitted to the President of the Ontario College of Physicians and Surgeons. Members of this professional body, which serves a licensing and disciplinary function for physicians in the province, reviewed each case to determine whether, in their opinion, the death could have been prevented.

Physical Function: Specific "outcome" measurements were applied to the same patients (drawn by random sampling from each of the families in the study and designated the "interview cohort") both before and at the end of the experimental period, to permit "paired" comparisons in which patients could serve as their own controls. The measurement of physical function determined the patient's mobility, vision, hearing and ability to execute activities of daily living. The three indexes of physical function were [1] the proportion of patients with unimpaired mobility, vision, and hearing on the day of the interview; [2] the proportion of patients able to execute their usual daily activities during the 14 days before the interview; and [3] the proportion of patients free from an illness or injury requiring them to remain in bed for all or part of a day during the 14 days before the interview.

These indexes of physical function were determined both before and at the end of the 1-year experimental period.

Emotional Function: It was necessary to develop measures of emotional and social function that were positive in their orientation, clinically valid, and capable of mass application and scoring by nonclinicians; they were developed in an independent Health Index Study (5, 6). Briefly, in the Health Index Study an interview containing questions judged to relate to important dimensions of emotional and social function was conducted on a random sample of patients, who were simultaneously assessed by a physician for their functional status. In work to be published elsewhere, various analytic strategies, including discriminant function analysis, identified a subset of these questions, which correlated with the clinician's clinical assessment of function, and these questions were applied in the Burlington Trial to the interview cohort at the end of the experimental period*.

The emotional function questions were concerned with feelings of self-esteem, feelings toward relations with other individuals, and thoughts about the future. By using weighting factors derived from the Health Index Study, the responses to each question were combined into a composite emotional function index for each of the Burlington Trial patients in the interview cohort at the end of the experimental period. This index runs from 0.0 (poor emotional function) to 1.0 (good emotional function).

Social Function: A composite index of social function was derived from each member of the Burlington Trial who was in the interview cohort at the end of the experimental period. This composite index, also developed in the Health Index Study (5, 6), considered the patient's interaction with others (as manifested by visits with, or telephone calls from, relatives, friends, social agencies, or other individuals); subjective feelings of happiness; and interactions with police, the courts, or welfare agencies. As in the case of emotional function, the answers to individual social-function questions were weighted and combined into a composite social-function index running from 0.0 (poor social function) to 1.0 (good social function).

Statistical Analyses

Similar to the pharmacologic randomized clinical trial, in which a new drug is compared with a "standard" drug in widespread current use, in our trial clinical outcomes among patients in the RNP group were compared with those of patients receiving "conventional" or "standard" care in the RC group. Since it was our thesis that the outcomes of RNP care would be equivalent to those resulting from RC care, the hypothesis that the RNP care was effective and safe would be supported if *no* statistically significant differences could be shown between the outcomes of the RNP and RC groups. In the analysis of these data, as in the testing of a phenotypic genetic model against a set of observations, the investigator wishes to minimize the chances of accepting the null hypothesis (no difference in outcomes) when it is false. Accordingly, the "alpha" level of the test of statistical significance, used when one wants to show "true" differences between comparison groups, is replaced in prominence by the "beta" level of the test of significance, a particularly important measure

---

*See NAPS Document # 02178 for 228 pages of questionnaire instruments in this project. Order from ASIS/NAPS, c/o Microfiche Publications, 305 East 46th St., New York, NY 10017. Remit, with order, $1.50 for microfiche or $34.70 for photocopies. Make cheques payable to Microfiche Publications.

TABLE 14:1

Comparison of the RC and RNP Interview Cohorts at the Start of the Trial*

	RC	RNP
Number of patients in the interview cohort	614	340
Mean number of persons per family	2.8	2.7
Males, %	42	43
Females, %	58	57
Age in years, %		
0 to 4	5	4
5 to 9	5	5
10 to 14	8	7
15 to 19	5	8
20 to 39	33	29
40 to 59	31	35
60 to 69	7	8
70 and over	6	4
Annual household income, %		
Less than $4000	4	4
$4000 to $7999	15	13
$8000 to $9999	13	12
$10 000 to $13 999	28	24
$14 000 to $17 999	15	14
$18 000 or more	16	23

* RC = patients receiving conventional care; RNP = patients receiving care from nurse practitioners.

of the possibility that one is "missing" a true difference. In assessing observed differences between the RNP and RC groups, we have indicated the results of tests of statistical significance in terms of the probability with which we have "missed" a true difference between the groups, in either direction, of 5% or more at the start of the experimental period (a "two-tailed" test). At the end of the period we have applied a more precise "one-tailed" beta level of the test to determine the likelihood that we have missed a true deterioration among RNP patients, one in which they are less healthy by 5% or more than RC patients.

RESULTS

Of 1598 families, only 7 refused their assignments (2 families from the RC group and 5 from the RNP group). Furthermore, during the 1-year experimental period, only 0.9% of RC families and 0.7% of RNP families left the practice because of dissatisfaction. By the final two months of the experiment, the proportion of RNP patient visits managed entirely by the nurse practitioners had stabilized at 67%.

Comparability of the RC and RNP Interview Cohorts at the Start of the Trial

Table 14:1 summarizes the distributions of family size, sex, age, and annual household income for the RC and RNP cohorts just before the 1-year experimental period. The groups are highly similar, and none of the observed differences approach statistical significance. The initial similarity of the RC and RNP groups is further supported in Table 14:2, which summarizes the physical function of members of the RC and RNP groups just before the 1-year experimental period. Large and identical portions of patients in the RC and RNP groups had unimpaired mobility, vision and hearing on the day of the interview. Similarly large and comparable proportions of patients in each group had been able to carry out their usual daily activities throughout the 14 days before this interview. A review of the "beta" levels for the differences between RC and RNP patients, given in the third column of Table 14:2, shows that RNP patients may have been less healthy than RC patients, in terms of bed disability, before the start of the experimental period.

Mortality

It was anticipated during the design of the trial that the number of deaths during the experimental period would be small. As shown in Table 14:3, there were only 18 deaths in the RC group and 4 deaths among RNP patients. The mean age at death was similar for decedents in the RC and RNP groups, and the difference in crude death rates for the two groups was not statistically significant. On the two occasions when the clinical records of decedents were reviewed by appointees of the Ontario College of Physicians and Surgeons, no deaths of RNP patients were judged to have been preventable.

TABLE 14:2

Physical Function Prior to the Experimental Period

	RC*	RNP*	B*
		%	
Unimpaired mobility, vision, and hearing	86	86	0.03
Unimpaired in usual daily activities	87	89	0.09
Free from bed-disability	86	83	0.22

* RC = patients receiving conventional care; RNP = patients receiving care from nurse practitioners.

† Indicates probability that we have failed to detect a *real* difference of $\geq$ 5% in physical function between RC and RNP patients.

TABLE 14:3

Mortality During the Study

	RC Group*	RNP Group*
	no.	
By cause of death		
Cancer	8	2
Myocardial infarction•	4	1
Other cardiovascular disease	4	—
Other	2	1
By age at death		
10 to 29 years	2	—
30 to 49 years	3	1
50 to 69 years	7	2
70 years and over	6	1
Mean age at death	59.3 years	57.0 years
Total deaths	18	4
Death rate per thousand	6.0	2.7

*RC = patients receiving conventional care; RNP = patients receiving care from nurse practitioners.

Includes sudden death.

TABLE 14:4

Physical Function at the End of the Experimental Period°

	RC Group	RNP Group	β†
Unimpaired mobility, vision, and hearing	88	86	0.10
Unimpaired in usual daily activities	90	90	0.02
Free from bed-disability	87	86	0.05

* RC = patients receiving conventional care; RNP = patients receiving care from nurse practitioners.

† Indicates probability that we have failed to detect a *real* deterioration of physical function among RNP patients of > 5%.

Physical Function at the End of the Experimental Period

Table 14:4 summarizes the measurements of physical function for 521 patients in the RC group and 296 patients in the RNP group at the end of the experimental period. The proportions of individuals in the two experimental groups with unimpaired physical function, unimpaired usual daily activities, and freedom from bed disability were again virtually identical, and a similar pattern emerges when this analysis is limited to

FIGURE 14:1

Emotional Function at the End of the Experiment

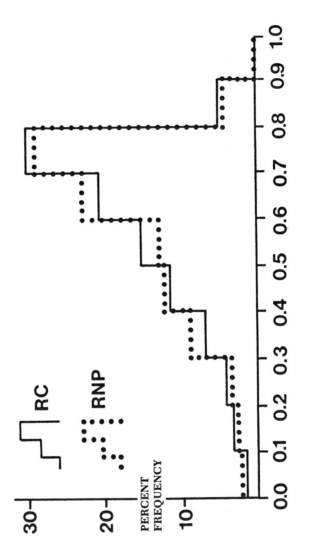

EMOTIONAL FUNCTION INDEX VALUE

RC = patients receiving conventional care; RNP = patients receiving care from nurse practitioners.

those members of the interview cohort who had these measurements both before and after the 1-year experimental period. The last column in Table 14:4 indicates the probability that patients in the RNP group are less healthy by 5% or more, in terms of physical function, than those in the RC group, and it is seen that we are unlikely to have missed a deterioration among RNP patients, had it occurred during the trial.

Emotional Function at the End of the Experimental Period

Figure 14:1 is a histogram of the distribution of emotional function indexes for patients in the RC and RNP groups. The mean emotional function index for RC patients at the end of the experimental period was 0.583 (SD, 0.187) and for the RNP patients, 0.577 (SD, 0.187). These results indicate closely similar levels of emotional function in the two groups of patients; the likelihood that we have missed a deterioration of 5% or more among RNP patients is shown by the beta value of only 0.068.

Social Function at the End of the Experimental Period

Figure 14:2 is a histogram of social function index values for RC and RNP patients; the respective mean social function index values are 0.832 (SD, 0.249) and 0.839 (SD, 0.274). The likelihood that a drop of 5% or more in the social function of RNP patients has been "missed" is 0.008.

DISCUSSION

The close comparability of mortality rates and of measurements of physical, social, and emotional function between the RC and RNP patients supports the conclusion that patients randomly assigned to receive first-contact primary care from a nurse practitioner enjoy favorable health outcomes, which are comparable to those of patients receiving conventional care. Before concluding that the nurse practitioner is both effective and safe, however, it is important to consider three potential pitfalls in the design and execution of this randomized trial, which may have created these favorable findings in a spurious fashion.

The first potential pitfall results from the absence of a "no treatment" control group. It could be argued that neither the nurse practitioner nor the family physician have any clinically significant impact on health outcomes and that this trial has merely compared equally ineffective, "neutral" alternatives for the delivery of primary care. We have deliberately excluded a "no treatment" control group for two reasons. First, we concluded with our collaborators that it would be unethical to withhold clinical services from a control group of patients in this investigation, just as it has been judged unethical to withhold treatment

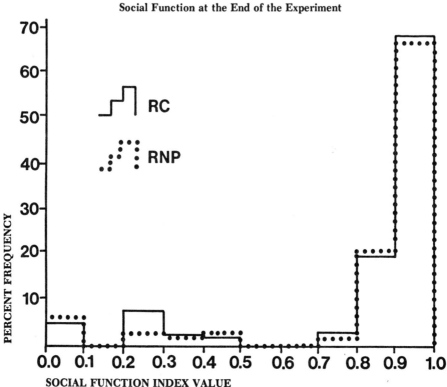

FIGURE 14:2

Social Function at the End of the Experiment

RC = patients receiving conventional care; RNP = patients receiving care from nurse practitioners.

from control groups in randomized clinical trials of surgical and chemotherapeutic approaches to cancer (7). Our trial is analogous to the trial in which therapy with a new pharmacologic agent is compared with current "standard" therapy. Second, primary care practices of this magnitude, studied over this duration of time, generate a volume of clinical conditions (both statistically and clinically significant in number) whose outcomes are profoundly affected by the skill of detection and the appropriateness of management. This is substantiated, for example, by the numbers of patients identified as requiring the diagnosis and treatment of occlusive cardiovascular and infectious disorders, both in this and in other investigations of primary care* (8, 9).

* Spitzer WO, Sackett DL, Sibley JC, et al: The Burlington randomized trial of the nurse practitioner. Methods and principal results. *N Engl J Med.* In press.

TABLE 14:5

Paired Comparisons of Physical Function Among Patients Assessed Both Before
and at the End of the Experimental Period

	RC Group*		RNP GROUP†	
	no.	%	no.	%
Patients impaired at start who were unimpaired at end of the trial				
Mobility, vision, hearing	39/71	55	18/41	44
Usual daily activities	58/67	87	27/34	79
Bed disability	55/73	75	39/51	76
Patients impaired at end who were unimpaired at start of the trial				
Mobility, vision, hearing	32/64	50	19/42	45
Usual daily activities	42/51	82	23/30	77
Bed disability	51/69	74	28/40	70

*Patients who continued to receive primary clinical services from a family physician working with a conventional nurse.
†Patients receiving care from nurse practitioners.

The second potential pitfall, "volunteer bias," was avoided by incorporating random allocation into the experimental design, and the comparability of the RC and RNP groups at the start of the trial, as shown in Tables 14:1 and 14:2, attests to the success of this procedure. Furthermore, as indicated by the extremely high rates of participation and follow-up, it is appropriate to compare the RC and RNP patients throughout the experimental period.

However, a third major potential pitfall remains: the measurements and indexes of function we used to assess health outcomes among patients. It is theoretically possible that our measures of physical, social, and emotional function may be insensitive to small but clinically significant changes in health status, which could have occurred during the experiment. If so, this insensitivity could mask a deterioration in the health status of patients assigned to the RNP group; for example, these indexes of function may remain fixed at relatively high levels until a substantial deterioration in health status has occurred and only then begin to show discernable declines.

The "paired" comparisons of physical function in the same patients, both before and at the end of the experimental period, suggests that this third potential pitfall has also been avoided. These paired comparisons (Table 14:5), indicate that the majority of patients with impaired physical function at the start of the trial no longer were impaired at the end of the experimental period; similarly, from 45% to 82% of patients whose physical function was impaired at the end of the trial were free of impairment at its start. We have therefore concluded that these measures of physical function are quite sensitive to short-term variations in physical function. It is extremely unlikely that a clinically important deterioration in health status of the RNP group could go undetected.

This search for answers to questions of effectiveness and safety in using the nurse practitioner as a provider of primary clinical services required the measurement of health outcomes among patients, and the development and application of such measures may be difficult. This is not the case if the end-result is a "hard" one, such as the death of a study subject. Although disagreement and a resulting misclassification can occur in assigning a cause of death, the fact of death is indisputable. The measurement of health outcomes becomes more difficult as one moves toward "softer" end-results, such as discrete clinical events. Despite the slow evolution of strategies and tactics for clinical measurement, sufficient experience has been gained to indicate the feasibility of measuring clinical outcomes*.

Outcome measurement becomes quite formidable, however, when the innovative clinical maneuver results in the multidimensional, functional state the World Health Organization defines as health. Not only are well-developed and easily applied health-outcome indexes very few in number, "observer variation" and disagreement extend to the rationale, definitions, and justification for the indexes themselves, as well as to the subsequent measurement process.

Nonetheless, the high degree of patient cooperation and the successful measurement of physical, social, and emotional function by nonclinicians have reinforced our earlier conviction that it is possible to design and execute randomized clinical trials of innovations in the delivery of broad categories of clinical services. These favorable and comparable health outcomes, besides answering the questions of effectiveness and safety, are a solid base from which to analyze other data collected before, during, and after the experimental period. The quality of clinical care provided, the attitudes of clinicians and patients toward this innovation, and the economic issues affecting the introduction of nurse practitioners as providers of primary clinical care can now be explored.

---

*Sackett DL: Design, measurement and analysis in clinical trials. Presented at the Symposium of Platelets, Drugs and Thrombosis, Hamilton, Ontario, Canada. October 16-18, 1972. In press.

ACKNOWLEDGEMENTS

The authors acknowledge, with thanks, the enthusiasm, patience, and persistence of Mrs. Betty Bidgood and her team of household interviewers in the Health Sciences Field Survey Unit, who carried out the measurements of physical, social, and emotional function used in this trial.

Grant support: DM34 and PR146, Ministry of Health, Ontario, Canada.

Received 5 November 1973; accepted 19 November 1973.

Address reprint requests to Dr. D. L. Sackett, Department of Clinical Epidemiology and Biostatistics, McMaster University Medical Centre, 1200 Main St. West, Hamilton Ontario, Canada L8S 4J9.

Notes

1. Bruett TL, Overs RP: A Critical Review of 12 ADL Scales. *Physical Therapy* 49:857-862, 1969.

2. The Staff of the Benjamin Rose Hospital: Multidisciplinary study of illness in aged persons. I. Methods and preliminary results. *J Chron Dis* 7:332-345, 1958.

3. Holland WW: Health services in London. *Br Med Jr* 2:233, 1972.

4. Spitzer WO, Kergin DJ: Nurse practitioners in primary care. I. The McMaster University Educational Program. *Can Med Assoc J* 108:991-995, April 21, 1973.

5. Macpherson AS: The Measurement of Mental Health in a General Population (M.Sc. dissertation). Hamilton, Ontario. McMaster University, 1972.

6. Chambers LW: An Index of Social Function (M.Sc. dissertation). Hamilton, Ontario. McMaster University, 1973.

7. Glaser EM: Ethical aspects of clinical trials, in *The Principles and Practice of Clinical Trials*, edited by Harris EL, Fitzgerald JD. Edinburgh, E. & S. Livingstone, Ltd., 1970, pp. 23-30.

8. Fry, J: *Profiles of Disease*. Edinburgh, E. & S. Livingstone, Ltd., 1966.

9. McFarlane AH, Norman GR, Spitzer WO: Family medicine: the dilemma of defining the discipline. *Can Med Assoc J* 105:397-401, 1971.

Chapter 15

Perinatal Care of Low-Risk Mothers and Infants: Early Discharge with Home Care

Mark J. Yanover, Deloras Jones and Michael D. Miller

A family-centered perinatal-care program featuring collaboration by nurse practitioners, obstetricians, pediatricians, and paramedical personnel was developed to enhance family participation and achieve a shorter but safe hospital stay. Discharge from the hospital was permitted as early as 12 hours after delivery. A perinatal nurse practitioner made daily home visits. The program's safety, feasibility, and acceptability to patients was studied by comparison of 44 patients so treated (study group) with 44 receiving traditional care (controls). Twenty-one study families, but no controls, went home within 24 hours. The study and control groups had no significant differences or trends in numbers or types of morbidity during hospitalization or the six-week post-partum period. The expense of the program is approximately equaled by hospital costs saved through early discharge. The results indicate that early discharge with home-care follow-up observation as described is safe, economically feasible, and well accepted by patients. (N Engl J Med 294:702-705, 1976)

The low-risk patient who receives obstetric care at Kaiser-Permanente Medical Center is offered two alternative modes of management: traditional care or the Family Centered Perinatal Care Program, described in 1972.[1] As one step in the development of the alternative program, we made the comparative study reported here. Its purpose was to determine whether such a program would prove medically safe, economically feasible, and well accepted by participating families.

From the departments of Obstetrics, Pediatrics and Nursing, Kaiser-Permanente Medical Center, San Francisco (address reprint requests to Dr. Yanover at Kaiser-Permanente Medical Center, 2200 O'Farrell St., San Francisco, CA 94115).
Supported by Kaiser Foundation Research Institute, General Research Support, under a grant (5 501 RR05521-10) from the U.S. Public Health Service.

Reprinted with permission from *The New England Journal of Medicine*, Vol. 294, pages 702-705, March 25, 1976.

SUBJECTS AND METHODS

Subjects

The patients were selected from the prenatal population of the Kaiser-Permanente Medical Center, San Francisco. All the full-time attending obstetricians participated in the evaluation. Each infant received care from one of the pediatricians or pediatric nurse practitioners at the Center.

The criteria for admission to the evaluation study were as follows: parity must be 0 or 1; the mother must be between 19 and 35 years of age, be at low risk medically, and have at least a 12th-grade education; the father must be willing to attend prenatal education classes; and the prospective parents must be living together, both able to communicate well in English, and residing within 32 km of the hospital. The obstetrician of each patient who fulfilled these criteria ascertained that her pregnancy did indeed fall into the low-risk category, and gave his formal written consent before those performing the evaluation study first made contact with the mother. The patient co-ordinator (described below) asked each such patient whether she would like to participate in a study concerned with delivery of health care to low-risk prenatal patients. She interviewed those who accepted, and explained the program to them.

Of 362 mothers screened, 271 were interviewed; 143 were not enrolled because of lack of interest (38 patients), residence farther than 32 km from the hospital (37), inability to communicate well in English (28), or inability to attend prenatal classes (14), or for other reasons (26). The remaining 128 families were enrolled and randomly assigned to the study (alternative-care) or control (traditional-care) group. Forty did not complete participation, because of change in medical status before delivery (15), inability or unwillingness to attend classes (10), lack of interest in research (six), or removal from area (five), or for other reasons (four). The changes in medical status were stillbirth (four), pre-eclampsia (four), premature labor (two), conditions necessitating cesarean section (two), or other (three). The types and frequencies of these disorders did not differ between the study and control groups.

Of the 88 remaining patients, 44 completed their perinatal care in the new mode, described below (the study group), and 44 in the traditional mode, also described below (the control group). There were no statistically significant differences between the two groups in age, race, father's occupation, planned pregnancy, duration of marriage, length of time to conceive, mother's and father's education, presence of another child in the home, or mother's preference regarding enrollment in prenatal education classes, natural childbirth, or breast feeding.

Methods

Traditional care. In our medical center, traditional perinatal care included the following items: father present in labor and delivery rooms with permission; observation of the infant in the nursery for 24 hours, followed by transfer to rooming-in; classes several times weekly on breast feeding, infant nutrition, skin care, etc.; discharge home not earlier than 48 hours post-partum; pediatric visit at two weeks; and obstetric visit at six weeks.

Family Centered Perinatal Care Program. The alternative represents an endeavor to respond to the wishes of numerous families interviewed in depth by one of us (D.J.), to enhance family participation, and to achieve a shorter, yet safe, length of hospital stay. Its features were as follows: collaborative perinatal care by nurse practitioners, obstetricians, pediatricians, and paramedical personnel; continuity of care from prenatal classes through hospitalization, with post-partum home care, provided by perinatal nurse practitioners; father's participation in prenatal education and his support during labor and delivery, and at home after delivery; prenatal education through classes offering orientation to the Family Centered Perinatal Care Program, and preparation for childbirth and early discharge; release from the hospital as soon as the mother and infant recover from the birth and the family is ready; and home visits by the perinatal nurse practitioner to provide health surveillance and to teach parentcraft.

Specifically, the Family Centered Perinatal Care Program was as follows: nursery personnel observed the infant more frequently than in the traditional mode during the first six hours after birth; if mother and infant had recovered appropriately, the infant was transferred to rooming-in six hours after delivery; the Program's staff evaluated mother and infant 12 hours after birth to determine whether the discharge criteria had been met (Table 15:1); if they had been met, the medical staff approved, and the family was ready, the mother and infant were discharged at that time; and the perinatal nurse practitioner made daily home visits for health surveillance and teaching of parentcraft through the fourth post-partum day,* with additional visits as needed. Families who did not fulfill the discharge criteria at 12 hours were not eligible for release before 24 hours. The nature of the variance determined the length of additional hospitalization.

---

*After completion of this study, experience with a larger number of patients showed that it was unnecessary to continue routine home visits after the third post-partum day.

TABLE 15:1

Criteria for Early Discharge (Events that Preclude Discharge Earlier than 24 hours after Delivery)

Intra-partum:
  Maternal:
    Prolonged rupture of membranes ($\geq$ 24 hr)
    Precipitous labor ($\leq$ 3 hr)
    Blood pressure $\geq$ 140/90 mm Hg
    Temperature $\geq$ 38°C (100.4°F)
Post-partum:
  Maternal:
    Temperature $\geq$ 38°C (100.4°F)
    Blood pressure < 90/60 or > 140/90 mm Hg
    Excessive vaginal bleeding
    Difficulty with ambulation or voiding
Infant:
    Birth weight < 2.7 or > 4.05 kg (6, 9 lb)
    Gestation age < 38 or > 42 wk
    Apgar score $\leq$ 7 at 1 min
    Abnormal vital signs:
      Heart rate < 110 or > 150
      Respiratory rate < 30 or > 60
      Temperature < 36.1° or > 37.2°C (97°, 99°F)
    Abnormal laboratory findings:
      Coombs test positive
      Hematocrit reading < 45 or > 65%
    Failure to void
    Feeding difficulty

The perinatal nurse practitioner who was assigned to a family was available to that family during the first two weeks post-partum. During the home visits, the nurse practitioner examined the mother for evidence of post-partum hemorrhage, subinvolution of the uterus, problems relating to the episiotomy, urination, the breasts, and for phlebitis, as well as for other infections, and hypertension, examined the infant for jaundice, and for signs of infection or other disease, and drew appropriate specimens for routine laboratory studies (maternal hematocrit, infant blood sample for phenylketonuria) and for others deemed necessary (such as urinalysis or blood count in the mother and bilirubin in the infant). The nurse practitioner discussed at length the parents' questions and problems, and helped them adapt to their new infant. The nurse practitioner reported unusual findings to a physician; the patient was then followed by the nurse practitioner at home or referred to a physician at the office or hospital for further evaluation.

The couples of both groups attended formal classes in preparation for childbirth. The families of the study group also attended sessions preparing them for early discharge.

Numerous data were collected at various times during the pregnancy and hospital stay, and for several months after delivery, by interview, chart review, and questionnaire. We sent a questionnaire concerning satisfaction with the length of hospital stay to the members of each group within two months after delivery. Statistical analysis was performed by the chi-square method.

Personnel trained especially for the alternative program were two perinatal nurse practitioners and a patient co-ordinator. The perinatal nurse practitioners completed four months' training, comprising 12 hours weekly of didactic sessions by attending obstetricians and pediatricians, and many hours of interviewing and examining patients. A four-hour written examination covered prenatal care, labor and delivery, and neonatal care, and emphasized problems that might arise after hospital discharge. Performance in this examination was comparable to that of several resident physicians who took the same examination.

The patient co-ordinator, selected from the hospital's auxiliary personnel, was trained to perform various functions in addition to her clerical tasks. She screened all prenatal patients for eligibility for the study, explained to prospective parents the nature of the alternative program's research and interventions, assigned enrollees randomly to the control group or to the study group with a specific nurse practitioner, and ascertained that all families of both groups had access to and attended prenatal education classes at this medical center or elsewhere. After delivery, the patient co-ordinator checked the mother's and infant's charts to determine that all discharge criteria were met, and then co-ordinated the discharge with the medical staff, the nursery staff, and the family's perinatal nurse practitioner.

RESULTS

The study and control groups showed no significant differences in medians and distributions of the length of labor, or amounts and frequency of administration of oxytocin or an analgesic (meperidine hydrochloride). The routes of anesthesia required are shown in Table 15:2 (mepivacaine was used for paracervical or epidural block). Significantly more study than control patients had local or no anesthesia, and fewer study than control patients had epidural block. Six of the 10 study patients having epidural anesthesia remained in the hospital more than 24 hours beyond the median for their group; only five of the 34 study patients who did not have epidural block had prolonged stays by this definition (P < 0.02). There were more spontaneous deliveries among the study patients (30) than among the control patients (22), but this difference was not statistically significant.

The ranges and median lengths of post-partum hospital stay are shown in Table 15:3.

TABLE 15:2

Types of Anesthesia Used for Delivery

Type of Anesthesia	No. of Patients*	
	Study	Control
None	4	0
Local only	12	3
Pudendal block	14	16
Epidural block	10	19
Saddle block	4	6
Totals	44	44

*These differences were significant at P< 0.02; chi-square = 12.74 (with 4 degrees of freedom).

TABLE 15:3

Length of Post-Partum Hospital Stay

Length of Stay (Hr)	No. of Patients	
	Study	Control
12-24	21	0
25-48	11	5
49-72	10	22
73-96	2	12
> 96	0	5
Totals	44	44
Range	12-86	31-167
Median	26	68

No significant differences or trends were observed in the numbers and types of morbidity occurring during hospitalization or during the first six weeks after delivery in mothers or infants of the study and control groups. The 13 cases of morbidity, in 10 infants, are listed in Table 15:4. The two study infants with elevated bilirubin were readmitted to the hospital for phototherapy; the two control infants with hyperbilirubinemia had prolonged hospital stays. All the superficial skin infections cleared with local therapy. The two control newborns with pneumonia had a prolonged nursery stay. The mothers' complications included precipitous or prolonged labor, midforceps delivery, obstetric laceration, post-partum infection, and post-partum hemorrhage. No mother in either group was readmitted to the hospital during the six-week post-partum period.

TABLE 15:4

Morbidity (13 Cases in 10 Infants)

Type of Morbidity	No. of Cases	
	Study	Control
Apgar score < 7 at 5 min	0	2
Total bilirubin ⩾ 15 mg/dl	2	2
Superficial skin infection	2	3
Pneumonia:		
Aspiration	0	1
Intrauterine	0	1
Totals	4	9

TABLE 15:5

Responses to Questionnaires Regarding Satisfaction with Length of Hospital Stay*

Questionnaire	Study	Control
Did you feel your hospital stay was		
Too long	5	9
Too short	2	1
Appropriate length	34	30
No answer	0	1
Would you participate in the Family Centered Perinatal Care Program in a subsequent pregnancy?		
Yes	39	—
No	2	—
Would you recommend this program to your friends?		
Yes	41	—
No	0	—
If you were to have another baby, would you elect to participate in a program in which you would be prepared for early post-partum discharge with home care follow-up?		
Yes	—	24
No	—	17

*41 of 44 patients in each group responded.

The responses to the questionnaire concerning satisfaction with the length of hospital stay are shown in Table 15:5.

The results of our screening procedures indicated that about 25 per cent of our prenatal population of 160 women per month would be eligible for participation in the Family Centered Perinatal Care Program. Extended experience has shown that one perinatal nurse practitioner in a half-time position, making daily home visits through the third post-partum day, can care for 15 families per month. We estimate that the cost of providing our program's services is approximated by the immediate saving derived from early discharge. The expenses include salaries of nurse practitioners, paramedical personnel, and medical consultants, as well as automobile expenses and home-care supplies. The immediate saving related to early discharge is about 30 per cent of the daily costs of providing inpatient care for mother and baby, including food, linen, supplies, and nursing care. If the vacated beds and rooms are used for other patients or purposes, considerable additional savings will accrue. Evaluation of admissions to the maternity floor at this medical center over the last few years shows such a changing pattern, with increased utilization of beds for high-risk prenatal patients.

DISCUSSION

Early discharge of maternity patients is not new. Hellman et al.,[2] in 1962, reported early discharge with little morbidity; however, few of the patients were released earlier than 24 hours post-partum, and concern about jaundice and other neonatal disorders has increased in recent years. Most previous reports have indicated that the authors had resorted to early discharge to alleviate overutilization of post-partum beds,[2,4] and that patients' acceptance was less than wholehearted. We endeavored to respond to the wishes expressed by a sector of the low-risk families, and designed the program to enhance family participation as well as to minimize unnecessary hospitalization.

The desires expressed by many of the low-risk families closely resembled those reported by Haire in 1972[5]; they reflect a changing attitude toward childbirth. Most of these young people viewed pregnancy and delivery as a normal variation of health, and wanted their physician and hospital to manage it as such. They asked for individualized attention, prepared childbirth, breast feeding, increased participation by the father, and adequate information, then a role in decisions about analgesics in labor and delivery, about infant feeding and circumcision. Many desired minimal separation of the infant from the mother, and of both from other family members. They believed that the principal benefit of hospitalization after the first post-partum day was the opportunity to learn to care for the infant, and questioned the need for the traditional stay of three or more days.

During the initial 15 months reported earlier[1] as a pilot phase, we found that most infants of low-risk mothers completed their transitional period[6] within six hours after delivery, and we discharged about 40 mothers and infants between 24 and 48 hours after delivery. Our criteria for 12-hour discharge (Table 15:1) were developed on the basis of experience in the pilot phase.

The markedly shorter post-partum stay of the study families than of the control families demonstrates their willingness to receive post-partum care at home after recovery from birth. We assume that the program's preparations for childbirth and early release and its continuing support were important to a good birth experience, rapid recovery, and successful early discharge.

The capacity for mother-infant attachment appears to be remarkably sensitive in the earliest hours and days after birth and its development may have profound long-term effects.[7-10] Many parents of our study group stated that they got to know their infants better by being at home without the disturbance of a hospital environment. It is our impression that many of the study-group fathers have a feeling of closeness to their infants resembling the engrossment described by Greenberg and Morris.[11]

Because the alternative program was based in part on the expectations and needs of prospective parents, it was essential to determine whether it had fulfilled their needs, and whether families gave evidence that they were willing to accept a nontraditional approach to perinatal care.[12][13] The study group's responses to the questionnaire (Table 15:5) suggested that a population similar to them would desire and accept this approach.

All complications that occurred at home after early discharge were managed expeditiously by the perinatal nurse practitioners and the consulting physicians; no complication was believed to be related to early discharge. The hyperbilirubinemia in the two study infants readmitted to the hospital for phototherapy probably would have been noted in the nursery if they had stayed the traditional three days, but might have been missed if they had been discharged at 48 hours.

Since the completion of this formal study, we have enrolled more than 400 families in the program, 34 participating for a second time. Three hundred and eighty-five families have successfully completed their participation, 178 (46 per cent) being discharged within 24 hours of delivery, 155 (40 per cent) between 24 and 48 hours post-partum, and 52 (14 per cent) more than 48 hours after delivery. Review of the medical records of these families reveals no case in which the mother was readmitted to the hospital. Several mothers were followed at home by the nurse practitioner or were referred to their physician's office for consultation regarding urinary retention (four cases), hypertension (three), anemia (one), episiotomy separation (two), infected episiotomy (two), endometritis (one), cystitis (one), vaginitis (one), or unexplained fever (three). Fifteen of the infants were readmitted to the hospital. Thirteen of them were admitted for observation and treatment of hyperbilirubinemia (total bilirubin $\geqslant$ 15 mg per deciliter), all after 72 hours of age. One infant was readmitted because of cyanosis and poor feeding, and one because of fever. The symptoms resolved soon after admission, and both were discharged within 48 hours. A number of other infants were followed at home by the nurse practitioner because of hyperbilirubinemia, superficial skin infections, or poor feeding, and several were referred to the physician's office for consultation.

The data regarding complications in the formal study, augmented by this larger experience, support the premise that this method of perinatal care is as safe as that traditionally provided at our medical center. The data also confirm our hypothesis that the Family Centered Perinatal Care Program is economically feasible, and highly acceptable to our patients. We advocate further exploration of perinatal care of low-risk patients that individualizes care, emphasizes good health, and facilitates parent-infant attachment.

We are indebted to Henry R. Shinefield, M.D., George Calderwood, M.D., Mikael Peterson, Peter Bigelow, Linda duTemple, and Ruth Straus for support and assistance. Our special gratitude to Robert Burnip, M.D., Betty Cahill, R.N. (PNNP), who cared for many of the study patients, and to William A. Silverman, M.D., without whose guidance and enthusiasm this project could not have been contemplated.

Notes

1. Yanover MJ, Miller MD, Jones DJ: A family-centered perinatal care program: a preliminary report, Program of the Ambulatory Pediatric Association Twelfth Annual Meeting, May 22-23, 1972, Washington, DC, p. 21.

2. Hellman LM, Kohl SG, Palmer J: Early hospital discharge in obstetrics. Lancet 1:227-232, 1962.

3. Theobald GW: Home on the second day: the Bradford experiment: the combined maternity scheme. Br Med J 2:1364-1367, 1959.

4. Day GA: Early discharge of maternity patients. Nurs Outlook 11:825-827, 1963.

5. Haire D: The cultural warping of childbirth. Int Childbirth Educ Assoc News 11:5-35, 1972.

6. Desmond MM, Rudolph AJ, Phitaksphraiwan P: The transitional care nursery: a mechanism for preventive medicine in the newborn. Pediatr Clin North Am 13:651-668, 1966.

7. Rubin R: Maternal touch. Nurs Outlook 11:828-831, 1963.

8. Klaus MH, Jerauld R, Kreger NC, et al: Maternal attachment: importance of the first post-partum days. N Engl J Med 286:460-463, 1972.

9. Kennell J, Jerauld R, Wolfe H, et al: Maternal behavior one year after early and extended post-partum contact. Dev Med Child Neurol 16:172-179, 1974.

10. Ringler NM, Kennell JH, Jarvella R, et al: Mother-to-child speech at 2 years: effects of early postnatal contact. J Pediatr 86:141-144, 1975.

11. Greenberg M, Morris N: Engrossment: the newborn's impact upon the father. Am J Orthopsychiatry 44:520-531, 1974.

12. Schroeder OC Jr: Health consumers and medical practitioners: is conflict inevitable? Postgrad Med 53(4):203-205, 1973.

13. Bailey DR: Hospitals can, must influence change. Hospitals 47(17):55-59, 1973.

Chapter 16

Medical Care by Nurses in an Internal Medicine Clinic: Analysis of Quality and Its Cost

Reynold Spector, Patricia McGrath, Joseph Alpert, Phin Cohen
and Helen Aikins*

● The quality and cost of medical care provided by specially trained nurses in an internal medicine clinic was evaluated prospectively during a three-month period. Clinic physicians referred patients to these nurses when they believed that the nurse could contribute to the patient's overall health care.

Nurse care was judged to be adequate in dealing with 98% of old problems (defined by the physician) and 85% of new problems (detected by the nurse). Scheduled visits to the physician and unscheduled visits decreased significantly $(P < .05)$ during the period of nurse care vs a control period, but the overall cost of health care per patient was increased significantly during the nurse care period $(P < .01)$ because of a disproportionate increase in visits to the nurse. We conclude that nurse care was feasible and of adequate quality. However, it was not cost-effective.

(*JAMA* 232:1234-1237, 1975)

Thoughtful proponents of direct nurse participation in the care of patients do not propose that nurses provide care in vacuo.[1] Instead, they suggest that nurses complement rather than replace the physician and that nurses work under a physician's supervision.[1] Several recent studies have suggested that well-trained nurses can participate in quality patient care at a reasonable cost.[2-5] However, these studies involved only one or two nurses who may not have been representative of nurses in general.[2-5]

*From the Department of Medicine, Harvard Medical School (Drs. Spector and Alpert), the Department of Nutrition, Harvard School of Public Health (Dr. Cohen), and the Medical Clinic, Peter Bent Brigham Hospital, Boston.

Reprint requests to Peter Bent Brigham Hospital, 721 Huntington Ave, Boston, MA 02115 (Dr. Spector).

Moreover, in one case, the providers of the care evaluated their own performance.[3]

The purpose of the present study was to see if high-quality, cost-effective care could be provided by nurses for *carefully selected patients* in an internal medicine clinic. In this study, we have shown that (1) clinically trained nurses could be integrated into the patient care system in our internal medicine clinic; (2) these nurses could provide adequate patient care under the supervision of the referring physician; (3) the patient care provided by the nurse could be effectively monitored; and (4) the cost to the patient of the care provided by the nurse could be measured.

METHODS AND MATERIALS

The basic structure of the Peter Bent Brigham Internal Medicine Clinic and the quality of care provided by the physicians have been previously described in detail,[6,7] Briefly, approximately 115 house staff, junior and senior staff physicians, each working one afternoon or evening a week, handle approximately 25,000 patient visits per year. In this setting, four offices for five clinic nurses were set aside for the visits described in this study as well as for the nurses' other duties. Each registered nurse underwent, at the hospital's expense, a three-month postgraduate training program that emphasized diagnostic, therapeutic, and supportive medical care. Each nurse was assigned to work with a group of physicians. When consulted, she would see any patient belonging to a physician in her assigned group. After this procedure had been in effect for approximately a year, a three-month study period was begun on Oct 1, 1973.

All physicians in the clinic were offered the opportunity to refer patients to a nurse for a scheduled visit if the physician thought the nurse could aid in that patient's overall care. Specifically, the patient had to have a subacute or chronic illness with a problem that had been previously diagnosed at least in part. The population served by the nurses was highly selected. Two hundred forty-five patients with hypertension were referred to the nurses; 87 for a medication check; 85 with diabetes mellitus; 59 with social or psychiatric problems; 17 with dietary problems; and 95 with other problems. Moreover, it was required that the physician have a definite plan for further diagnosis and therapy before a referral was considered appropriate.

After the initial nurse referral, both the nurse and the physician jointly cared for the patient. Initially, the physician was asked to fill out a referral form listing the patient's problems, medications, specific instructions for care, as well as a telephone number where he could be reached during nonclinic hours. The physician was expected to discuss the problem with the nurse at the time of referral. When the nurse saw the patient, she was asked to fill out a short form showing the date and length of time of the visit, defining new problems found and new tests or procedures ordered, and noting any consultations with the referring or other physician. (Data forms are available from us on request.) All patients referred to the nurses between Oct 1, 1973, and Dec 31, 1973, were the subjects of the study, and each patient in the study was followed up for three months following the initial nurse visit after Oct 1, 1973. Visits to the nurse were termed "nurse interim care" (NIC) visits.

At the end of the study period, records of the visits of all referred patients as well as the nurse's forms were reviewed by three of us (R.S., J.A., and P.M.) who were not directly involved in the care of these patients. The quality of the diagnostic, therapeutic, and supportive patient care was determined by consensus of the three of us after careful discussions. Our standards were T. R. Harrison's *Principles of Internal Medicine* (New York, McGraw-Hill Book Co., Inc., 1970) and the *Standard Practical Manual* of the Peter Bent Brigham Hospital (1973). Moreover, it was expected that the following information be appropriately recorded in the patient's chart: history, physical examination, interpretation of pertinent laboratory data (with consultation with the physician as necessary), as well as the appropriate data base and conclusions. Data and conclusions not in the record were considered to be not done or inadequate.[7]

Each patient served as his own control in measurements of the cost of individual patient care during the three-month period before a nurse was involved in the patient's care as compared with the three-month period of the study. The number of visits to the physician, cancellations and no visits to the physician and nurse, the number of nonscheduled visits as to the emergency room, and admissions to the hospital were the variables compared for the two three-month time periods.

RESULTS

A total of 403 NIC visits by 174 referred patients were studied, yielding an average of 2.3 visits per patient during the three-month study period. Ninety-three percent of NIC visits were handled by the five regular clinic nurses. Although an attempt was made to have each patient see the same nurse at each visit, 43 of the 107 patients with more than one visit to the nurse during the period of the study saw more than one nurse. Of the 59 patients with more than two visits to the nurses, seven saw more than two nurses. Seventy-eight of 115 clinic physicians referred patients for NIC visits. The types and problems referred for NIC visits are listed in

TABLE 16:1

No. and Cost of Visits per Patient

	Before Study	During Study
Scheduled visits to physician	1.63	1.18*
Nonscheduled visits	0.68	0.34*
Visits to nurse	—	2.32
Total visits	2.31	3.84†
Total cost of visits	$53.94	$66.76†

*Difference from previous column: $P < .05$ by both the Sign test and the paired t test.
†Difference from previous column: $P < .01$ by both the Sign test and paired t test.

the previous section. In 59% of all NIC visits, the nurse consulted either the referring physician (49%) or another physician (10%) such as the clinic director.

Quality of Care

We analyzed whether the nurse carried out the physician's orders as written and whether new problems were found and recorded. Our judgment was not involved in the analysis of these two questions. In the former case, 98% of the physician's orders were performed correctly, including one order that was obviously an error. In the latter case, 107 new problems were identified. The commonest new problem identified (13 of 107) was the incorrect taking of medications.

Questions involving judgment on our part included the appropriateness of the physician's referral and plan, the appropriateness of action taken on a new problem uncovered by the nurse, the soundness of the rationale used by the nurse for ordering tests on her own initiative, and the overall quality of care at a particular visit. Employing the strict criteria outlined above, physician's referrals were appropriate in 98% of NIC visits. Appropriate action was taken in 85% (91 of 107) of new problems uncovered by the nurse. This 85% figure for new problems differs significantly ($P < .001$; proportion comparison) from the 98% figure for old problems when appropriate action was taken on the physician's written plan. On 91 visits, the nurse ordered new laboratory tests. Thirty-five of these tests were ordered on the nurse's sole initiative, and only two of these were judged to have been unnecessary. Evaluation of overall quality of care at each visit suggested that the care was without detectable fault in 89% of the visits and inadequate in 11% of the visits. Inadequate care occurred for a variety of reasons: the physician's referral or plan were judged inappropriate, the physician's orders were not carried out correctly, or appropriate action was not taken on a new problem. In only 5 of 403 NIC visits was the quality of care judged poor.

Cost of Care

To measure the cost of caring for these patients before and during the nurse's involvement in the patient's care, only visits to the nurse, to the medical clinic physician, and nonscheduled visits (eg, to the emergency room) were included. The cost to the patient of visits to the physician was $23; to the nurse, $13; and for nonscheduled visits (as to the emergency room), $25. As indicated in the Table, the number of visits to the physician as well as nonscheduled visits both decreased significantly ($P < .05$) during the period of NIC care. However, the total number of visits and the total cost (charge) of caring for the 174 patients increased ($P < .01$). Since there was no significant difference in hospitalizations and in no-visit-plus-cancellation rates in the two study periods, these data were not included in the cost analysis.

The average length of time spent by the nurse per patient visit was 41 minutes, as determined from the forms filled out by the nurse.

COMMENT

This study has shown that nurses can be integrated into direct patient care in a large teaching hospital internal medicine clinic without difficulty, when there is close physician supervision. The nurse has been accepted by the clinic physicians, as shown by the 65% (75 of 115) of physicians who referred patients to the nurse during the three-month period of the study. The use of a physician's referral form, which listed the patient's problems, medications, and plan of care, allowed for a flexibility that would have been impossible with algorithms. On the other hand, the referral form committed the physician and nurse to a definite course of action.

Analysis of quality of care at each NIC visit employed judgmental as well as objective criteria. Questions involving no or minimal judgment by us included those concerned with whether or not the nurse carried out the physician's orders properly and whether new problems were uncovered. Questions involving judgment included those concerned with whether the nurse ordered laboratory tests on a rational basis, whether new problems were handled appropriately, and whether the overall quality of care was adequate. The answers to the latter questions depended on the presence or absence of data in the record or in the nursing forms.

The validity of such an analysis, however, is open to multiple potential criticisms. First, the nurses studied, although not volunteers, were aware that this study was in progress and, consequently, may have been excessively cautious. The very high consultation rate with the physicians (59%) may reflect this caution as well as the complexity of the patients' conditions or the lack of confidence by the nurses in themselves. Second, no comparison was made with care provided by the medical clinic physicians. This was not possible since the nurse provided only a part of the patient's overall care, and hence her role was not comparable to that of the physician. The quality of care provided by the physician at the clinic has been previously reported.[7] Third, *clinical outcomes were not measured* except for hospitalizations. The lack of feasibility and difficulty of such measurements in this type of study has been previously discussed.[4,5] For example, the commonest condition referred to the nurse was hypertension. To demonstrate differences in morbidity or mortality for groups of patients with hypertension followed up by either physicians or nurses might require years, given that the differences in quality of care between the two groups were small.[8,9] Moreover, current evidence suggests that long-term morbidity and mortality in hypertension are related to blood pressure control.[8] Therefore, observations on the adequacy of blood pressure control, such as those monitored in the present study, should correlate with outcome.

These reservations notwithstanding, certain conclusions were possible. In 98% of NIC visits, the nurses were able to carry out the physician's plan without detectable fault, including the ordering of laboratory tests, when necessary, on a rational basis. However, only 85% of visits during which the nurse detected a new problem for which there was no written plan by the physician were adequately handled. One unexpected problem with the referral system that may have caused some of the inadequate visits was the finding that 40% (43 of 107) of the patients who had more than one visit to the nurse saw different nurses.

To measure the cost (charge) to the patient (or society) of medical care in the period before and during the study, we assumed that our study population behaved as all other patients visiting the Peter Bent Brigham Hospital. If this assumption was correct, the differences in visit rates reported in the Table could not be explained by seasonal variations, and the decrease in the number of scheduled physician and nonscheduled visits can be ascribed to the new variable in the study period, the nurse.

The overall increase in the number of patient visits during the study period (Table 16:1) could be due to the discovery of the 107 new problems in the 174 patients, or to the insecurity on the part of new providers of care, whose anxiety over patient welfare resulted in a high return appointment rate, or to a relatively primitive state of trust between physicians and nurses. The data obtained in this study do not allow one to decide which, if any, of the above possible explanations was operative. Others have reported similar increases in patient visits.[2,9]

The cost of outpatient care to the patient (Table 16:1) in the study period was significantly greater (24%) than during the control period. The increased costs of care to the patient (or society) in the study period, as noted in Table 16:1 do not include the cost of the postgraduate training program (approximately $2,400/nurse), the cost of nursing supervision, the time spent by physicians in consultation with the nurses, or the relatively expensive cost of hospital overhead for nurse clinic areas. These costs were absorbed by the hospital but ultimately must be passed on to the consumer. Unless combined nurse-physician care was unequivocally superior to physician care, such an expense would not seem to be justified in our University Hospital if the cost of medical care is the only criterion employed. Although we did not specifically study this, other have shown that nurse-physician care is not superior to routine physician care.[4,5,9]

It is possible that the increased costs of patient care by nurses in this setting might be reduced by a change in the clinic organization or in the physicians' attitudes. However, even if the costs cannot be reduced, these increased costs may be justified if the goal of such nurse-clinician programs is to train nurses who will work in the clinic for a period of time in a capacity analogous to an internship, and then leave the hospital setting to work in areas where medical care is presently inadequate.

Michiko Spector aided with the data analysis and Madeline Faunce helped prepare this article.

Notes

1. Burrows B, Traver GA: Nurse practitioner programs. *Ann Intern Med* 80:268-269, 1974.

2. Lewis CE, Resnick BA: Nurse clinics and progressive ambulatory patient care. *N Engl J Med* 277:1236-1241, 1967.

3. Schulman J Jr, Wood C: Experience of a nurse practitioner in a general medical clinic. *JAMA* 219:1453-1461, 1972.

4. Spitzer WO, Sackett DL, Sibley JC, et al: The Burlington randomized trial of the nurse practioner: *N Engl J Med* 290:251-256, 1974.

5. Sackett DL, Spitzer WO, Gent M, et al: The Burlington randomized trial of the nurse practitioner. Health outcomes of patients. *Ann Intern Med* 80:137-142, 1974.

6. Walker JEC, Murowski BJ, Thorn GW: An experimental program in ambulatory medical care. *N Engl J Med* 271:63-86, 1964.

7. Goetzl EJ, Cohen P, Downing E, et al: Quality of diagnostic examinations in a university hospital outpatient clinic. *Ann Intern Med* 78:481-489, 1973.

8. Taguchi J, Freis ED: Partial reduction of blood pressure and prevention of complications in hypertension. *N Engl J Med* 291:329-331, 1974.

9. Gordon DW: Health maintenance service: Ambulatory patient care in the general medical clinic. *Med Care* 12:648-658, 1974.

Chapter 17

The Memphis Chronic Disease Program: Comparisons in Outcome and the Nurse's Extended Role

John W. Runyan, Jr.

IN PREVIOUS communications, the service program in Memphis and Shelby County (Tennessee) for the continuing care of patients with selected chronic diseases has been described.[1-3]

Since the report in 1970,[2] more than 140,000 patient-visits to the decentralized facilities have been made, and patients under regular care now exceed 9,000. The number of urban and rural neighborhood and satellite clinics, which are operated by the Health Department, has been increased to 20, with several more planned.

Although the main efforts have been service oriented and directed toward meeting the medical needs of a large chronically diseased population, some measurements of the effectiveness and acceptability of continuing care to patients in the program and its effects on the course of the chronic illness have been presented recently.[3] This report extends these observations but is primarily concerned with making certain comparisons between patients receiving care in decentralized facilities staffed by specially trained nurses and those rendered care in a more conventional manner in the outpatient clinics of the City of Memphis Hospital.

PATIENTS AND CLINIC SETTINGS

These observations were made on two groups of patients with combinations of three conditions: diabetes mellitus, hypertension, or cardiac disease. The group who received their maintenance medical care principally

in the decentralized facilities is called the "study group" and those who received their care in the hospital outpatient clinics are referred to as the "control group." Included in the first group were the 1,006 patients transferred from the hospital clinics to the decentralized facilities located closest to their home over a period of a year beginning Sept 1, 1969; the 498 patients who comprised the second group included all patients who met the following criteria: they had adequate records, sufficient duration of observations, the observations had been made in the same period in a hospital outpatient clinic for chronic disease, and the clinic was staffed by internists. Patients in the hospital outpatient clinic (the medical facility most convenient to their home) had been referred for continuing care after their conditions had been stabi-

Table 1.—Population Characteristics

	No. of Patients	
	Study Group* (n = 1,006)	Control Group† (n = 498)
Men	231	124
Women	775	374
Diabetes‡	797	410
Hypertension‡	515	409
Cardiac disease‡	555	226

*Maintenance care principally in decentralized facilities; mean age of patients, 59 years (range 12 to 93).
†Maintenance care principally in the hospital clinic; mean age of patients, 64 years (range, 15 to 94).
‡The sum of these numbers exceeds the total patients because of multiple diseases in the same patient.

Table 2.—Diabetes-Cardiac Disease-Hypertension Category— Diastolic Blood Pressure in the Study and Control Groups (mm Hg)

Age Group, yr	Study Group					Control Group				
	Mean Before Transfer	SE	Mean† Change	SE	P‡ Value	Mean Before Transfer	SE	Mean Change	SE	P Value
30-39 No.	92.0 3	3.4	18.7	4.7	NS	... 1	...	...	...	...
40-49 No.	103.0 17	3.8	−13.6	4.2	<.01	95.0 8	3.9	−2.3	3.5	NS
50-59 No.	95.8 45	2.1	−7.1	2.7	<.02	95.9 35	2.8	0.5	2.7	NS
60-69 No.	92.4 52	1.7	−7.3	2.1	<.01	88.5 38	1.8	0.3	2.6	NS
70-79 No.	84.1 27	2.7	−6.2	2.9	<.05	86.1 44	2.4	0.8	2.4	NS
Over 80 No.	90.0 6	6.7	−18.7	8.2	NS	80.4 15	4.1	−0.8	3.8	NS
Mean age, yr No.	61.2 162	0.9				66.4 143	0.9			

*No patients in age group 10 to 29 years had blood pressure data analyzed.
†Probability of a mean change this different from zero; NS indicates not significant at the .05 level.
‡Mean change derived from after-transfer minus before-transfer blood pressure, mm Hg.

From the Division of Health Care Sciences, departments of medicine and community medicine, University of Tennessee College of Medicine, Memphis.
Reprint requests to 800 Madison Ave, Box GA150, Memphis, TN 38163 (Dr. Runyan).

Reprinted from the *Journal of the American Medical Association*, January 20, 1975, Volume 231. Copyright 1975, American Medical Association.

Table 3.—Analysis of Age-Adjusted Changes in Diastolic Blood Pressure and Blood Glucose—All Patients

Disease Categories	No. of Patients		Blood Pressure		Blood Glucose	
	Study	Control	F Value*	P	F Value	P
Diabetes only	94	20	...	...	13.11	<.001
Hypertension only	139	36	31.14	<.001	...	...
Diabetes-cardiac disease	14	26	...	...	0.05	NS†
Diabetes-hyper-tension	132	17	...	...	4.37	<.05
	158	26	6.87	<.025	...	...
Cardiac disease-hypertension	216	194	21.27	<.001	...	...
Diabetes-cardiac disease-hyper-tension	123	114	...	...	0.17	NS
	150	141	15.87	<.001	...	...

*With significant F values, the study group reductions in blood glucose and blood pressure were always greater than those in the control group.
†NS indicates not significant at the .05 level.

Table 4.—Hospital Days per 1,000 Patients per Year

	Study			Control		
	Before	After	% Change*	Before	After	% Change
Diabetes	3,319	1,680	−49.4	1,261	2,107	+67.1
Hypertension	2,509	1,196	−52.3	1,966	2,671	+35.9
Cardiac disease	3,074	1,560	−49.3	2,129	3,084	+44.9
Total	3,439	1,603	−53.4	2,499	3,573	+43.0

*Percent change = ([after value − before value]/[before value]) × 100.

Table 5.—Total Hospital Days—Analysis by Age Decades, Study vs Control

Age Decade	Study			Control		
	Before	After	% Change	Before	After	% Change
10-29	204	77	−62.3	60	155	+158.3
30-39	486	210	−56.8	80	169	+111.3
40-49	864	256	−70.4	271	167	−38.4
50-59	1,370	725	−47.1	504	471	−6.5
60-69	1,383	680	−50.8	602	707	+17.4
70-79	797	365	−54.2	597	1,199	+100.8
Over 80	321	138	−57.0	236	274	+16.1

RESULTS

Clinic Visits and Professional Contacts

As previously reported, professional contacts increased in frequency in the study group after transfer from the medical center to decentralized facilities with home visits. In contrast, clinic visits were found to decrease after the transfer date in the control group, with 6,488 visits/1,000 patients/yr before transfer and 5,503 visits after transfer. Accurate information on emergency room use is not available for the control group, but in the study group this use decreased.

Blood Glucose and Diastolic Blood Pressure Levels

We analyzed the data relating to diastolic blood pressure and blood glucose for patients in the following disease groups: hypertension only, diabetes only, diabetes-cardiac disease, diabetes-hypertension, hypertension-cardiac disease, and diabetes-cardiac disease-hypertension.

The method of analysis of the data relating to diastolic blood pressure and blood glucose is illustrated by Table 2, which gives the data on diastolic blood pressure for the diabetes-cardiac disease-hypertension category of patients. The mean blood pressures prior to transfer and the mean changes in blood pressure following transfer are shown by age decades. The mean change in blood pressure is calculated from the patients' distribution of after-transfer values minus before-transfer values. Hence, a negative (−) value for mean change shows that the patients, on the average, had a lower blood pressure after transfer. The standard errors (SEs) of the means are also shown. The P values indicate whether the mean changes within a particular

lized in various other clinics in the hospital. Some had been participants in phase three drug-evaluation studies (antihypertensive and antidiabetic drugs) in the past. None of the patients was a participant at the time of these evaluations. The first clinic visit in the year beginning Sept 1, 1969, was considered the reference date or point of "transfer" of the patients. Observations extend for two years before and after transfer. As the need arose, both study and control patients were referred to the various hospital speciality clinics or to the General Medicine Clinic if a detailed reevaluation was indicated.

The two populations were of similar socioeconomic backgrounds, with comparable men-to-women ratios (Table 1). Hypertension was more prevalent in the control group while cardiac disease was more prevalent in the study group. The mean age of the study group was 59 years and of the control group, 64 years. Because of the frequent occurrence of multiple diseases in the same patients and in-

complete data on some patients, the totals in the analysis of blood pressure and blood glucose vary from the figures given in Table 1.

STATISTICAL METHODS

Preliminary testing indicated minimal base-line variable differences between the study and control groups and also few differences by sex. Consequently, all comparisons were made with men and women combined. However, there were significant differences in age in some of the patient subgroups and to allow for these, age-adjusted comparisons were made. Our major interest was in the analysis of variable changes, ie, after-transfer values minus before-transfer values in the study and control groups. The significance of these variable changes within the two groups by decades of age was tested with the paired t test. Age-adjusted comparisons of variable changes in the study and control groups were made by the analysis of covariance with patient age as the control variable.

age decade differ significantly from zero.

Table 2 shows that the study group of patients in all age decades except the 30- to 39-year-old age group (only three patients) had lower blood pressures after transfer and that these reductions were significant in all ages except among those 30 to 39 and over 80 years of age. In the control group blood pressures were reduced among those 40 to 49 and over 80 years of age, but none of the changes differed significantly from zero. Overall, the control group was significantly older than the study group ($P < .05$).

The data for the variable changes in Table 2 and for the other five disease groups listed above are summarized in Table 3, which shows the age-adjusted comparisons between the study and control groups.

Table 3 shows that study patients with hypertension disease always experienced significantly greater age-adjusted reductions in diastolic blood pressure as compared to the control subjects. Reductions in blood glucose levels were found in the study group in all disease categories that included diabetes when compared to control subjects, but the F values were only significant in two disease categories: diabetes and diabetes-hypertension.

Hospital Inpatient Utilization

The number of hospital days/1,000 patients/yr for patients in each disease category in the study group for the two-year period before transfer was greater than in the control group (Table 4). In the two-year period after transfer, the study group, who were provided maintenance care in decentralized facilities, utilized approximately 50% fewer hospital days, while the control group showed an increase in hospital days for each disease category. The data relating to total hospital days in the study and control groups by age decades are shown in Table 5 and the age-adjusted changes are shown in Table 6. The analysis of the changes in hospital utilization (Table 6) after transfer in the study group showed that utilization was reduced in all age decades, whereas the control group only experienced reductions in the 40- to 59-year-old age groups.

For an overall comparison of the two groups, we tested the age-adjusted changes in hospital utilization by the analysis of covariance with the age of each patient as a control value (Table 5). The changes consisted of the number of hospital days after transfer minus before transfer hospital days in the study and control groups. This calculation showed that in all three main disease categories, the study patients had significantly reduced hospitalization compared to the controls.

Primary Causes for Hospital Utilization

The three major disease categories—hypertension, diabetes, and cardiac disease—were examined without regard to associated diseases (Table 7). We analyzed the data in these broad categories because of the relatively small numbers of patients hospitalized when broken down into the previously analyzed categories plus cardiac disease only. For the study group, some of these data in a different form have been presented but without the control group data. In the study group with *diabetes*, hospital days devoted to the categories of (1) diabetic acidosis and severe infections, and (2) peripheral vascular disease and amputations declined (61% and 68%, respectively) after transfer, while in the control group the number of hospital days for the first category

increased 17% and for the second category, decreased 13%. Number of hospital days resulting from vascular and renal diseases increased in both study and control groups but increased to a greater extent in the control group. In the study group with *hypertension*, hospital days for stroke, organic heart disease, and congestive heart failure decreased after transfer, while an increase occurred in the control group. Both study and control groups showed an increase in hospital utilization after transfer for patients with renal insufficiency and myocardial infarction. In those with *cardiac disease*, hospital utilization in the study group for organic heart disease and congestive heart failure decreased after transfer, while a significant increase in hospital utilization occurred in the control group. Also, hospital days for

Table 6.—Total Hospital Days— Analysis of Age-Adjusted Changes, Study vs Control

Disease Group	No. of Patients		F* Value	P
	Study	Control		
Diabetes	223	103	24.73	<.001
Hypertension	271	170	17.09	<.001
Cardiac disease	205	181	18.44	<.001

* The F values reflect a greater decrease in hospital utilization in the study patients following transfer.

Table 7.—Hospital Days per 1,000 Patients per Year

	Study			Control		
	Before	After	% Change	Before	After	% Change
Diabetes						
All causes	3,319	1,680	−49.4	2,728	4,838	+77.3
Diabetic acidosis-infections	900	350	−61.1	587	688	+17.2
Peripheral vascular disease and amputation	626	201	−67.9	436	379	−13.1
Renal, cardiovascular	388	505	+30.2	355	1,523	+329.0
Hypertension						
All causes	2,509	1,196	−52.3	2,395	3,238	+35.2
Stroke	281	102	−63.7	72	201	+179.2
Myocardial infarction	54	56	+3.7	80	239	+198.8
Renal	56	139	+148.2	0	93	...
Organic heart disease and congestive heart failure	136	131	−3.7	411	699	+70.1
Cardiac disease						
All causes	3,074	1,560	−49.3	2,594	3,739	+44.1
Myocardial infarction	89	87	−2.2	80	269	+236.3
Renal	87	216	+148.3	0	60	...
Organic heart disease and congestive heart failure	366	221	−39.6	465	857	+84.3

myocardial infarction increased in the control group.

Mortality

Although a two-year period of observation has limited value in terms of mortality data, 7% of the study population and 11% of the control population died in this period. As would be expected, those 70 years of age and older had the higher death rates in both study and control populations. However, there were no statistically significant differences in death rates in the two populations when examined by age decades.

COMMENT

A number of factors may have contributed to some of the differences in the measurements, observations, and patient-care experiences in the two populations with combinations of the three conditions: diabetes, hypertension, and cardiac disease. Were the study and control populations dissimilar enough to account for these differences? The mean age in the control group was significantly higher than that in the study group. However, comparisons were made by age decade and analysis of covariance that removed age differences as a factor in the observed outcome. On the other hand, in examining some of the clinical features of the diabetic population in the preceding two years, it was seen that incidence of a history of diabetic acidosis and amputations was higher in the study group than in the control group; also, the study group had higher blood glucose levels before transfer and more days spent in the hospital. In both the *hypertensive and cardiac disease* populations, hospital utilization was greater for the two-year period before transfer in the study group than in the control group. Hospital utilization for renal disease with its recognized relationship to both diabetes and hypertension was more prevalent in the study population before transfer. Although the problems of relating two populations with multiple risk factors are recognized, the data do not suggest that the study population were at less risk than the control population, and there is evidence that the opposite may have been the case.

Those in the study group received maintenance care in decentralized facilities by nurses, and therefore, several factors were introduced that are considered to have favored the outcomes observed. Professional care and advice are easier for the patients to obtain when the barrier to care of a rigid appointment system, characteristic of the hospital clinic, is removed. Patients are given the opportunity to call, if in need of medical assistance, and appropriate advice is given or home visits are made, if found advisable. During 1973, more than 8,000 home visits to these chronically diseased patients were made. The same medical protocols and opportunities to obtain selected laboratory tests prevail whether the patient is seen in the decentralized clinic or home. Missed appointments are followed up. Drugs are actually dispensed directly to the patient when being seen by the nurse, which gives the opportunity for patient education and counseling, and it is believed that patient compliance is greatly enhanced as a result. Goals of therapy for hypertension and diabetes and the means to achieve them are stipulated in the protocols used by the nurses. Physicians' attitudes toward hypertensive therapy have been commented on,[6] even though the benefits of therapy have generally been recognized since reports of the Veterans Administration study on hypertension conducted by Freis.[7,8] In in-service training sessions and the protocols, the early recognition of cardiac failure and digitalis intoxication with appropriate follow-up action is emphasized to the nurses, and this factor may contribute to the favorable experience with patients with cardiac disease in the study group. Prevention of diabetes and essential hypertension is not a reality at present. Control of these diseases, which is possible but not always attained in a public hospital setting, leads to a reduction in those complications that are associated with increased mortality, morbidity, and hospital utilization.[9] The Memphis Chronic Disease Continuing Care Program makes available to patients in a systematic manner the basics of good medical practices: accessibility

to care, patient education and counseling, follow-up, home visits, selected effective medications, laboratory test monitoring at intervals, realistic goals of therapy, and appropriate referrals and contacts with the back-up physicians and the medical center.

The observations in this report give further support to the concept introduced nearly 12 years ago that nurses can effectively share a large and increasing responsibility in chronic disease care. In the EDITORIAL in THE JOURNAL[3] relating to the Memphis Program, the question was asked "should the nurse, even after special training, have this much autonomy in the regulation of uncontrolled glycosuria, the delicate balancing of blood pressure between too high and too low with potent antihypertensive drugs and the adjustment of digitalis dosage?" With detailed protocols and physician and medical-center back-up, the data presented here indicate that this question can be answered in the affirmative.

These investigations were supported in part by a grant from the Robert Wood Johnson Foundation.

George S. Lovejoy, MD, Director of the Memphis and Shelby County Health Department and the staff of City of Memphis Hospital, helped in program development and collection of data. Marion G. Baker assembled the data. Harry Robinson, ScD, assisted with statistics.

References

1. Guthrie N, Runyan JW, Clark J, et al: The clinical nursing conferences: A preliminary report. N Engl J Med 270:1411-1413, 1964.
2. Runyan JW, Phillips WE, Herring O, et al: A program for the care of patients with chronic diseases. JAMA 211:476-479, 1970.
3. Physician's assistant or assistant physician?, editorial. JAMA 212:313, 1970.
4. Runyan JW: Physicians' assistants: Nurses as physicians, letter to the editor. JAMA 213:1037, 1970.
5. Runyan JW: Decentralized medical care of chronic disease. Trans Assoc Am Physicians 83:237-244, 1973.
6. Stokes JB, Payne GH, Cooper T: Hypertension: The challenge of patient education. N Engl J Med 28:1369-1370, 1973.
7. Effects of treatment on morbidity in hypertension: Results in patients with diastolic pressures averaging 115 through 129 mm Hg, Veterans Administration Cooperative Study Group on Anti-hypertensive Agents. JAMA 202:1028-1034, 1967.
8. Effects of treatment on morbidity in hypertension: II. Results in patients with diastolic blood pressures averaging 90 through 114 mm Hg, Veterans Administration Cooperative Study Group on Anti-hypertensive Agents. JAMA 213:1143-1152, 1970.
9. Miller LV, Goldstein J: More efficient care of diabetic patients in a county-hospital setting. N Engl J Med 286:1388-1391, 1972.

Chapter 18
Nurse-Staffed Decentralized Care of Diabetes at Frontier Nursing Service: Clinical Outcomes

Karen A. Gordon and Gertrude Isaacs

Cost, inaccessibility and the discontinuous nature of medical services remain unresolved problems for many chronically ill persons. Complications of chronic illnesses account for a substantial proportion of costly hospitalization throughout the nation—a situation that might be changed by providing ongoing ambulatory care and health maintenance.

This chapter describes decentralized services provided primarily by nurses at Frontier Nursing Service (FNS)* in Southeastern Kentucky and their impact of reducing the hospitalization rate of diabetic patients. The findings of significantly reduced average hospitalization for such patients at the Frontier Nursing Service support the results reported in studies of decentralized ambulatory services in Los Angeles County and Memphis (Shelby County), Tennessee.[1]

THE FNS DECENTRALIZED SYSTEM OF HEALTH CARE

Fifty years ago, FNS was developed as a decentralized health care system to bring basic medical care to an economically depressed area of Appalachia where none existed.

FNS consists of the new 40-bed Mary Breckinridge Hospital in Hyden and six satellite clinics each serving 300-400 families. The total population served of approximately 15,000 is widely scattered throughout a mountainous two-county region. Once reached only by horseback, the satellite clinics are now within a 40-60 minute jeep ride from Hyden. The district health care system was established in 1925 by Mary Breckinridge, to meet the county's basic health needs in maternal and child health and infectious diseases. Traditionally, FNS has been

*FNS is assisted by a PRIMEX Grant No. HS 00885 by the National Center for Health Services Research, USPHS, DHEW, Rockville, Maryland; and through a grant from The Robert Wood Johnson Foundation, Princeton, New Jersey. The opinions, conclusions and proposals are those of the authors, and do not necessarily represent the National Center for Health Services Research or The Robert Wood Johnson Foundation.

staffed by nurse-midwives who still form the nucleus of the service. In 1969, a Family Nurse Practitioner (PRIMEX) program was initiated to augment the training in midwifery. The backbone of the system is the FNS *Medical Directives,* first written in 1928 by physicians and nurses and now in its seventh edition.[2] These detailed protocols for a variety of illnesses enable the nurse to diagnose, treat and dispense medication through the FNS pharmacy system. The *Medical Directives,* used by nurses and physicians alike, contribute to consistency in care.

A recent study of the distribution of FNS services until 1975 showed approximately 40 percent provided in an outpatient hospital clinic, 30 percent in district clinics, and 30 percent in home health services.[3] In 1974 there were a total of 29,969 district clinic and home visits and 24,535 hospital clinic visits. Preliminary findings from a 1974 utilization study indicate that essentially similar services are provided in district clinics and in the hospital, but that hospital services are sought more frequently for acute problems and complications resulting from chronic ailments.

available through a 24-hour telephone or two-way radio consultation and referral with the hospital and monthly physician-conducted clinics at each outpost. Medical problems requiring the attention of a specialist are referred to medical centers such as the University of Kentucky Medical Center. Notable features of the FNS system are the on-call coverage, flexible clinic schedules and home visiting—all adopted to eliminate a rigid appointment system.

Each outpost satellite clinic is a self-contained living and health care facility. Each outpost staff consists of family nurses and/or RNs, a secretary and a health aide. The aide is from the local community but receives her training at FNS. Each clinic has a stockroom, waiting room, laboratory, office, and one or more examining rooms. Sufficient drugs, supplies and equipment are provided for simple diagnostic treatment and laboratory procedures. The nurses are supplied with jeeps, which are needed to reach the most remote families located in the narrow hollows. In this part of Kentucky the majority of residents do not have telephones or transportation. Thus, home visiting is a vital feature of the decentralized system, and a major element in the follow-up of chronically ill patients. For example, of 2,271 outpatient diabetic visits in 1974, 78 percent were conducted in the district outpost clinics or in the home (see Table 18:1). The larger proportion of home visits have proved to be an important ingredient in providing continuity of care.

Since there are no nursing homes in the area and only a few extended care facilities in neighboring Harlan and Hazard, these home visits permit accessible continuous service for the elderly chronically ill patient. In

1974 alone, 60 percent of the medical care for the elderly was provided through home visits, with only 12 percent having to be hospitalized. The nurses make home visits to follow up on routine problems, administer specific treatment in unusual situations when the individual cannot come to the district clinic or when a patient fails to show for an appointment.

DECENTRALIZED CARE OF DIABETICS

During home or clinic visits by diabetics, routine procedures include a partial physical, urine check, and discussion of any medical problems and diet. For permanently home-bound patients, periodic blood samples are drawn as required. For more extensive laboratory work, the patient must go either to the hospital outpatient clinic or have a sample sent into the central laboratory, where the results can be telephoned to the district nurse.

Although the average diabetic has approximately 11 clinic or home visits per year, diabetics with multiple chronic diseases or chronic acute infections have 15-20 annual encounters. Much of the treatment, regardless of the complexity of the diabetes, is directed at coping with day-to-day problems of being chronically ill. The importance of the nurse's visit in the clinical management of diabetes lies in the social support provided and in the early recognition of abnormal developments that require referral to more extensive medical facilities. Patients with debilitating problems are visited every two to three weeks. The majority of diabetics are scheduled for routine six-week check-ups. The time of a home visit ranges from 45 minutes to 1-1/2 hours during which social conversation and support-giving are important features in the FNS approach to care for the chronically ill. In an activity study undertaken in 1974, "social conversation" and "therapeutic listening" appeared in 86 percent of the home visits sampled.[4] Social conversation may include discussion of the individual and his family, the garden and news of other neighbors. How well the patient is following a diet or medication regimen is often determined in this manner. Because the patient is in familiar surroundings, open communication is more readily established with the nurse who is able to observe the conditions under which the patient lives. Embarrassing explanations of limited personal resources or incapacity for managing health problems can be avoided. This kind of communication is important in building rapport with the patient, an essential component in helping patients feel confident to assume greater responsibility for the management of their diabetes.

METHODOLOGY

The method used in this study to obtain information about the effectiveness of decentralized ambulatory care of diabetics was the tracer condition, which looks at how well the needs are met of an identified population with a clinical disease.[5] Diabetes was selected as the tracer condition for this study because the diabetic requires continuous, comprehensive care; and the treatment requires a discrete set of services, resources and personnel. Although diabetes cannot be cured, morbidity and mortality from related complications can be reduced. For example, if services are not very effective or utilization is poor, one can expect an increase in diabetes-related complications and a progression of functional disabilities such as blindness. On a broader level, assessing the effectiveness of services for a given chronic disease can have implications for other chronic disease programs.

The study population was defined as those diabetics who had at least one FNS encounter in 1974. Data on ambulatory patients were collected through computerized encounter records. At each encounter, the provider filled out a form that described the status, location, type and reason for the visit; diagnosis; treatment, services and drugs prescribed; type of provider(s) and source of payment. Twenty-five percent of all medical records of the diabetic patients were abstracted to verify the information on the encounter form, and 89 percent of those abstracts were found to verify pertinent data on the encounter forms. Data on the hospitalized patients were obtained through the Professional Activity Study (PAS) system. All 25 medical records of persons admitted with diabetes mellitus or diabetic acidosis were reviewed for verification, and 23 of the PAS abstracts were found to reproduce the data in the medical records.

The record system is uniform with one medical record number assigned to each patient for district outpatient clinics and the hospital. If a patient who is registered at one of the district clinics is seen at the hospital outpatient clinic, a copy of the clinic notes are sent to the district nurse who places them in the patient's chart. A separate chart for the patient is kept at the hospital. Both the medical and nursing staff use a modification of the problem-oriented SOAP (subjective, objective, assessment, plan) record.

RESULTS

The Diabetic Population at FNS

At FNS, diabetes is the third most common chronic illness (the other two are arteriosclerotic heart disease and hypertension). A total of 239

TABLE 18:1

Ambulatory Encounters for Diabetics by Location, 1974

Location	Number of Encounters	%
Total	2,271	100
Hospital clinic	507	22.3
District clinic	1,508	66.4
Home	256	11.7

persons were treated for diabetes through FNS in 1974. Since FNS is virtually the only source of primary care, this number was determined to be a rough estimate of the number of diabetics in the FNS area. An additional 30 persons were being followed by two other clinics located on the periphery of the FNS area, ten of whom also used the services of FNS. Since the total population in the FNS area is approximately 15,000, the estimated prevalence rate of 2 percent is comparable to the national figure.

The FNS diabetic population has a two-to-one ratio of women to men; the mean age of both groups is 58 years with a range of 6-91 years. The majority of the 239 diabetics had one other chronic disease; of all encounters, 43.3 percent were for multiple problems including acute illnesses. Thirty-seven percent had hypertension, 16 percent had obesity, and 3.3 percent were both hypertensive and obese. Nineteen percent of the diabetics also had arteriosclerotic heart disease.

The most frequent type of diabetic encounter in the district and outpatient facilities was for routine checkups with the majority (84 percent) seen in district clinics. A total of 2,271 visits directly related to the diabetic condition were made in all three ambulatory settings (hospital clinic, district outpost clinic, or the home). A majority of diabetics was seen by a team or combination of providers; thus 14 percent were seen by a physician and nurse or family nurse, while 77 percent were managed by nurses and aides only. Physicians were present at 50 percent of encounters in the hospital outpatient clinic, but in district clinics physicians were present during only 0.03 percent of the encounters. (Table 18:2).

Reduced Hospitalization for Diabetes

A total of 63 diabetics were hospitalized in 1974. Within this group, 22 were hospitalized with the primary diagnosis of diabetes mellitus and three with the diagnosis of diabetic acidosis. Thirty-eight diabetics were hospitalized with other primary diagnoses. Together, these diagnoses

TABLE 18:2

Encounters for Diabetes by Type of Provider, 1974

Type of Provider Present	Number	%
Total	2,271	100.0
Physician/Nurse Team	310	14.0
RN and/or Family nurse, aides	1,741	77.0
Other provider (e.g., social worker, pharmacist)	210	9.0

TABLE 18:3

Age Distribution of all Diabetics, and all Hospital Discharges Compared
with Diabetics Discharged, 1974

	Age Distribution of Diabetics		Total Hospital Discharges		Hospital Discharges for Diabetics	
	No.	Percent	No.	Percent	No.	Percent
Total	239	100%	2,088	100%	63	100%
Years						
0-15	6	3%	623	30%	3	5%
16-64	149	62	1,211	58	33	52
65+	84	35	254	12	27	43

constituted 3 percent of 2,088 discharges at the Mary Breckinridge Hospital in 1974 and 367 days of care (3.7 percent of total patient days). Three diabetic patients, one a pregnant mother, were transferred to other hospitals for more extensive treatment or rehabilitation, and 22 were discharged with specific plans of care to be carried out under home health care supervision by the district nurses.

The average length of stay for diabetic patients with single and multiple problems was 6 days with a range of 1-22 days. Patients discharged with the single diagnosis of diabetes mellitus averaged 4.3 days compared to the national average of 7.2 days; patients discharged with multiple problems averaged 8.7 days, compared to the national average of 11.2 days.[6] Forty-three percent of the discharged diabetics were 65 years and over. Five percent of the discharged diabetics were under age 15. (Table 18:3).

The days of hospitalization for diabetics averaged 1.6 days per diabetic patient at FNS in 1974, which is about the same as the average number of hospital days per year for the general population nationally.[7] The low hospitalization for FNS diabetic patients compares favorably with the results achieved at the University of Southern California Los Angeles Medical Center, which reported an average number of 1.7 days in hospital per year for each diabetic clinic patient[8] and is exactly the same as the figure for diabetic patients served by nurse practitioners in the Memphis Chronic Disease Program[9] in contrast to the national average of 5.4 days of hospitalization for the diabetic patient.[10] These results indicate that programs providing accessible decentralized ambulatory nurse-staffed services effectively reduce hospitalization, whether in rural or urban areas.[11] Good follow-up and continuous care appear to reduce unnecessary and lengthy hospitalizations.

Cost for Care

Another benefit of decentralized nurse-staffed care may be cost savings. The average cost to the patient in a district clinic or in the home, of $5.80 is considerably less than the $13.63 at the average hospital outpatient clinic. Average visit costs are slightly higher for diabetics—$10.69 at district clinics and $12-14 at the hospital outpatient clinic where more extensive laboratory work and dispensing of medications from the central pharmacy account for the higher charges.

Through achievement of low hospitalization of diabetics, a considerable saving is made both to the institution and to the patient. On a yearly basis, the average cost per diabetic at FNS is $309 (11 outpatient visits at $11/visit/year plus an average of 1.6 days of hospitalization at $118/day = $309). The average of 1.6 days of hospitalization per diabetic per year at FNS is 70 percent lower than the national diabetic average of 5.4 days.[12] This represents a savings of $448 in hospitalization alone,* excluding the cost of outpatient medical care. Such savings should be of interest to third-party payers, state or federal agencies, to diabetics who pay for their services, and to institutions—frequently rural agencies that are reimbursed at less than cost.

DISCUSSION AND CONCLUSIONS

The achievement of lower hospitalization for diabetic patients through nurse-staffed service programs in Los Angeles County, Memphis (Shelby County), and at FNS illustrate the effectiveness of medical services when organized into a comprehensive system. In the Los Angeles program,

---

*$118/ hospital day was compared to the cost/hospital day in community hospitals.

marked reductions in admissions for diabetics were noted after the implementation in 1969 of a program of patient education, a telephone answering service, and the screening of potential admissions by a nurse-practitioner and a hospital resident. In Shelby County a program was initiated in 1963 to provide care for diabetics, and others with selected chronic illnesses, in decentralized clinic facilities, using nurse practitioners working with medical protocols and medical facility backup.[13]

The experience at FNS and the achievements of the Memphis and Los Angeles programs highlight a number of misconceptions concerning the organization and provision of primary and specialty medical services. First, the distinctions often made between urban and rural populations when designing programs are questionable when one looks at clinical needs. Whether they live in urban or rural areas, chronically ill patients have similar health care needs and similar difficulties in obtaining readily accessible services at prices they can afford. Both rural and core urban areas traditionally face shortages of primary health care manpower, and these shortages have a greater impact on those with limited resources. Second, as demonstrated by the FNS and Memphis programs, indigent patients with chronic disease need not receive less comprehensive care nor experience more frequent and lengthy hospitalizations than the general population—a situation frequently excused as inevitable and at high cost to the tax payer. Third, the FNS and Memphis programs demonstrate that effective day-to-day health care can be managed by specially trained nurses who are supported by medical backup and protocols. Fourth, the Memphis and FNS experiences suggest that decentralized care is viable in urban and rural areas alike. Common factors in the achievement and maintenance of low hospitalization rates are the organization of resources, personnel and services into a unified system of primary care, referral, and health education.

Broader issues requiring the attention of providers and legislators are reimbursement and funding policies of governmental, third party and voluntary organizations. Current reimbursement mechanisms are organized and categorized in a manner that perpetuates sporadic medical services. The categories of care which may be reimbursed are highly restrictive. Thus it becomes difficult for an agency dependent on reimbursement to remain responsive to the continuing needs of the chronically ill patients. Furthermore, categorical funding promotes programs that are unwieldy to implement and costly to manage.

FNS is one demonstration of a decentralized nurse-staffed system as an effective method of reducing costly hospitalization and bringing primary care services closer to the public.

Notes

1. J. W. Runyan, "The Memphis Chronic Disease Program," *JAMA* 231 (1975), 264-267; L. Miller, and J. Goldstein, "More Efficient Care of Diabetic Patients in a County-Hospital Setting," *New England Journal of Medicine* 84 (1973), 237-1391;

   J.W. Runyan, "Decentralized Medical Care of Chronic Disease," *The Transactions of the Association of American Physicians* 84 (1973), 237-44.

2. *Medical Directives* (7th edition), Hyden, Kentucky: The Frontier Nursing Service, Inc., 1975.

3. G. Isaacs, "The Dilemma of a Primary Health Care Agency in a Medically Oriented Society," Paper Presented at the International Health Conference, the National Council for International Health; 1975 (publication forthcoming).

4. F. Golladay, and K. Smith, "Efficient Health Manpower Utilization Project: A Description of Practice Activity at the Frontier Nursing Service," Health Economics Research Center, University of Wisconsin, 1974.

5. D.M. Kessner, and C. Kalk, "A Strategy for Evaluating Health Services," *Contrast in Health Status,* Volume 2, Health Services Research Study, (Washington, D.C.; Institute of Medicine, National Academy of Sciences, 1973), p. 5.

6. Commission on Professional and Hospital Activities, *Length of Stay in PAS Hospitals, United States, 1974,* Ann Arbor, Michigan, October, 1975.

7. Ibid.

8. Miller and Goldstein, op. cit.

9. Runyan, "The Memphis Chronic Disease Program," op. cit.

10. United States National Center for Health Statistics, Washington, D.C.: Government Printing Office, 1967, *Characteristics of Persons with Diabetes: United States—July 1964—June 1965* (Publication No. 1000, series 10, No. 40), p. 9.

11. Runyan, "The Memphis Chronic Disease Program," op. cit., and "Decentralized Medical Care of Chronic Disease," op. cit., and Miller and Goldstein, op. cit.

12. United States National Center for Health Statistics, op. cit., p. 9.

13. Runyan, "Decentralized Medical Care of Chronic Disease," op. cit., and "The Memphis Chronic Disease Program," op. cit.

Chapter 19

Quality of PA Performance at a Health Maintenance Organization

Jane Cassels Record, Arnold V. Hurtado and Joan E. O'Bannon

The unmarked trails and hazards of the quality landscape are widely respected by students of health care. Yet the very concept of substitutability assumes that a shifting of services from MDs to PAs does not result in quality deterioration. The five PAs who practice in the Medical Department of the Kaiser-Permanente system in metropolitan Portland, Oregon are fully credentialed. All five are graduates of the Duke University PA program and are licensed under the Oregon state PA law. For a description of the setting in which they practice, see the earlier chapter entitled, "Physician Supervision of PAs: How Much is Enough and What Does it Cost?"

To test the PAs' performance, comparative data have been developed on processes, outcomes, and patient complaints. The process and outcome data will be discussed first.* For selecting the morbidities to be studied, the following criteria were used: (1) having high frequency, (2) being within the PA competence range, (3) being sufficiently easy to define so that nonhomogeneity probably could be reduced to a satisfactory level, (4) having well-established diagnosis and treatment procedures, and (5) having measurable outcomes reasonably well related to the quality of diagnosis and treatment. Four morbidities which seemed to meet these criteria were chosen: strep throat, coryza-upper respiratory infection (URI), bursitis and bronchitis. Data in the 5 percent sample include information about patient characteristics, the kind of patient encounter and its setting, the diagnosis and treatment procedures (process indices) used and certain kinds of outcomes. Data were retrieved on age

*The authors are indebted to Merwyn R. Greenlick, Ph.D. for general counsel. The process and outcome measures used here were chosen primarily by Dr. Hurtado, as preface to a more comprehensive, long-term study of quality which Dr. Hurtado, Dr. Greenlick and J. David Bristow, MD, are developing at the Center. The research described here was funded by HMEIA Contract No1-MD-44173(P), Bureau of Health Manpower, Health Resources Administration, HEW.

and sex of the patient; type of appointment—whether regularly scheduled, walk-in or emergency room (ER); status of the provider— whether the patient's regular provider or not; status of the diagnosis on the first visit—whether unknown, tentative or established; whether the episode started with a phone call or a visit; the number of associated morbidities; the number of laboratory tests and X-rays ordered; whether a throat culture or urine culture was among the lab procedures used; whether chest X-ray was among the X-rays taken, whether injections were given; whether there were adverse effects from antibiotics, analgesics or other medication; whether complications occurred such as sinusitis, otitis media, pneumonia and bronchitis as a complication for the other three morbidities; and whether there was a hospital admission. These various kinds of information related to the first Outpatient Visit (OV) of the episode. (See Chapter 12 for a description of the 5 percent sample.)

The data were retrieved within the frame of episodes of illness; that is to say, all of the contacts with the system by a patient for a given morbidity were treated as a unit. The great majority of cases were one-visit episodes. Unfortunately, although the criteria used to select the four morbidities to be studied were reasonable, given their purpose, there was a price. More complicated morbidities (e.g., some of the chronic diseases) would have permitted with multiple visits study of management processes and outcomes for an illness over a longer period.

The number of episodes in the 5 percent sample for each of the four morbidities selected, together with the number of one- and two-visit episodes in each group, are seen in Table 19:1

TABLE 19:1

Morbidity by Number of Episodes

Morbidity	MD Episodes			PA Episodes		
	Total	One-visit	Two-visit	Total	One-visit	Two-visit
Strep throat	133	90%	8%	42	95%	5%
URI	529	89	9	131	95	3
Bursitis	93	60	18	19*	79	10
Bronchitis	236*	79	11	29	76	17

*Data missing for three bronchitis visits and one bursitis visit; the percentages are calculated for the totals shown.

For three of the four morbidities, a larger portion of the patients who saw an MD had at least one associated morbidity than was true for the patients of PAs. The PA-MD differential was greater in URI and bronchitis than in the other two. The percentages of cases where *no* associated morbidity was recorded are seen in Table 19:2.

The comparison suggests that MDs' patients were sicker, perhaps because they tended to be somewhat older (see Table 19:3).

Both MDs and PAs were able to diagnose the illness on the first visit in a high percentage of episodes except for strep throat, where it is the throat culture which usually fixes the diagnosis and the lab results are not always immediately available (see Table 19:4).

TABLE 19:2

Morbidity by Provider

Morbidity	MD	PA
Strep throat	89%	86%
URI	74	88
Bursitis	83	90
Bronchitis	74	93

TABLE 19:3

Distribution of Morbidity

	Age Group			
Morbidity	0-19	20-44	45-64	65+
Strep throat				
MD	19%	72%	8%	2%
PA	26	71	2	0
URI				
MD	9	66	21	4
PA	20	66	13	1
Bursitis				
MD	3	48	40	9
PA	5	45	45	5
Bronchitis				
MD	3	49	35	13
PA	10	62	24	4

Note: Figures rounded off.

TABLE 19:4

Establishment of Diagnosis on First Visit, by Provider

Morbidity	MD	PA
Strep throat	65%	64%
URI	99	100
Bursitis	86	90
Bronchitis	97	96

TABLE 19:5

Provider Use of Lab and X-Rays for each Morbidity

Diagnostic Tests	Strep throat		URI		Bursitis		Bronchitis	
	MD	PA	MD	PA	MD	PA	MD	PA
X rays of any kind								
0	99%	95%	93%	93%	80%	80%	69%	41%
1	1	5	6	6	16	20	30	59
2 or more	0	0	1	1	4	0	1	0
Chest X ray	*	*	6	7	*	*	31	59
Lab tests of any kind								
0	15	2	66	58	82	95	84	48
1	77	73	31	34	6	5	13	44
2 or more	8	24	3	8	12	0	3	8
Throat culture	84	98	31	41	*	*	10	24
Urine culture	*	*	1	1	*	*	**	0

* Not included in inquiry
**Less than .5%

There is very little distinction between MDs and PAs in this comparison. The morbidities are relatively uncomplex by definition, and it should be remembered that a large percentage of the episodes are one-visit cases.

Figures concerning use of lab and X-ray services for these particular morbidities suggest that the PAs tend to practice more conservatively; that is, they rely somewhat more heavily upon supportive diagnostic services,* especially lab tests (see Table 19:5).

---

*Comparison of MDs and PAs with respect to use of supportive diagnostic services over a wider range of morbidities showed little difference between the average MD and the average PA.

The outcome data, though far from conclusive, are useful and interesting. For all four morbidities, with a total of 1,216 episodes, only 7 instances of adverse drug effects were recorded. Moreover, the other complication rates were practically zero for all but URI (see Table 19:6).

The force of these figures as outcome indices is diminished by the fact that they do not distinguish between those episodes in which the complications were present on the first visit and those in which they developed later. This is especially important if sicker patients tend to be triaged to MDs (see Table 19:1 and 19:3 for age and number of associated morbidities). Moreover, the overwhelming percentage of URI cases were one-visit episodes (89 percent for MDs and 95 percent for PAs).

To improve the data's usefulness, the URI episodes in which the complications were not presented on the first visit were separated; specifically, only those episodes were included—390 (74 percent) for the MDs and 115 (88 percent) for the PAs—where there was no associated morbidity on the first visit. Adverse drug effects were looked at in addition to the four complications listed above. The results, shown as a percentage of those episodes where the first visit had no associated morbidity, are seen in Table 19:7.

TABLE 19:6

Complication Rate, by Provider

Morbidity	MD	PA
Sinusitis	1%	0%
Otitis media	3	2
Pneumonia	1	1
Bronchitis	5	1

TABLE 19:7

Adverse Drug Effects and Complication Rates

	MD	PA
Adverse drug reaction (antibiotic)	0%	0%
Adverse drug reaction (other)	.3	0
Sinusitis	.5	0
Otitis media	1.0	0
Pneumonia	.3	.9
Bronchitis	1.3	0

These figures show the percentage of URI cases where complications developed after the first visit. Even allowing for the fact that MDs still may have received sicker patients (as defined by factors other than associated morbidities) and for the fact that many of the above cases were one-visit episodes, the record is impressive. Because Kaiser-Permanente is a pre-paid system, with a fixed population to whom comprehensive care is given, most patients presumably would have come in again had complications occurred; the absence of a second visit suggests that the first was adequate.

Although quality cannot be read directly and conclusively from the data presented in this discussion, the findings strongly suggest that within the stated frame of reference PA performance compares quite favorably with that of physicians. Particularly with respect to URI, the total number of episodes is large enough for the low rate of complications to be taken seriously. Certainly there is no evidence that PAs provide inferior services.

Quality of service must be measured at least in part by patient reaction, and one index of patient dissatisfaction is the complaint rate. The Health Plan not only investigates all complaints but keeps detailed records, and the complaints are sorted into categories: general attitude of the provider, including quality of communication, diagnosis and treatment proficiency, time spent with the patient, patient waiting time in the clinic, return of telephone calls, and so on. Overall, for the calendar year of 1975 the average number of patient complaints about a PA was only 58 percent of the average number of patient complaints about an MD in the Department of Medicine. The percentage figure varied among the complaint categories. With respect to general attitude, for example, the PA complaint rate was only 47 percent of the MD complaint rate, whereas with diagnosis and treatment the average PA rate was nearer (67 percent) that of physicians. The overall absolute numbers are small, and because of the MDs' more complicated cases and longer work week, they might be expected to receive more complaints. Yet, here again the PA performance appears to stand up well under comparison.

In summary, the data presented here suggest that the PAs practice conservatively within the Kaiser-Permanente system, and that PA performance compares well with MD performance within the range of the non-complex, routine cases which define the PA practice at Kaiser-Permanente.

Editors' Note

Subsequent research on PA practice at Kaiser-Permanente has addressed the outer limit of PA substitutability for physicians. In proposing a Maximum Substitution Model, the researchers developed four criteria to be used in triaging patients to a physician or a PA. Patients were to be referred to an MD: (1) if their condition was immediately life-threatening; (2) if there was a risk of missing the diagnosis, with serious consequences; (3) if there was a risk of rapid deterioration in the patient's condition; or (4) if case management was judged too difficult by the PA. (See J.C. Record et al., "What Physician's Assistants Can Do: Probing for the Outer Limits of Substitution." Presented at the American Public Health Association Annual Meeting, October 1976, Miami, Florida.

Part IV

Evaluative Research on NHPs

In the Preface, research was listed as a major "determinant" of practice, and preceding chapters of the book have stressed new health practitioner research on patient outcomes. Because of the importance of evaluative research a review of its pitfalls may help the reader to sort fact from fantasy and objectivity from subjectivity.

Central to the evaluation of medical decision-making—whether by physicians or NHPs—is clinical judgment. Feinstein's chapter presents a composite of principles which guide clinical judgment. As he has said elsewhere:

> The practice of clinical medicine involves two different types of decisions about the phenomena that doctors observe in patients. In a series of explanatory decisions, doctors give names to the observed phenomena, and provide concepts to account for the causes and mechanisms that presumably created the phenomena. In a series of managerial decisions, doctors choose strategies of intervention to prevent the phenomena from occurring or to alter them after they have occurred. The explanatory decisions lead to intellectual conclusions about ideas such as diagnosis and pathogenesis of disease: the managerial decisions lead to therapeutic actions, in which the patient is treated to thwart what might happen or to remedy what has occurred.[1]

Feinstein who has written numerous articles on diagnostic reasoning, refers to this process as a sequence of intellectual stations through which patients' symptoms are transferred en route to the diagnostic entities that emerge as explanatory conclusions. He discusses here the series of steps in the process of clinical decision making and patient management, through the construction of clinical algorithms.*

---

*Appendix F presents the findings of several HEW funded studies on the use of algorithms in PA training.

261

The chapter by Gavett et al. presents a classification scheme of ambulatory care utilization as a way to analyze the efficiency of health manpower resources allocation. Gavett introduces the concept of justification for the type of primary care problem to be handled by the physician rather than the usual approach of justifying task delegation to the nurse practitioner or the physician's assistant.

Kessner and his coauthors are among the pioneers in developing methods by which the quality of patient care for a specific disease can be measured. Inasmuch as the ultimate test of efficacy of medical care is its impact on the health of patients, it is of critical importance to measure end results and to identify clinical methods for carrying out such research. The tracer method refined by Kessner, also has been used by Sackett and his colleagues in evaluating nurse practitioner care. In addition to the classic paper on the tracer method, Kessner and his colleagues provide an epilogue based on continued research using this particular approach to evaluation. "The Tracer Concept Revisited" reminds the researcher continually to reexamine methods on the basis of study findings.

Kane and Olsen offer a candid view of the problems in program evaluation. The review of one MEDEX program's impact points out the various pitfalls in evaluation and is intended to help the reader assess the generalizability of findings beyond the settings and circumstances in which a given study is conducted. It further stresses the desirability of using existing sources of data, whenever practicable, to reduce the costs of program evaluation. The chapter by Gaus, Morris, and Smith serves two purposes. It provides an outline of the various steps of the Social Security Administration Physician Extender Reimbursement Study and also underscores the difficulty in undertaking research in which numerous intervening variables require continuous adjustment in the research design. Ott and Knox address yet another important component of evaluative research on new health manpower resources: the cost of education. They enumerate many factors to consider in computing and comparing program costs.

These chapters provide methodological approaches and insights which might serve to inspire research on the impact of NHPs on the health care system—in particular the clinical outcomes of NHP care. At the same time the lessons learned from previous studies should alert the researcher to the inherent difficulties in documenting such impact.

Note

1. Alvin Feinstein, *Yale Journal of Biology and Medicine,* 46 (1973), 212-232.

Chapter 20

An Analysis of Diagnostic Reasoning: III. The Construction of Clinical Algorithms[1]

ALVAN R. FEINSTEIN[2]

Department of Medicine, Yale Medical School, Veterans Administration Hospital,
West Haven, Connecticut 06510

Received October 23, 1972

As "input" data are converted to "output" conclusions, diagnostic reasoning traverses a complex series of intermediate decisions, each of which is intended to identify and preferably to explain the entities cited in the preceding stages (1, 2). Because these intermediate decisions are ignored during the formulation of Bayesian and other statistical theories (3–11) about the diagnostic process, a purely statistical approach to diagnosis has two insurmountable handicaps (2). For purposes of identification, calculations of statistical probability cannot provide the precise diagnostic evidence that is desired in modern science and that can often be obtained with suitable technologic tests. For purposes of explanation, current statistical strategies do not delineate the sequence of morbid anatomic and pathophysiologic entities that act as "proximate causes" for the observed clinical manifestations. The statistical conclusions may produce the name of a "disease" as a likely candidate in diagnostic nomenclature, but they do not demonstrate the disease, or explain what has happened.

The statistical strategies, however, have a powerful intellectual attraction. Because the input data are specified, and because their manipulation with Bayesian or other calculations is also specified, statistical strategy offers the scientific advantage of expressing a rational process in mathematical symbols. This advantage would be lost if clinicians, trying to preserve their customary "art" in diagnostic reasoning, were to renounce the new statistical formulations in favor of traditional methods of branching logic. The total rejection of computational tactics in diagnosis would deprive clinicians of a unique scientific opportunity to elevate their mode

[1] From the Cooperative Studies Program Support Center and the Department of Medicine of the West Haven Veterans Administration Hospital, and the Departments of Medicine and Epidemiology of the Yale University School of Medicine. This investigation was supported by PHS Grant Number HS 00408 from the National Center for Health Services Research and Development.

[2] Professor of Medicine and Epidemiology, Yale University School of Medicine, New Haven, Connecticut; Chief, Clinical Biostatistics and Cooperative Studies Program Support Center, Veterans Administration Hospital, West Haven, Connecticut.

Reprinted with permission, from the *Yale Journal of Biology and Medicine*, Volume 1, pp. 5–32, 1974.

of reasoning from its current state of amorphous "judgment." Without a delineated expression of strategy in clinical reasoning, the clinician would remain scientifically inarticulate, knowing what he thinks, and knowing that his thoughts are important, but having no mathematical equations or other coherent techniques with which to display the logic of his rational pathway.

Until recently, a clinician who wanted to retain the traditional "art" of diagnostic reasoning could not avoid its concomitant scientific aphasia. Having no symbols, no structures, and no tactics with which to demonstrate his patterns of thought, he could not attempt to express his reasoning with any of the traditional oral, written, or graphic patterns of scientific communication. A chemist could use chemical formulas, drawings, and arrows to show the path of an enzymatic transformation; a physicist could use photographs to show the path of an electron's movement; but a clinician had no substance or method that could show the path of a rational sequence.

A sublime paradox of the age of inanimate digital computers is the solution it provides for this long-standing intellectual dilemma. Although computational "hardware" can perform the calculations that might allow statistical conjectures to become substitutes for human thought, computational "software" provides the concepts and diagrams with which thought itself can be maintained, discerned, expressed, and dignified. Not by using the computer itself, but with the graphical notation developed as a prerequisite to computation, a clinician can now, at long last, specify the flow of logic in his reasoning.

In this concluding paper of this series, I should like to outline some of the principles and applications of the algorithms, flow-charts, and decision tables with which diagnostic reasoning can begin to achieve the reproducibility and standardization required for science.

A. BASIC CONCEPTS AND NOMENCLATURE

1. Algorithm

The word *algorithm* is commonly used in computer activities to refer to the plan of strategy for solving a problem. People constantly use algorithms in daily life. We all have plans of strategy for deciding what to do about an impending traffic light, a ringing telephone, or a verbose writer. In the case of the traffic light, a traditional algorithm would be: if it is green, go; if it is yellow, slow down; if it is red, stop.

Despite an appealing simplicity and general utility, this algorithm would be inadequate for many situations that confront a driver approaching a traffic light. An ambulance on an emergency mission might not stop for a red light; a driver who sees people or another car occupying the intersection might stop although the light is green. Because so many variations can occur in the associated conditions, a complete algorithm for a particular problem must contain instructions that provide rules of action not only for the ordinary occurrence of the problem, but also for situations that are exceptions to the ordinary.

The recognition of the way that specific circumstances may modify a general principle is one of the hallmarks of good clinical judgment, and is a crucial distinction between the clinician's concern for the nuances of individual patients, and the statistician's concern with the average characteristics of a group. "The object of statistical methods," as R. A. Fisher (12) has said, "is the reduction of data." The statistician wants to reach decisions by compressing or obliterating individual details into the construction of a general case. The individual details, however, are often the essentials of clinical reasoning. A clinician will practice a poor brand of medicine if he makes decisions only on the basis of general formulations that ignore the distinctions of individual patients.

Nevertheless, a clinician must arrive at certain general formulations. He cannot practice medicine at all if he regards each patient as so unique that no general principles of decision can be established. Thus, in devising strategies for the decisions of clinical practice, a clinician must search for an operational balance. At one extreme is the intellectual chaos of excessive details that cannot be rationally formulated; at the other extreme is the futile imprecision of statistical generalizations that cannot be realistically meaningful. Between these two extremes lie the algorithms that describe good clinical reasoning: rules that are specific enough to manage the standard situations, broad enough to encompass the common exceptions, and flexible enough to allow separate decisions for the rare.

2. *Flow Charts*

The sequence of logic in algorithmic strategy is conventionally illustrated with a flow chart, which contains diagrams and graphic symbols for each act of reasoning in the strategy.

The flow chart for a "traffic-light" algorithm is presented in Fig. 1. A description and justification of the contents of this algorithm will be presented later. For the moment, let us consider the different graphic symbols that have been used in this portrait of rational thought.

Every flow chart must have a starting point, which is marked START in Fig. 1, and placed in an oval outline. Ellipses, ovals, or circles can be used for instructions about the beginning or end of an algorithm, and particularly for designating the sites of continuation when a flow chart extends beyond a single page. Even if the chart is confined to a single page, the flow may sometimes be broken and continued at another location on the same page in order to avoid the confusion of visual complexity that would occur if one set of directional lines crossed over a previous set of lines. No such continuations were necessary in the pattern of Fig. 1.

Two main types of "boxes" are used to indicate the logical activities within a flow chart. A *decision box* contains a statement of a question to be answered; an *execution box* contains a statement of a procedure to be performed. In Fig. 1, the decision boxes are shown as flat hexagons; the execution boxes are shown as rectangles. A decision box is followed by a branching in which the rational pathway takes the direction indicated by the answer to the question. Each box must have at least two outlet branchings (commonly YES and NO), but many other branchings (such as MAYBE, UNKNOWN, etc.) can be used according to the type of question and the possible answers. Arrows are used to indicate the exits and pathways leading from one decision or execution box to the next. When several different exits all lead to the same pathway, the arrows join in a common flow, as shown in the far right of Fig. 1.

The symbols employed in flow-charts are not sacrosanct, and may vary from one user to the next. In fact, as long as arrows were maintained to

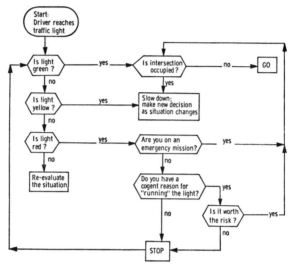

FIG. 1. Flow chart for traffic-light algorithm (for details, see text).

show the directional flow of logic from one question or statement to the next, the entire chart could be constructed without any kind of oval, hexagonal or rectangular boxes. Like digitalis preparations, any collection of these graphic symbols can work effectively provided that they are used in a well-defined, consistent manner. Readers who are familiar with the conventional graphology of flow-charts will note that I have used flat hexagons instead of the customary diamond shape for decision boxes. In constructing such boxes, I prefer the graphic and esthetic convenience of writing out the question and then enclosing it in a flat hexagon, rather than to squeeze the writing into a predrawn diamond, or to waste the unused space occupied at the upper and lower poles of a diamond that is drawn afterward. In some of the illustrations to be shown later, the decision and execution boxes all appear as rectangles, and in other illustrations, no boxes are used.

3. Decision Tables

The same strategies outlined in Fig. 1 could have been portrayed alternatively in a *decision table,* which is a tabular array of sets of conditions, and of the decisions selected as a response to each set of conditions. In a conventional form, such a table has four major sections (13, 14). The *condition stub* section shows the conditions under examination, and the *condition entry* section shows the presence or absence of each of the conditions under scrutiny. An *action stub* section shows the possible actions (or decisions) that can be taken for the various conditions that are present, and an *action entry* section shows the responses for each combination of conditions. The illustration in Fig. 2 shows an example of a decision table that contains exactly the same strategies portrayed in Fig. 1.

	Condition Entry										
	1	2	3	4	5	6	7	8	9	10	11
Is light green ?	Y	Y	N	N	N	N	N	N	N	N	N
Is light yellow ?	N	N	Y	N	N	N	N	N	N	N	N
Is light red ?	N	N	N	Y	Y	Y	Y	Y	Y	Y	Y
Emergency mission ?				Y	Y	N	N	N	N	N	N
Cogent reason to "run light" ?						N	Y	Y	Y	Y	Y
Good excuse if caught ?							N	Y	Y	N	N
Is it worth risk ?								N		Y	Y
Is intersection occupied ?	N	Y		N	Y			N	Y	N	Y
GO	X			X				X	X		
WAIT		X	X		X					X		X
STOP							X	X			

Action Entry

FIG. 2. Decision table for traffic-light algorithm. (The letters Y and N represent *yes* and *no*. The letter X shows the action to be taken for each set of conditions. For further details, see text.)

Like flow-charts, decision tables can be constructed in various ways, and certain principles of logical design can be used to enhance simplicity and eliminate redundancy (13, 14). Since any well constructed decision-table can be converted into a flow-chart, and vice versa, either procedure can be chosen for portraying a logical pathway. The correspondence between the two procedures is indicated by the occasional use of the name *decision tree* for what has here been called a *flow chart*.

In general, flow charts are preferred by computer programmers, since the chart shows the direct sequence of the path of logic, and can be easily translated into a computer program. The sequential arrangement may often save space because it can allow several decisions to terminate in a common sequence, and because it can eliminate the repetition of components that are necessary for some decisions but unnecessary for others. Thus, in comparison to the decision table of Fig. 2, the flow chart of Fig. 1 contains no blank spaces for situations in which the particular condition was not applicable. On the other hand, a decision table might be more convenient than a flow chart for portraying certain diagnostic decisions that depend on a particular array of information, rather than on the specific sequence in which each component of the array was noted.

Because I am more familiar with flow charts than with decision tables, the illustrations in the rest of this dissertation will be based on flow charts. Regardless of whether the components of clinical strategy are portrayed in flow charts or in decision tables, however, the potential value of these graphic media should now be apparent. They offer a method of depicting rational processes that cannot be expressed in the conventional equations, parameters and calculations of mathematics, and that cannot be demonstrated visually with the photographs or conventional diagrams of science. Furthermore, these new graphic media are both strict enough to provide exactness in expressing the main paths of thought for a decisional process, and flexible enough to allow the construction of branching paths when the main path requires modifications or diversions.

B. PROCEDURES IN JUSTIFICATION

A requirement of scientific or logical reasoning is not merely that decisions be reached, but that each decision be justified. The justification can consist of diverse

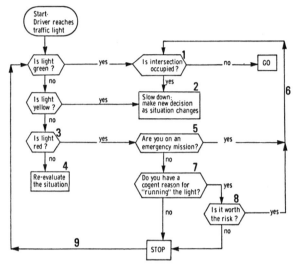

FIG. 3. Points of justification in traffic-light algorithm (for details, see text).

forms of factual evidence and conceptual principles. For example, the justification procedures used as "proofs" for theorems in grade school geometry contain a cohesive pattern of logic, making sequential use of accepted axioms and of previously proved theorems.

The decisions of clinical reasoning, however, can seldom be justified with neat patterns of mathematical logic, and a suitable substantiation will require reference to different types of data and principles, derived from practical observations in the world of clinical reality. The addition of suitable justification, containing citations of data or principles to substantiate each decision, is the activity that converts a flow chart from an arbitrary set of rules into a scientific document.

To illustrate a procedure of justification, the flow-chart of Fig. 1 is repeated in Fig. 3, with appended numbers that will be used as references in the following discussion of the reasons for the decisions made in the "traffic-light" algorithm.

1. With a green light, a driver would ordinarily proceed ahead with unchanged speed unless he sees that he may crash into an object (such as an automobile, person, or construction) that occupies the intersection. The state of the intersection must therefore be assessed before he continues.

2. This execution box could be entered in two different ways, each of which calls for the driver to "slow down" and then make a new decision as the situation changes. If the intersection is occupied by a moving object, the driver can anticipate its time of departure, and can plan to proceed accordingly. If the situation does not change because the object is stationary, separate decisions are needed. The other entrance to this box occurs if the light is yellow. The decision to "slow down"

is based on the awareness that such lights are usually brief, and followed by red lights. The next decision would be based on the driver's plan of response to the red light.

3. Connoisseurs of flow-charting will recognize that this decision box is redundant here. Instead of including the question, "Is light red?", we could have assumed that when a traffic light is neither green nor yellow it must be red. Accordingly, the red light question could have been eliminated, and the "NO" exit from the yellow-light box could have led directly to the box asking about an emergency mission, thus sparing us the need for the diversion that follows in point 4.

4. At this step in the algorithm, the driver has decided that the traffic light is neither green nor yellow nor red. He must therefore reevaluate the situation. Has he suddenly entered a strange new land that uses unconventional colors for traffic lights? Has he mistaken some other type of light for a traffic signal? Has he become color blind?

5. We are now thinking about breaking the law by "running" a red light. Since we shall, as noted later, always assess the risk of injury before crossing the intersection, our main deterrent to law-breaking is the fear of arrest. Although the term "emergency mission" is not defined here, it would refer to a situation (such as an ambulance urgently racing to a hospital, or a fire truck enroute to a fire) where a universally acceptable excuse exists for "running" the light.

6. This line represents a common pathway for the ending of several situations in which a driver, planning to take the legal risk of crossing against a red light, is first led to check that occupancy of the intersection does not create the additional risk of a crash or other injury.

7. In this situation, the driver does not have a mission that would be universally accepted as an "emergency." He now contemplates whether he has some other "cogent" reason (i.e., one that he thinks would be acceptable to a policeman) for crossing against the light.

8. He believes his reason is "cogent," but before the algorithm allows him to proceed, we caution him about the consequences. Suppose the policeman does not accept the excuse? Even if the excuse is accepted, would being stopped by a policeman be worth the time wasted in giving the explantion? (Connoisseurs of red-light running will probably suggest that the driver, before all this soul searching, should have checked to see whether any policeman are present to note the contemplated malefaction. If no policeman is evident, a "cogent" excuse may be unnecessary. Since our goal is to provide justification, however, this example will stay within the bounds of order and law).

9. The arrow here demonstrates the recursive quality of many sequential thought processes. After the driver stops, he constantly rechecks to see whether the light has turned green. If it has not changed, he continues his mental "loop" through the "nongreen" pathway until the light turns green.

After noting the extensive justification procedure needed for so simple a decision as what to do at a traffic light, the reader may now begin to appreciate the enormous complexity involved in trying to create and to justify algorithms for the intricate problems of clinical diagnosis. The activities will require several types of major intellectual effort:

1. To compose flow charts whose contents are adequate for typical clinical situations as well as for exceptions to the typical.
2. To arrange each chart into a diagram that is logically clear, esthetically attractive, and intellectually economical. (An example of such "economy" in the traffic-light flow chart would have been the removal of the extraneous "red light" decision, as noted in the third paragraph of the justification).
3. To provide a clinically convincing account of the reasons for each of the decisions that require justification. The justifying statements for many minor decisions may not be wholly necessary and can be omitted. For many other minor decisions, however, and for all major ones, the justification is the crux of scientific "proof" for the procedure. After a justified algorithm has been established and generally accepted, its flow-chart can be used thereafter without the appended "proof," in a manner similar to the way that a new laboratory test, having had its basic validity demonstrated, can then be employed without constant recourse to the methodologic documentation.

Justifications have been omitted from all of the flow-charts that will be shown later, but can usually be found in the text of the reference where the charts first appeared.

C. THE CAPACITIES OF DIGITAL COMPUTERS

Because the operation of digital computers has been the prime stimulus for attention to the development of algorithmic procedures, and because computers depend on different kinds of algorithms, a knowledge of the functions performed by computers will be useful background in contemplating the diverse algorithms needed for clinical activities.

A computer ordinarily operates with two sets of information: one set contains a program[3] of the algorithmic instructions for "processing" a collection of data; the other set of information provides the data subjected to the processing. For these activities, the computer has four main "intellectual" capacities: it can acquire, store, retrieve, and interpret data. The distinctions of these capacities, which are not well understood by most clinical readers, will be defined and illustrated in the paragraphs that follow.

1. *Acquiring Data*

Since data are human artefacts, rather than natural phenomena, data must be created as a result of observation, description, and communication. A patient may have an oppressing sensation under his breastbone, but the sensation does not become the data of "substernal chest pain" until he has communicated its description. Another patient may feel warm, but he does not have a rectal temperature of 103°F

---

[3] A computer "program" consists of an algorithm that has been "translated" into the symbols of a "language" that the computer can "understand." Many such languages have been constructed (15). Among the most popular ones in use today are FORTRAN, ALGOL, COBOL, and PL/I.

until a thermometer has been shaken down, inserted in his rectum, removed, inspected, and had its results recorded.

The acquisition of data thus refers to the process of converting an observed phenomenon into a reported description. The process is either transferred or direct, according to whether or not the observer's reported description has been transferred through another observer enroute to the formation of data. For example, the data recorded after a clinician takes a history are transferred from the patient's account of his sensations; whereas the data of physical examination are usually a direct account of what the clinician observed himself. Similarly, data are acquired by transferral when a clinician reads a printed value of 130 from a line marked "130" on a graphic scale of serum sodium levels, but the acquisition is direct when the clinician looks at a series of electrocardiographic wiggles and decides that the P–R interval is 0.12 sec. In many medical applications of computers, the machine acquires the data by transferral through an external observer. In certain new medical approaches, however, the clinician or other intermediary observer is eliminated, and the computer acquires data directly by "taking" a history from a patient, or by "determining" the P–R interval and other measurements from a suitably prepared electrocardiogram.

2. Storing Data

The storage of data refers to the way a computer maintains the information it has received. For example, the computer may not store temperature data in degrees Fahrenheit. In such circumstances, the user of the computer might be asked to convert Fahrenheit results into Centigrade before entering the data, or the computer might perform the conversion itself, with an "internal" set of programmed calculations that will translate Fahrenheit input into Centigrade storage.

3. Retrieving Data

For retrieval of data, the computer is asked to return the information it has stored. In a simple retrieval, the data would be displayed in the exact form of the storage. In the most common situations of retrieval, however, the computer is asked to sort and count the information, and to print out certain enumerated results. For example, a computer that contains data for the histories of a large population of patients might be asked to indicate how many of those patients had substernal chest pain. The computer would then "sort" through the data for each case, looking for patients with substernal chest pain. Whenever it finds a patient with this symptom, it would add one unit to a special "counter." After the sorting of cases has been completed, the sum on this counter would represent the total number of people with substernal chest pain. In an analogous manner, the computer could perform more complex sortings, such as finding the number of children who had substernal chest pain and a temperature of 103°F.

4. Interpreting Data

No subtle judgmental decisions were needed for any of the activities just described in acquisition, storage, and retrieval of data. The computer received information that is preserved and then returned after counting specified classes of data. In addition to these elementary capacities, however, a computer can be instructed to perform interpretations of data. Some of the interpretations are trivial, such as the decision that one number is larger than another. Other interpretations require a designated numerical background, such as the decision that a particular number falls within a certain "range of normal." The interpretations that are especially interesting to clinicians, however, involve sophisticated value judgments about such concepts as *improving* or *worse,* and the intricate subtleties of diagnostic, therapeutic and other clinical decisions.

Since a computer does only what it is commanded to do, it must receive a specific program for each of these decisions, and the person who composes the program must establish suitable strategies and criteria for the decisions. Thus, the computer can store and retrieve the fact that a patient's temperature was 103°F, but it cannot tell us that he had "fever" until a value has been established for the temperature to receive this interpretation. The computer can store and retrieve "substernal chest pain," but it cannot make the interpretation that the pain is "angina pectoris" or due to "coronary artery disease," unless appropriate additional data and specific decisional strategies have been provided for the interpretations.

D. ELEMENTARY CLINICAL APPLICATIONS OF ALGORITHMS

Since diagnostic reasoning is composed of numerous interpretive decisions, the conversion of these decisions into diagnostic algorithms is a formidable task. In view of the difficulties, it is not surprising that some of the relatively successful current applications of "computers in medicine" have been based on algorithms that deal with processes much more clinically simple than diagnostic reasoning.

1. *Acquisition of Data in History-Taking*

To acquire data by "taking" a patient's history, a computer program depends on algorithms for the logical branchings that expand to additional questions when certain routine questions are answered "Yes," and that progress to the next routine question when the reply is "No." The contents of some of the associated algorithms and flow charts have been displayed in reports of such programs (16, 17).

Although diagnostic purposes for the acquired data must be considered when such algorithms are constructed, most history-taking algorithms have been devoted almost exclusively to the logical sequence of getting the data. The type of branching clinical logic used for explanatory diagnostic reasoning has not been part of the strategy. For example, a history-taking algorithm might contain the entire sequence of branching inquiries needed to obtain all the descriptive details about the severity, timing, duration, provocative factors, alleviating factors, and other features of a patient's dyspnea. A quite different algorithm with quite different strategies, however, would be needed to decide diagnostically whether the dyspnea is due to lung disease, to cardiac decompensation, or to other causes.

2. *Acquisition of Data for Visual Patterns*

During the history-taking just described, the basic phenomena were perceived and converted into data by the patient. The computer "acquired" these data by using an algorithm that contained suitable expressions for asking questions and anticipating answers, but the fundamental process of observation had not been "automated" into an algorithmic strategy. The phenomena described in the data were observed by the patient, not by the computer.

In computerized electrocardiography, however, an algorithm has been created for a computer to perform the basic process of observation. The actual perception of the voltages on the tracing is done by an electronic instrument, and an algorithm is used for converting these voltages into electrocardiographic data (18–20). For this process, the computer must receive instructions on how to scan the array of repetitive voltages, and identify them as P-waves, QRS complexes, etc. After these constituents of the tracing have been identified, the algorithm instructs the computer to calculate such data as measurements of cardiac rate, amplitude of various PQRSTU constituents, and intervals between constituents. When these activities are completed, the computer displays the data it has acquired as a basic description of the visual forms on the electrocardiogram. The interpretation of the data requires a different set of algorithms, to be discussed later.

The successful achievement of this type of automated observation is facilitated by the concurrence of several visual features that greatly simplify the optical pattern of an electrocardiogram. The first feature is that the image is two-dimensional, so that only an x and y coordinate need to be considered when the visual record is regarded as a voltage that changes with time. A second feature is that an electrocardiographic tracing, unlike the diverse images seen in a blood cell or a roentgenogram, is essentially linear; its observation thus requires a consideration of change in the pattern of voltage for only a single line, whereas a white blood cell or a roentgenogram has enormously greater visual complexity. A third feature is that the electrocardiographic image has a fixed axial orientation. Like a roentgenogram, the ECG tracing can always be arranged with a distinct top and bottom, whereas a white blood cell can emerge on a smear with its nucleus curving upward, downward, or in various lateral directions. Finally, the ECG pattern, unlike the two-dimensional, linear, axially oriented image on an electroencephalogram, usually shows temporal repetition; and the repetition of the pattern serves as a major aid in the automated recognition and labeling of the constituents.

Although this regularity of pattern has been a boon to the rapid development of automated electrocardiography, the problems of irregular patterns have not yet been solved. Certain simple irregularities in cardiac rhythm have been algorithmically mastered (19, 21, 22) but the gross irregularities of complex arrhythmias have not yet received suitable algorithms for automated identification. No computer can currently deal with complicated arrhythmias, and when they occur, the computer must be replaced by the superior pattern-recognition abilities of a human observer. Furthermore, for nonlinear visual patterns, as in white blood cells or roentgenograms, a satisfactory "recognition algorithm" is extremely difficult to create. Despite intensive efforts in the past few years, no thoroughly successful algorithms have yet been developed for these purposes, although considerable progress has recently been reported for direct computer (23) screening of cardiac roentgenograms.

3. Storage of Data in Clinical Examination

In the types of algorithm just described, the computer received its "input" of medical data without the intervention of a clinician. For data acquired during a clinician's examination of a patient, an algorithm can be developed to allow the clinician to "record" (or store) his findings in a computer (24–27). Such algorithms contain a series of branchings that continue the "routine" topics when the clinician's findings are "negative," and that provide appropriate expansions for "positive" results. The basic principle of the algorithms is similar to that used in history taking from a patient, except that the computer gets the information from a clinician; and the scope of the information may include results from the physical, roentgenographic, and other examinations, rather than from history taking alone. Such algorithms are used for entering and storing data in the computer system, but not for any type of diagnostic interpretations.

4. Retrieval of Laboratory Data

One of the most currently popular and medically effective uses of computers is for storage and retrieval of the vast amounts of data now being assembled in clinical laboratories. The basic data are usually obtained via the customary laboratory equipment and personnel, and entered into the computer by the personnel. The plan of storage allows the computer to maintain and retrieve an inventory of results for each patient, and to perform sortings, enumerations, and calculations with the data stored for a group of patients (28–30).

The composition of algorithms for these activities requires little or no clinicial sophistication, and excellent programs can be (and have been) developed by programmers familiar with the algorithms for "inventory" procedures, regardless of the type of data that constitute the inventory. Because improved methods of management are needed for the plethora of laboratory data now being produced at medical centers, and because the necessary algorithms can be created by a good computer programmer who has no medical background, the storage and retrieval of laboratory data has been a particularly successful application of computers in contemporary hospital practice.

Efforts are now being made to create systems in which the results of laboratory tests are entered directly into the computer, without human intervention (31). Most of these programs are based on automated recording of the voltages generated as "readings" by the laboratory instruments.

5. Interpretation of Clinical Data

Algorithms were needed for all of the procedures that have just been described, but none of the algorithms dealt with diagnostic *reasoning,* and none required any profound clinical experience or thought. Many of the algorithms could have been constructed by people with no clinical experience, or with no more than one or two student clerkships. That so little clinical knowledge was needed to construct the algorithms does not detract from some of the splendid achievements contained in the cited programs for acquiring, storing, and retrieving medical data. As the new technology of computers was introduced into the ancient traditions of clinical medicine, relatively simple challenges were obviously the first ones that could be approached effectively.

Despite the existing and often laudable progress, however, none of the cited algorithms has entered the higher realm of reasoning that distinguishes clinical activity. Almost all of the results achieved with the computer could have been accomplished without the computer, and are still so accomplished in most medical settings today. The described algorithms and computer programs can enable a clinician to automate his standard methods for maintaining and displaying medical data, but the activities have not affected the standard reasoning with which the data are interpreted and used. Unlike the data, the reasoning remains essentially undefined and unspecified. Its constituents and logical branchings are often relegated to the realm of "art," or consigned to a nondescript rationality called *clinical judgment* (32).

A paramount intellectual challenge for clinicians today is to identify the components and pathways of these judgments, and to express them in suitable algorithms.

If clinicians accept the lure of noninterpretive data processing while preserving the intellectual inertia of their own undelineated reasoning, the result will be merely an automation of the status quo. Because of many existing deficiencies in both the data and the scientific goals of the reasoning (33, 34), the status quo needs to be improved rather than merely automated. For the improvement, clinicians must begin to respect the importance of their own thinking, to explore its constituents and directions, and to convert its logic into algorithmic outlines.

E. ADVANCED CLINICAL APPLICATIONS OF ALGORITHMS

A clinician who begins to think about the way he thinks will soon discover that clinicial reasoning does not follow the simplistic schemes into which it is sometimes cast to illustrate the potential application of computers in medicine. An efficient practicing clinician, for example, does not usually go through a segregated sequence of exclusively history-taking, followed by exclusively physical examination, followed by laboratory tests. He often takes part of the history *while* he does the physical examination; or he may obtain certain laboratory data *before* any of the clinical examinations begin; or he may do parts of the clinical examination, obtain certain laboratory tests, and then complete the clinical examination later.

Another example of the difference between current algorithms and clinical practice is that a clinician interpreting an electrocardiogram seldom confines his attention exclusively to the configuration and measurements of the individual tracing. He compares the findings in the patient's previous tracings, and incorporates data from the concurrent history, physical examination, and laboratory tests. The clinician's final diagnostic decision is based on this mixture of information, not on the single electrocardiogram alone.

A particularly important departure from the contents of current algorithms is created by the diversity of decisions made during clinical reasoning. Although many existing algorithms are concerned with diagnosis alone, an efficient clinician regularly intermingles many other decisions with the diagnostic reasoning. The mixture of decisions includes prognostic estimations, choices of additional paraclinical tests, selection of therapeutic agents, and behavioral planning for the personal interchange with the patient. Algorithms that concentrate on only diagnostic identifications will seldom suffice for the diverse managerial decisions that are an integral, concomitant part of the reasoning used in clinical practice.

For these reasons, when clinicians undertake the rigorous intellectual challenge of describing the pathways of clinical reasoning, the horizon need not be constricted to diagnostic targets alone. The challenge is to contemplate what happens as clinicians think during clinical activities, and to describe the strategy. If the thought processes shift from one type of thinking to another and on to a third before returning to the first, and if this rational pathway can be justified either by valid logic or by documented evidence or by both, then these are the thought processes to be cited in the algorithms. As clinicians enter a new era in patterns of clinical thought, we need not limit the future to preconceptions about the past or to oversimplifications of the present. The object is to preserve the vitality of clinical reasoning while enhancing its scientific effectiveness.

In the remainder of this paper, I shall outline some of the diverse situations that provide challenges in the construction of clinical algorithms. In some of the situations, certain algorithms have already been formed and can be shown as examples. The existing algorithms may appear either primitive or highly developed, but almost all of them are new, unproved, and unaccompanied by the substantiating evidence of their validity. The further scientific development and justification of these algorithms, and the creation of the many required new algorithms will be major challenges for clinical research in the future.

1. *Diagnostic Analysis of Paraclinical Data*

Roentgenograms, electrocardiograms and the data of other paraclinical tests can often receive a preliminary diagnostic analysis without regard to the associated clinical information. After the clinical data are noted, the initial diagnostic decisions may or may not be modified. For example, certain disorders in cardiac conduction or rhythm (such as bundle branch block and supraventricular arrhythmias) are usually diagnosed exclusively from an electrocardiographic tracing, regardless of the patient's clinical signs or symptoms; whereas disorders in cardiac morphology (such as myocardial infarction or myocardial aneurysm) require diagnostic attention to clinical as well as electrocardiographic data.

Algorithms have now been developed for several types of diagnostic analysis that can be performed exclusively with paraclinical data. A series of flow charts for the electrocardiographic diagnosis of cardiac arrhythmias has been presented in recent publications by Lindsay and Budkin (22) and by Wartak et al. (35, 36). The latter authors have also demonstrated the use of decision tables for these diagnostic purposes. An example of one of the Lindsay-Budkin flow-charts is shown in Fig. 4, and a Wartak decision table is shown in Fig. 5. In radiology, Tuddenham (37) has begun to develop a series of algorithms for teaching "visual discrimination and search strategy." An example of one of Tuddenham's flow charts for radiographic diagnosis is shown in Fig. 6.

In the situations just described, the clinician had already ordered an electrocardiogram or a roentgenogram, and the purpose of the flow-chart was to help interpret the results. A different aspect of diagnostic strategy involves decisions about which tests to order. In contrast to a "diagnostic interpretation" algorithm, which deals with a fixed array of assembled data, a "diagnostic search" algorithm will branch into different types of tests and data, according to the results found in preceding tests. Since the "search" algorithms require considerations of the interpretation that will be given to each test and its predecessors, such algorithms can often be used both to demonstrate the direction of the search, and to indicate the diagnostic meaning of the results.

An example of a diagnostic-search algorithm for paraclinical chemical data is shown in Fig. 7. This flow chart, which is modified from the one prepared by Rabinowitz, Prout and Walker on page 1097 of the textbook (38) by Harvey et al., indicates the direction and interpretation of the tests that might be ordered after mellituria is discovered as a positive copper-reduction reaction in urine tested with Benedict's solution or Clinitest tablets.

A diagnostic-search algorithm for the laboratory data of acid-base disorders has been prepared by Bleich (39). The algorithm is entered with the results of measurements for a patient's serum sodium, potassium, chloride, and carbon dioxide. Additional measurements of blood pH and pCO_2 may then be requested. If all the solicited data are normal, the algorithm indicates that acid-base equilibrium is undisturbed; otherwise, the algorithm branches into a differential diagnosis of the disturbance.

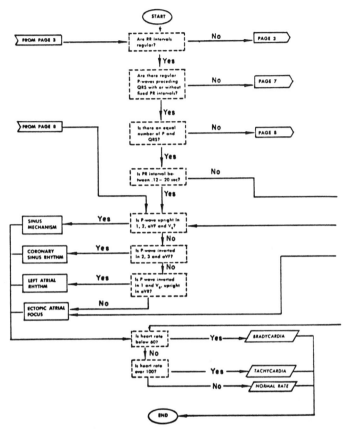

Fig. 4. Portion of flow chart for cardiac arrhythmias. Reproduced, with permission, from page 114 of textbook by Lindsay and Budkin (22).

2. *Diagnostic Analysis of Clinical Data*

During the process of obtaining clinical data in a patient's history and physical examination, a clinician constantly contemplates diagnostic possibilities. The directions that he chooses in the sequence of the examination are often intended to exclude or amplify these possibilities. During this process, the clinician works only with the clinical and demographic data obtained during clinical examination, before any paraclinical data have been obtained from ancillary tests.

An example of part of an algorithm for the clinical diagnostic analysis of chest pain is shown in Fig. 8. This segment of the flow chart shows only the paths of reasoning and data that might lead to the indicated diagnoses. The reader is invited to complete the unfinished parts of this algorithm, beginning at each place marked "continue to other topics."

DECISION TABLE FOR DIAGNOSING ELECTROCARDIOGRAMS	TABLE NAME CRUDE ANALYSIS	RULE NUMBER						
		1	2	3	4	5	6	
ALL QRS COMPLEXES ≥ 0.11 SEC		N	Y		N	N		
ALL QRS COMPLEXES ≤ 0.10 SEC		Y			N	Y		
AT LEAST 1/2 OF QRS COMPLEXES ≥ 0.11 SEC			N	Y	N	N		
RR INTERVAL REGULAR		Y	Y					
RR INTERVAL IRREGULAR		N		Y		Y		
AT LEAST 1/3 OF QRS COMPLEXES ≥ 0.11 SEC				Y				
SUPRAVENTRICULAR TACHYCARDIA (SVT)		X						
VENTRICULAR TACHYCARDIA OR SVT WITH ABERRANT QRS			X					
BIGEMINY OR MULTIPLE PVC'S				X				
TRIGEMINY OR MULTIPLE PVC'S					X			
SVT WITH VARIABLE AV BLOCK						X		
SYSTEM ERROR							X	
END OF ANALYSIS		X	X	X	X	X	X	

FIG. 5. Decision table for 'crude analysis' of electrocardiogram. Reproduced, with permission, from page 346 of paper by Wartak, Milliken, and Karchmar (35).

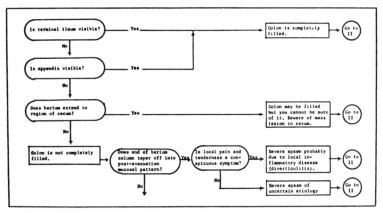

FIG. 6. Flow chart for examining part of a barium enema. Reproduced, with permission, from page 36 of Medical News section of JAMA (37).

D. A. W. Edwards (40) has prepared an extensive flow-chart, shown in Fig. 9, for the diagnostic analysis of dysphagia. The numbers appended to the chart indicate portions of the algorithm for which comments of explanation or justification are provided in Edwards' original paper. Because the logical sequence and

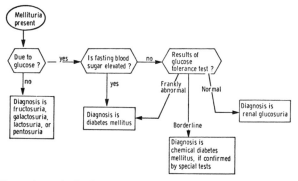

FIG. 7. Diagnostic-search algorithm for mellituria. Modified and redrawn from the original flow chart on page 1097 of Ref. (38).

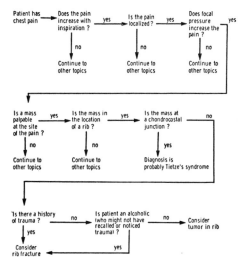

FIG. 8. Algorithm for diagnostic clinical analysis of chest pain (for further details, see text).

its clinical justification are so well organized, Edwards' work is an excellent model of this type of clinical diagnostic algorithm.

Another example of an algorithm for clinical diagnostic analysis is shown in Fig. 10. This flow chart, which deals with the search for causes of edema, represents the consensus of a symposium (41) sponsored by the journal PATIENT CARE, which has pioneered in the pictorial use of flow charts to summarize strategies of clinical diagnosis and therapy. The editors of that journal have created more than 100 flow charts for the analysis and/or management of diverse clinical conditions, and each new issue usually contains one or more additional charts. (A "Pa-

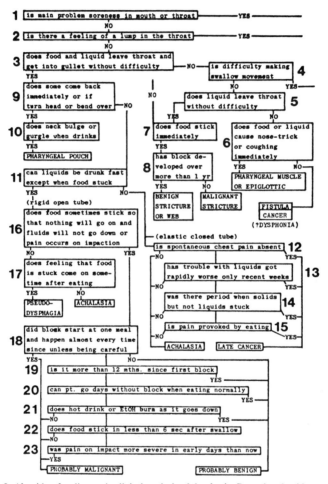

FIG. 9. Algorithm for diagnostic clinical analysis of dysphagia. Reproduced, with permission, from page 381 of Ref. (40).

tient Care Flow Chart Service," available by subscription, is offered by the Miller and Fink Publishing Corporation, 16 Thorndal Circle, P.O. Box 1245, Darien, Connecticut 06820.)

Flow charts of this type can be used to illustrate the difference between the way a novice and an expert approach issues in clinical examination. A flow chart prepared by Johns and Tumulty on page 17 of the medical textbook by Harvey *et al.* (38) shows that an expert who encounters jaundice on examination of the skin will usually not continue immediately with the rest of the cutaneous examination. Instead, the expert will branch into a series of questions that clarify the concomitant features and possible causes of the jaundice. When this branched deline-

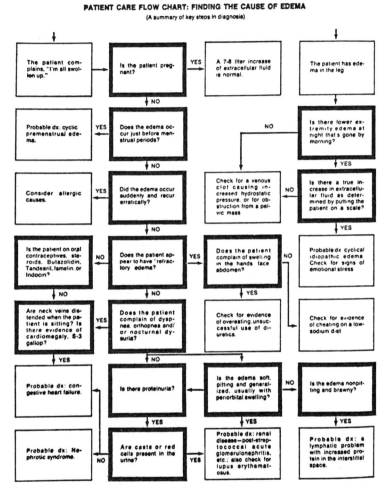

PATIENT CARE FLOW CHART: FINDING THE CAUSE OF EDEMA
(A summary of key steps in diagnosis)

Fɪɢ. 10. Algorithm for diagnostic analysis of edema. Reproduced, with permission, from page 50 of panel discussion in PATIENT CARE (41).

ation of the jaundice has been completed, the expert returns to the rest of the cutaneous examination. A neophyte, on the other hand, may not perform this branching, and may simply continue with the rest of the routine examination of the skin.

3. Planning the Diagnostic Work-Up

In the two types of analysis that have just been described, the reasoning was restricted to either clinical or paraclinical data. In many modern clinical situations, of course, the two types of data are intermingled during diagnostic activities. Thus, after the routine clinical examination and laboratory tests are performed, the clinician may decide about further clinical examinations and additional paraclinical tests. These results may then lead to further examination procedures, and so on.

The development of suitable algorithms for the strategy of diagnostic work-ups has become a critical challenge in modern medicine. The work-ups, which occupy increasingly large amounts of staff and facilities at any large medical center, are generally uncomfortable and often dangerous for patients, but the strategy of the work-ups has not yet been suitably investigated. Should certain tests be obtained sequentially, or as a simultaneous "battery"? If tests A and B are both to be done, should A always precede B, or vice versa?

Since ancillary tests can be ordered at each step in the flow of clinical or paraclinical examination procedures, a thoughtful clinician would like to know not merely the general costs, risks, and advantages of the individual tests, but the specific value of each test at each step in the sequence of examination. For example, the risks of esophagoscopy can be assessed from its consequences in a large series of patients exposed to the procedure, but this information is much too vague for direct clinical utility. What a clinician would really like to know is not the general risk of esophagoscopy, but its risk in individual situations. Such situations include the diverse circumstances of patients who have had an episode of hematemesis, with or without recurrent episodes, with or without persistent bleeding, with or without melena, with or without shock, with or without an antecedent history of gastrointestinal bleeding, with or without an associated history of peptic ulcer, with or without clinical evidence of liver disease, and so on. For patients with hematemesis, the clinician might also like evidence about the value of performing esophagoscopy and upper gastrointestinal roentgenograms immediately as an emergency procedure, as compared to deferring these procedures until a later point at various stages of the patient's management and clinical course. Another example of the need for sequentially specified evaluations occurs in the work-up of a patient with hypertension. In what clinical circumstances and at what stages of the work-up are the greatest diagnostic benefits attained from such hazardous procedures as intravenous pyelography and intra-arterial aortography?

As a prerequisite to such information, appropriate algorithms must be constructed to demonstrate the clinical and paraclinical sequence of a work-up for each of the cited conditions. After the algorithm has been prepared as an architectural outline for classifying and storing the subsequent information, the data obtained during the course of work-ups for many patients can then be suitably classified and analyzed for the desired appraisals. This type of evaluation is not available today for any of the many clinical conditions that are constantly worked up at modern medical centers. Despite the increasing costs and other problems of contemporary diagnostic work-ups (42), the sequential path of the work-ups has not been adequately outlined or documented. The few existing algorithms do not contain enough detail for satisfactory classifications of data; and the algorithms have not been suitably justified either with physiologic rationales or with empirical data derived from direct observation of patients.

Although many new formats and computer techniques have been proposed for storing the "data base" produced by the diagnostic technology of modern medicine, the technology itself has not been critically evaluated. The new formats and media for the medical record create a rearrangement and recataloging of the data that emerge from a medical work-up, but the sequence of the work-up is not denoted, the data are not "edited," and the results are not assessed. Since the unique pathway of decisions and judgments that characterize the work of a clinician has been omitted from the formats of data stored in both the old and the new media of medical records, the existing media cannot provide satisfactory information for appraising the diagnostic work-up.

The task will require attention, intellect, and effort not from computer experts, but from knowledgeable clinicians. A clinician's irreplaceable role in diagnostic activities is to make choices in clinical management, not just to prepare charts of information. His main job is to arrive at validated decisions, not just to arrange volumes of a "data base." To achieve validation for those decisions, clinicians must create the appropriate algorithms and collect the appropriate information for demonstrating which data are needed in a diagnostic work-up, in what sequence, and why.

4. Strategies of Clinical Management

In all of the foregoing clinical algorithms, the decisions were aimed at either attaining a diagnostic name or ordering a diagnostic test. In many common clinical situations, however, an act of therapy may interrupt the diagnostic reasoning before it is completed. The treatment may sometimes act as a diagnostic test or it may provide the ultimate clinical management before a precise diagnosis is achieved.

Consider a patient with a clinical condition manifested by a one-day history of malaise, low grade fever, an aching throat, and a stuffy nose. After finding nothing strikingly abnormal on physical examination, the clinician may regard the condition as a nonspecific viral illness, and may prescribe only minor supportive agents. If the illness promptly subsides, the patient will receive no further tests or treatment, and his "final" diagnosis may be nothing more specific than "flu" or "common cold." If the illness persists or worsens, however, the clinician will then reappraise the situation with additional examinations, tests, or treatment.

A different type of example is provided by an elderly patient with fever, inspiratory chest pain, hemoptysis, negative tests of sputum cytology, and a roentgenographic pulmonary shadow that could be due to pneumonia, to cancer, or to both. Reluctant to expose the patient to the discomforts of bronchoscopy, the clinician may use antipneumonia treatment as both a therapeutic procedure and a diagnostic test. If the roentgenographic shadow disappears completely after the treatment, the clinician may conclude that the diagnosis was pneumonia alone.

In both of the examples just cited, the diverse branchings of a diagnostic work-up were delayed to await results of a treatment that could provide both diagnostic assistance and therapeutic management. This type of delay for "exploratory therapy," or a more simple delay to await the action of time and nature alone, is a common managerial strategy in regular clinical practice, but the strategy is seldom considered in diagnostic activities at academic medical centers. Because of various peculiarities of clinical practice at such centers—the expensiveness and shortage of beds, the need to educate students and house officers, the unrepresentative character of the referred population, the focus on in-patient work-ups rather than out-patient treatment, and an "explanatory" rather than "managerial" scientific orientation (43)—the academic clinician seldom engages in the "watchful expectancy" and diagnostic-therapeutic mixtures of strategy that are used so often and so successfully by the family practitioner. These strategies are nevertheless an important part of the general tactics of clinical management for patients, and will require appropriate algorithms to indicate the roles of both time and treatment as diagnostic agents in clinical management.

Another important distinction between scholastic activities and clinical practice is the role of clinical data in strategies of therapy. For almost a century, medical students have been taught to believe that clinical data were used mainly for deducing a diagnosis, and that therapy then depended on the inferred diagnosis. This hoary custom of academic pedagogy is honored much more by its breach than by its observance in the realities of medical practice. As noted elsewhere (32), clinical data are often used as inferential guides to a diagnostic name, and the diagnosis may often determine at least one aspect of treatment, but many other acts of ordinary treatment depend directly on the clinical phenomena, not on a diagnostic name. Thus, if a patient has chest pain, shock, and a cardiac arrhythmia, we might diagnostically infer that he has acute myocardial infarction, but our only therapeutic act for the myocardial infarction itself is to put the patient to bed. All the other treatment depends on the associated clinical findings. Morphine is given for the pain, not the infarction; vasopressors are given for the shock, not the infarction; and digitalis is given for the arrhythmia, not the infarction.

Although this essay is generally concerned with diagnostic rather than therapeutic reasoning, the diverse algorithms of clinical medicine would be incompletely described without mention of their role in strategies of therapy. Clinicians who create such therapeutic algorithms will find that many critical decisions in treatment depend much more on clinical phenomena than on diagnostic names. An example of a therapeutic algorithm, again borrowed from the collection developed by the editors of PATIENT CARE (44), is shown in Fig. 11. There are 10 major decisions (bordered with thick-lined rectangles) that precede the therapeutic actions noted in the flow chart of Fig. 11. Each of those decisions depends mainly on clinical phenomena, rather than on diagnostic titles.

Not all clinicians will agree with the recommendations made by the panel of experts (44) whose consensus is reflected in the flow chart of Fig. 11. What the chart does provide, however, is a method of outlining a course of therapeutic strategy clearly enough and specifically enough for a reader to decide whether he agrees or disagrees. In contrast to the vagueness and ambiguity with which many therapeutic recommendations appear in free text, the flow-chart format provides a direct, precise demonstration of the observations, decisions, and actions entailed in therapeutic management.

Managerial clinical algorithms (45), sometimes called *protocols* (46), have also become a valuable tool in providing instructions for the patient care activities performed by physician assistants and other "medical extenders." With suitable arrangements of data, the flow chart format can be used both for indicating what to do and for auditing the performance.

5. Intellectual and Clinical Economy

The last type of algorithm to be discussed here deals with the problem of "economy" in the sequence of thoughts, tests, and decisions that occur in clinical reasoning. Every observant clinician has discovered that certain "short-cuts" or other maneuvers, either of intellect or of action, can increase the efficiency of his work

PATIENT CARE FLOW CHART: TREATING CHRONIC LUNG DISEASE
(A summary of key steps in managing mild-moderate disease)

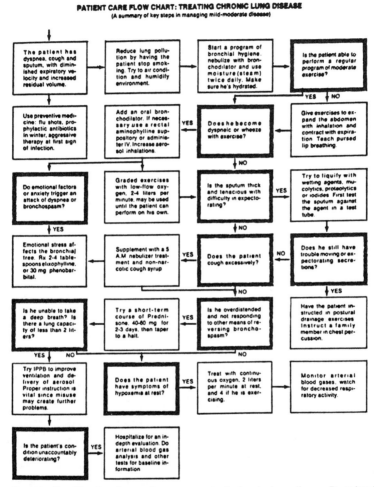

FIG. 11. Algorithm for therapeutic management of chronic lung disease. Reproduced, with permission, from page 62 of panel discussion in PATIENT CARE (44).

in clinical practice. A clearly outlined flow chart offers a method of discerning the relative efficiency or inefficiency of different sequences in the path of clinical decisions.

For example, on learning that the patient has a sore throat, an experienced clinician seldom goes through the traditional ritual of getting a complete account of the present illness, review of systems, past history, social history and other aspects of history-taking before he begins the physical examination. He usually looks at the throat immediately. Having noted the physical findings, or while noting them, he may ask about the symptomatic details of the sore throat and present illness.

At the same time, or slightly later, he may examine the gums and palpate the lymph nodes of the neck. While engaged in these physical procedures, or shortly thereafter, the clinician may ask about other details of the history that seem cogent for the array of clinical decisions that must be made.

These decisions may often be managerial before they are diagnostic. For example, if the patient with a sore throat also has a large pharyngeal mass and complains of rapidly progressive respiratory distress, the clinician may decide to do a tracheostomy before proceeding with any other examination procedures or diagnostic decisions. Similarly, if a patient with active gastrointestinal bleeding is hypotensive and in a cold sweat, the clinician may start an intravenous infusion, make preparations to administer blood, and alert the operating room staff, before he begins any of his exercises in history taking. (An algorithm for the above sequence would have included obtaining a statement about the bleeding, and then a physical examination of the skin and blood pressure before onset of the managerial procedures).

Even in nonemergency situations, many parts of the physical examination and laboratory tests are regularly performed before the total history is consummated. A gastroenterologist, for example, may regularly want to know the results of the array of paraclinical data that can be used to rule out "organic disease" before he concludes that the patient has "functional bowel distress" and begins a probing history about psychosocial-environmental features that may be causing or aggravating the distress.

The clinicians who practice in this sequentially mingled manner generally do so because they have found it more efficient than the tandem conjunction of isolated sequences that they were taught in medical school. The need for such mingling of sequences has been unofficially recognized by leading accreditation agencies such as the American Board of Internal Medicine, which allowed only 45 min for the performance of a complete history and physical examination when a candidate physician sought certification in the Board's oral examination. A candidate who had not learned to mingle sequences could seldom take a complete history and then do a complete physical examination and still be finished within 45 min.

Despite the constant admixture of history taking and physical examination in clinical practice, medical students are traditionally taught to perform the two procedures in an isolated manner, one following the other. This traditional sequence in techniques is probably pedagogically useful for instructing a beginning clinical student, who later learns to perform the mingling as he advances from neophyte to expert. Unfortunately, however, each physician does the mingling differently, ascribing his techniques to "judgment" and "experience," and almost no one can demonstrate exactly how the procedure is done when we want to study its efficiency, teach it to a student, or describe it to a machine.

Regardless of any instruction the delineations might provide for a computer, they are worth creating if only for their value in improving the efficiency of clinical examination, both in performance and in pedagogy. The creation of the appropriate algorithms cannot be done as an act of theoretical strategy. Knowledgeable clinicians will have to study their own activities, and then delineate the algorithmic flow and the rational justifications. In Figs. 12 and 13, I have indicated brief segments of intellectual sequences that can illustrate the managerial inefficiency of delaying certain critical examination procedures while pursuing the conventional sequence of history taking, followed by physical examination, followed by paraclinical tests.

A. Standard Sequence of History followed by Physical Examination

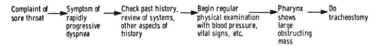

B. Intermingled Sequence of Examination

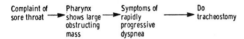

FIG. 12. Economy of intermingled vs standard sequence of examination in patient with sore throat and rapidly progressive dyspnea (for further details, see text).

A. Standard Sequence of Clinical Examination followed by Roentgenogram

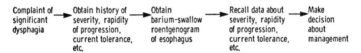

B. Intermingled Sequence of Examination

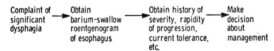

FIG. 13. Economy of intermingled vs standard sequence of examination in patient with significant dysphagia (for further details, see text).

The illustration in Fig. 12 shows the pathway between onset of clinical examination (with the patient's complaint of sore throat) and the clinician's therapeutic conclusion to perform tracheostomy. The pathway required six steps with the conventional sequence in Part A, but only four steps with the mixed sequence of Part B.

In Fig. 13, the clinician must make a decision about therapeutic management for a patient with the complaint of significant dysphagia. With the standard sequence of examination, in Part A, the clinician learns about severity and other descriptive details of the dysphagia before the esophagus is examined roentgenographically. After the roentgenogram is seen, all these symptomatic details must then be recalled for the managerial decision. With the mixed sequence, in Part B, the roentgenogram is obtained immediately after the main complaint is noted. Knowing the roentgenographic findings, the clinical then learns the other symptomatic details as a direct prelude to deciding about management. An extra step, the intermediate recall of symptoms, has been saved. Analogous "economies" are practiced by gynecologists who perform the pelvic examination before obtaining all the historical details in a patient with amenorrhea.

* * *

To avoid an overly prolonged discussion, I shall omit some of the many other important topics for which clinical algorithms are needed. Most prominent among these topics are the role of social, personal, psychic, and financial features in affecting clinical strategies. The relatively simple diagnostic and therapeutic problems illustrated here could be solved with algorithmic plans based mainly on clinical and paraclinical data. In the realistic practice of medicine, however, the algorithmic strategies will be inadequate unless they provide suitable, and often paramount, attention to a patient's demographic and behavioral data. After appropriate algorithms are established for strictly managerial decisions about the pathology of the disease, the algorithms can be modified to include the totality of decisions in the care of the patient.

SUMMARY

The plan of strategy used for solving a problem is called an *algorithm* and can be portrayed either in the sequential treelike structure of a *flow chart* or in the tabular array of conditions and actions that is called a *decision table*. An algorithm prepared for scientific purposes should be accompanied by statements of factual evidence or conceptual principles that provide its *justification*.

An enormous variety of algorithms is needed to describe the many decisions that occur in clinical activities. Some of these algorithms will depict processes that are clinically more simple than diagnostic reasoning. Such algorithms include the instructions for automated acquisition of data in history taking and for automated observation of paraclinical visual patterns. The "elementary" algorithms also include procedures for storage and enumerative retrieval of the data obtained during clinical and laboratory examinations.

The "advanced" clinical algorithms deal with the complex interpretations that occur during diagnostic, prognostic, and therapeutic reasoning. Diagnostic algorithms include the analysis of paraclinical data, the analysis of clinical data, and the plans for a diagnostic workup. Although purely diagnostic algorithms may be followed by separate algorithms for prognostic and therapeutic reasoning, these procedures may often occur in an intermingled sequence in clinical practice. The diagnostic process may be interrupted by treatment that acts as a diagnostic test or that eliminates the need for further diagnosis. The traditional diagnostic succession of history, physical examination, and paraclinical tests may also be performed in a sequence different from conventional pedagogic instructions.

The algorithmic portrayal of these processes is crucial for determining the intellectual "economy" with which they are performed, for improving the way in which they are taught, and for assembling satisfactory data to evaluate their costs, risks, and benefits to patients. The construction of justified clinical algorithms requires intimate familiarity with clinical activities and offers a major new scientific challenge in basic clinical research.

REFERENCES

1. Feinstein, A. R. An analysis of diagnostic reasoning. I. The domains and disorders of clinical macrobiology. *Yale J. Biol. Med.* **46,** 212–232, (1973).

2. Feinstein, A. R. An analysis of diagnostic reasoning. II. The strategy of intermediate decisions. *Yale J. Biol. Med.* **46**, 264–283, (1973).

3. Warner, H. R., Toronto, A. F., Veasey, L. G. and Stephenson, R. A mathematical approach to medical diagnosis: Application to congenital heart disease. *JAMA* **177**, 177–183 (1961).

4. Ledley, R. S. Computer aids to medical diagnosis. *JAMA* **196**, 933–994 (1966).

5. Manning, R. T. Signs, symptoms, and systematics. *JAMA* **198**, 1180–1184 (1966).

6. Cornfield, J. Bayes theorem. *Review International Statistical Institute* **35**, 34–49 (1967).

7. Hall, G. H. The clinical application of Bayes' theorem. *Lancet* **ii**, 655–557 (1967).

8. Lincoln, T. L., and Parker, R. D. "Medical Diagnosis Using Bayes Theorem." Health Services Research, pp. 34–45, 1967.

9. Peckham, R. H. Betting odds in medical diagnosis. *Amer. J. Med. Sci.* **253**, 35–37 (1967).

10. Lusted, L. B. "Introduction to Medical Decision Making." Charles C Thomas, Springfield, Ill., 1968.

11. Templeton, A. W., Bryan, K., Waid, R., Townes, J., Huge, M., and Dwyer, S. J. Computer diagnosis and discriminate analysis decision schemes. *Radiology* **95**, 47–55 (1970).

12. Fisher, R. A. On the mathematical foundations of theoretical statistics. *Phil. Trans. Roy. Soc. London, Series A*, **222**, 309–368 (1922).

13. King, P. J. H. Decision tables. *Comp. Journal* **10**, 135–142 (1967).

14. McDaniel, H. "An Introduction to Decision Logic Tables." Wiley, New York, 1968.

15. Galler, B. "The Language of Computers." McGraw–Hill, New York, 1962.

16. Mayne, J. G., Weksel, W., and Sholtz, P. N. Toward automating the medical history. *Mayo Clin. Proc.* **43**, 1–25 (1968).

17. Slack, W. V., and Van Cura, L. J. Patient reaction to computer-based medical interviewing. *Comp. Biomed. Res.* **1**, 527–531 (1968).

18. Pryor, T. A., Russel, R., Budkin, A., and Price, W. G. Electrocardiographic interpretation by computer. *Comp. Biomed. Res.* **2**, 537–548 (1969).

19. Caceres, C. A., and Dreifus, L. S. (Eds.) "Clinical Electrocardiography and Computers." Academic Press, New York, 1970.

20. Milliken, J. A., Wartak, J., Orme, W., Fay, J. W., Lywood, D. W., and Abrahams, V. C. Computer recognition of electrocardiographic waveforms. *Canad. Med. Assn. J.* **103**, 365–370 (1970).

21. Miyahara, H., Whipple, G. H., Teager, H. M., Webb, T. W., Theophilis, C. A., and Dohi, Y. Cardiac arrhythmia diagnosis by digital computer. Considerations related to the temporal distribution of P and R waves. *Comp. Biomed. Res.* **1**, 277–300 (1968).

22. Lindsay, A. E. and Budkin, A. "The Cardiac Arrhythmias. An Approach to Their Electrocardiographic Recognition." Year Book Medical Publishers, Chicago, 1969.

23. Hall, D. L., Lodwick, G. S., Kruger, R. P., Dwyer, S. J., and Townes, J. R. Direct computer diagnosis of rheumatic heart disease. *Radiology* **101**, 497–509 (1971).

24. Slack, W. V., Peckham, B. M., Van Cura, L. J., and Carr, W. F. A computer-based physical examination system. *JAMA* **200**, 224–228 (1967).

25. Juergens, J. L., and Kiely, J. M. Physician entry of cardiac physical findings into a computer-based medical record. *Mayo Clin. Proc.* **44**, 361–366 (1969).

26. Greenes, R. A., Barnett, G. O., Klein, S. W., Robbins, A., and Prior, R. E. Recording, retrieval, and review of medical data by physician-computer interaction. *New Engl. J. Med.* **282**, 307–315 (1970).

27. Weed, L. L. "Medical Records, Medical Education, and Patient Care." Year Book Medical Publishers, Chicago, 1970.

28. Hicks, G. P., Gieschen, M. M., Slack, W. V., and Larson, F. C. Routine use of a small digital computer in the clinical laboratory. *JAMA* **196**, 973–978 (1966).

29. Lindberg, D. A. B. "The Computer and Medical Care." Charles C Thomas, Springfield, Ill., 1968.

30. Walsh, J. M., and Goldblatt, S. A. A punch-card laboratory reporting system with a cumulative summary format. *JAMA* **207**, 1671–1678 (1969).

31. Kinney, T. D., and Melville, R. S. Automation in clinical laboratories. The present state and future uses of automation. Proceedings of a workshop conference. *Lab. Invest.* **16**, 803–812 (1967).

32. Feinstein, A. R. Clinical Judgment. Williams & Wilkins, Baltimore, 1967.
33. Feinstein, A. R. Clinical judgment in the era of automation. *Ann. Otol. Rhinol. Lar.* **79**, 728–737 (1970).
34. Feinstein, A. R. Quality of data in the medical record. *Comp. Biomed. Res.* **3**, 426–435 (1970).
35. Wartak, J., Milliken, J. A., and Karchmar, J. Computer program for pattern recognition of electrocardiograms. *Comp. Biomed. Res.* **3**, 344–374 (1970).
36. Wartak, J. "Computers in Electrocardiography." Charles C Thomas, Springfield, Ill., 1970.
37. Tuddenham, W. J. The use of logical flow charts as an aid in teaching roentgen diagnosis. *Am. J. Roentgenol., Rad. Ther. and Natl. Med.* **102**, 797–803 (1968) [The flow chart in Fig. 6 appeared in Medical News section, *JAMA* **196**, 36 (1966).]
38. Harvey, A. M., Cluff, L. E., Johns, R. J., Owens, A. H., Jr., Rabinowitz, D., and Ross, R. S. The Principles and Practice of Medicine. 17th ed. Appleton–Century–Crofts, New York, 1968.
39. Bleich, H. L. Computer evaluation of acid-base disorders. *J. Clin. Invest.* **48**, 1689–1696 (1969).
40. Edwards, D. A. W. Flow charts, diagnostic keys, and algorithms in the diagnosis of dysphagia. *Scot. Med. J.* **15**, 378–385, 1970.
41. Panel Discussion. (Bulger, J. J., Hellerstein, S., LeBauer, E. J., Smith, R. A., Maddock, R. K., Jr., Reeves, J. E., Roland, A. S. and Scribner, B. H.) The patient with edema: Searching for the cause. *Patient Care,* 21–52 (1969).
42. Schimmel, E. The hazards of hospitalization. *Ann. Intern. Med.* **60**, 100–110 (1964).
43. Feinstein, A. R. What kind of basic science for clinical medicine? *New. Engl. J. Med.* **283**, 847–852 (1970).
44. Panel Discussion. (Egan, D. F., Gray, F. D., Jr., Kaiser, H. B., Noehren, T. H., Petty, T. L. and Sanchez, R. C.) What more can you do for your chronic lung patients? *Patient Care* 18–63 (1970).
45. Sox, H. C., Jr., Sox, C. H., and Tompkins, R. K. The training of physician's assistants. The use of a clinical algorithm system for patient care, audit of performance and education. *New Engl. J. Med.* **288**, 818–824 (1973).
46. Komaroff, A. L., Black, W. L., Flatley, M., Knopp, R. H., Reiffen, B., and Sherman, H. Protocols for physician assistants. Management of diabetes and hypertension. *New Engl. J. Med.* **290**, 307–312 (1974).

Chapter 21

Physician Judgments and Resource Utilization in a Private Practice

J. William Gavett, Arthur R. Jacobs and Christine L. Thurber

A study of 419 visits to a group of internists was conducted in a semi-rural private practice in upstate New York. The purpose of the study was to obtain physician value judgments about the appropriate level of care for each visit. Each patient visit was judged by a single physician immediately after the physician attended the visit. Judgments about the "complexity of the visit," the appropriate level of manpower to manage the visit, the urgency of the visit, the number of visits required for management of the problem, the diagnostic classification of the problem, and other variables were judged by a physician for each of the sampled visits. These were supplemented with objective data about the patient. Thirty per cent of the visits were judged to be manageable by a physician expander. These visits were distributed among the short-term episodic illnesses as well as the chronic cases. Finally, the value judgments were used to classify the visits on a scale of "complexity" with focus on the definition of the non-complex or simple case. Eighty-three per cent of the cases were judged as "relatively easy to diagnose and treat."

METHODS ARE NEEDED for analyzing ambulatory care in order to provide physicians, consumers, and communities with information that will aid in improving the effectiveness and efficiency of ambulatory health services.[1, 4] The results of a study of patient visits in a semi-rural private group practice are presented to illustrate the relationship between patient characteristics and resource utilization. Appropriate levels of resource utilization are based upon the judgments of the practicing physicians. Similar analyses of the utilization of services should be an important input for the reorganization of ambulatory services.

The authors have previously suggested a first order classification of ambulatory utilization, as measured by patient visits, that differentiates in terms of the "complexity" of the visit.[2] Case complexity is defined by measures of the type and quantity of resources required to manage the visit. The classification scheme centers around a four-category classification of the visit as follows:

* Associate Professor, Department of Preventive Medicine and Community Health, and Graduate School of Management, University of Rochester, Rochester, N. Y.

† Assistant Professor, Department of Community Medicine, Dartmouth Medical College, Hanover, N. H.

‡ Research Assistant, Rochester Regional Medical Program, Rochester, N. Y.

Reprinted with permission from *Medical Care*, Volume II, pp. 310-319, 1973.

Class	Description of Visit
A	Acute, life-threatening; involving significant pathophysiologic disturbance; may require intensive care.
B	Complex case visit, possibly involving multiple problems, requiring extensive diagnosis, evaluation, and management. Typically organized around a chronic pathophysiologic process by medical specialization. Return visits required. Continuity of records and personnel is often important.
C	Relatively easy to diagnose and treat; requires non-complex facilities and medical techniques. Psychologic support may be an important component of therapy.
D	Other; such as physical exams.

The general purpose of such a classification is to suggest where innovations in manpower, equipment, and organization might be appropriate and also to provide a means of categorizing the demand for a given ambulatory service. It should be noted that the above classification scale can also characterize the episode of illness as well as the visit. Individual visits must be classified to plan for future services. For example, if the C visit is an infrequent event and the A visit, a frequent event, a different constellation of resources is needed than for a service that renders mostly C visit care.

Purpose

The specific goal of this study was to measure the level of resource utilization for a sample of visits to a semi-rural group of private internists. Criteria of what was appropriate included measures of physician judgment as well as objective facts about the visit. A second purpose of the study was to provide some empirical data for the classification of patient visits by the "intensity of the resources" applied to the visit. A third purpose of the study was to gain information that would be useful to the practitioners regarding the need for allied health personnel in their practices. The term "physician expander" is used generically to label the kind of person that would be used in providing direct patient care in the practice (e.g., nurse, nurse practitioner, physician's assistant, Medex, etc.). No attempt was made in this study to differentiate among these kinds of personnel.

Method

The method consisted of the physician answering some questions about patient visits at the time that he actually saw the patient. The information about each visit was supplemented with information from the patient record, i.e., age, sex, etc.

The setting for the study was a group practice consisting of 10 physicians practicing in an office building in a small city (population 10,000). The group owns the building and shares a central reception area, record and billing system, secretarial pool, and answering service. Physicians have separate examining rooms, waiting and reception areas. The individual physicians have their own patients who are seen by another physician only on the weekends, in emergencies, or when their own physician is unavailable. At least one member of the group practice is on call in the evenings and weekends. The group is composed of five internists, two general surgeons, one pediatrician, one obstetrician, and one anesthesiologist. This study relates only to the five internists. A sample of 419 visits from the practices of the five internists was made. The ages of the internists range from 35-50 years. Two of the internists are board-certified. The internists serve as "family" physicians as well as

TABLE 1. Episodic Nature of the Visit

Classified	No.	Per cent
One visit required	77	18.38
Two visits required	52	12.41
Short-term episodic	129	30.79
Three or more visits required	87	20.76
Long-term chronic care	173	41.29
Hospitalization	5	1.19
Physical examinations	23	5.49
No answer	2	0.48
TOTAL	419	100

"referral" physicians. The sample was taken between April and June, 1971. Each sampled visit was selected systematically from the group practice log book in which each patient entering the building is registered. Every *seventh* patient registered in the log was selected, regardless of the internist seen. A questionnaire accompanied the patient's record to the physician's office. At the completion of the visit, the questionnaire was completed by the physician rendering care. Subsequent to the visit, additional factual information about the patient and the visit was added to the questionnaire by the physician's office staff.

No attempt has been made to consider the reliability of the value judgments made by the physicians. Reliability in this case refers to the degree of repeatability of the response by the physician to the question given the same set of circumstances (patient, illness, etc.). It also refers to the degree of agreement among physicians regarding a given visit. When a physician made a judgment on the questionnaire regarding appropriate care for a particular visit, it would have been interesting to know if one or more of the other physicians would have agreed. However, this kind of study was not feasible.

Results

Results of the study that are particularly relevant to the question of appropriate utilization of resources will be discussed.

Episodic Nature of the Visit. A first order classification of the relationship of the sampled visit to other visits for the same episode of illness was made. Each visit was classified by the physician on a scale representing the number of visits the physician thought was required to manage the episode of illness for which the visit being evaluated was a part. Table 1 shows the results of this classification that provides a basic picture of the practices. Thirty-one per cent of the visits were judged short-term, episodic, requiring only one or two visits for management. One might categorize these visits as a set of C type *cases* where both the episode and the visit(s) are non-complex. In contrast, the longer term episodic and chronic cases would constitute the B-type case. This hypothesis will be examined later.

Visit Complexity. The physicians were asked to categorize the visit on a scale of A, B, C, D complexity. Table 2 shows the questions and the results by physician respondent and for the total sample of 419 visits. The last row shows the number of the visits seen by each physician. Only one case was classified as acute and life threatening, while 83 per cent were classified by the internists as relatively easy to diagnose and treat. The data conflict with the stereotype internist as a provider of care to B-type cases. While this "gestalt" classification of the visit is interesting it provides little information upon which to generalize about the nature of the visits in each class, particularly the attributes that distinguish complex from non-complex visits.

Use of the Physician Expander. One specific indicator of visit complexity might be reflected in the willingness of the physician to delegate the visit or portions of it to a physician expander. Therefore, the physician was asked to determine the appropriate manpower level required to treat the visit. Table 3 indicates the results of

TABLE 2.   Physician's Judgment of Visit Complexity

Visit Complexity Classification	Physician Respondents													Total	
	1		2		3		4		5		N.A.				
	No.	Per cent	No.	Per cent	No.	Per cent	No.	Per cent	No.	Per cent	No.	Per cent		No.	Per cent
Acute, life threatening; involving significant pathophysiologic disturbance; may require intensive care	0	0	0	0	0	0	0	0	1	1.7	0	0		1	0.24
Complex case visit, possibly involving multiple problems, requiring extensive diagnosis, evaluation, and management. Typically organized around chronic pathophysiologic process, by medical specialization, return visits. Continuity of records and personnel is often important	20	21.9	7	7.8	4	3.8	0	0	4	6.9	0	0		35	8.35
Relatively easy to diagnose and treat; requires non-complex facilities and medical techniques. Psychologic support may be an important component of therapy	69	75.9	79	87.8	86	81.9	67	94.4	49	84.5	2	50.0		352	83.53
Other or not available (N.A.)	2	2.2	4	4.4	15	14.3	4	5.6	4	6.9	2	50.0		31	7.88
Total visits seen in sample	91	100	90	100	105	100	71	100	58	100	4	100		419	100

TABLE 3. Physician's Judgment of Appropriate Skill Level

Appropriate Skill Level for Treatment	Physicians Respondents										N.A.	Total	
	1		2		3		4		5				
	No.	Per cent	No.	Per cent	No.	Per cent	No.	Per cent	No.	Per cent	No.	No.	Per cent
This visit should most appropriately (least specialized level of care) be treated by:													
Multiple specialist team-physician, nurses, corpsmen, technician	0	0	0	0	0	0	0	0	0	0	0	0	0
Specialist M.D., D.D.S.	5	5.5	2	2.2	16	15.2	0	0	16	27.6	0	39	9.31
General M.D.	67	73.6	49	54.5	47	44.8	56	78.9	33	57.9	1	253	60.38
Specially trained nurse, nurse practitioner, physician's assistant, or corpsman	19	20.9	39	43.3	42	40.0	15	21.1	9	15.5	1	125	29.83
Not available (N.A.)	0	0	0	0	0	0	0	0	0	0	2	2	0.48
TOTAL	91	100	90	100	105	100	71	100	58	100	4	419	100

that question by physician respondent. No attempt was made to advise the respondents before the study on the characteristics of the various kinds of physician expanders. Nurses were the only other health personnel used in the practices. Almost 30 per cent of the visits would have been delegated to a physician expander for treatment but with considerable variation among the physicians. For example, physicians 1 and 2 saw about the same number of patients yet exhibited significantly different judgments in willingness to delegate visits to a physician expander. The variation might be explained by differences in style of practice, differences in patients and their illnesses in the respective practices, or some combination thereof. A subsidiary question was asked relative to the use of the physician expander for the visit in question. Table 4 indicates the alternatives and the results. No physician thought he needed to be in the room while treatment was being administered and, in only 12 visits, did the physician feel it necessary to be on the premises; 10 of these were responses by physician 1. In 30 per cent of the visits classified, it was not deemed necessary for the physician to be advised that treatment was being administered. The physician expectations regarding the role of physician expanders are greater than the role presently permitted by some state medical licensure authorities.

Table 5 provides data on the use of the physician expander as related to the class of episodic illness. Only 41 per cent of the one-visit episodes were delegated to the physician expander indicating that the single visit episode is not always a non-complex case if the use of the physician expander for treatment is a criterion of non-complexity. Thirty-five per cent of the chronic visits were delegated to the physician expander thus emphasizing the notion that the C-type visit is a component of the set of visits comprising the chronic

TABLE 4. Respondent Proximity to Physician Expander during Treatment of Visit

	Respondent					Total	
Proximity	1	2	3	4	5	No.	Per cent
1. In the room while treatment is being administered	0	0	0	0	0	0	0
2. On the premises while treatment is being administered	10	2	0	0	0	12	10.9
3. Consulted about or notified that treatment is being administered	2	23	29	9	3	66	60.0
4. Not necessary to notify or consult the physician that treatment is being administered	6	14	4	5	3	32	29.1
TOTAL	18	39	33	14	6	110	100.0

Fifteen other visits were unclassified.

B-type case. The data suggest that physician expanders have an appropriate role in the care of C-type visits in single visit episodes of illness and in chronic illness.

Distribution of Charges. Table 6 indicates the distribution of charges for services rendered. Almost 79 per cent of the patients were charged only for the office visit ($9), and less than 12 per cent of the visits were charged for office visit plus ancillary services. The charge data also illustrate that tests and complex procedures are not generally being performed in the office.

Need for Patient Record. The need for the patient record both for the treatment of the visit in question and preservation of information for the future management of the case would be another indicator of the case complexity. Therefore, the physicians were asked to make a judgment about the record. Table 7 shows the results of this question. The important figure is the number of visits for which the record was not needed for future care of the patient. This subject is also contained in the subset of 80 visits for which the history was not required for treatment of the visit. Continuity of records appear to be important in the ambulatory care delivered by the physicians.

Non-complex Visit and Case. It has been hypothesized by the authors that the non-complex, C visit to a primary ambulatory care organization is large in numbers, but that the organization is often overly

TABLE 5. Visits Judged Treatable by Physician Expander as a Percentage of Visits in Episodic Class

	No. Visits		
Class of Episode of Illness	In episodic class	Delegated to PX	Percentage of episodic class
One-visit episode	77	31	41.0%
Two-visit episode	52	12	23.0%
Three or more visits	87	17	19.5%
Chronic care	175	62	35.4%
Other	28	3	10.4%

TABLE 6. Distribution of Total Charges

Charge	Percentage of Visits
$0–8	10.28
$9	78.76
$10–15	5.02
$16–20	1.43
$21–30	2.87
Greater than $30	1.44
TOTAL	100

equipped to manage such visits. Also, from the patient's point of view, accessibility of service might be an important factor in C visits if such visits constitute minor, but patient-perceived, urgent problems. In terms of organizational innovation, this implies the possible justification of "convenience" facilities such as are currently being inefficiently met by emergency departments ("non-emergencies") and physicians' offices ("walk-ins"). Therefore, it would appear useful to both define the non-complex, C visit and measure its occurrence in a given organization of health care.

Figure 1 is a composite subclassification of the sample designed to segregate characteristics of the visit that could define the C visit and case. The total sample consists of 416 rather than 419 visits due to three incomplete questionnaires.

The first order classification is by factual information, i.e., whether or not the visit had been scheduled. A non-scheduled

category gives some information for the ultimate evaluation of the convenience attribute of a service. The high percentage (46.4) of the non-scheduled visits may imply a measure of patient-perceived urgency and an important parameter for the design of ambulatory care delivery systems.

Both the scheduled and non-scheduled sets are partitioned in terms of the urgency of the visit. Urgent visits were classified by physician judgment as requiring treatment either "immediately" (1.3 per cent of the sample) or "within a few hours" (12.0 per cent of the sample). The non-urgent visit could be seen by a scheduled appointment. Note that only 49, or about 25 per cent, of the non-scheduled visits were classified as urgent by the physician.

In the case of the non-scheduled visits, the physician was asked if this visit could be initially screened by a physician expander (PX) or should it be screened by an M.D. $(\overline{PX})$. Screening meant the ability to decide when the patient should be seen in the case of a telephone contact and who should see the patient. Of the subset of 193 non-scheduled visits, 61 (31.5 per cent) could have been screened by other than the M.D., while 132 (68.5 per cent) would have required the physician to decide on the disposition of the visit. Decision rules should be developed so that the physician expander can play an active role in the triage of patients in ambulatory care settings, as Weinerman has done in New Haven.[3]

TABLE 7. Need for Patient Record

	Yes		Maybe		No		N.A.		Total	
	No.	Per cent	No.	Per cent	No.	Per cent	No.	Per cent	No.	Per cent
Is the medical record history important for proper treatment of this visit?	320	76.37	17	4.06	80	19.09	2	0.48	419	100.00
For the future care of this patient is the record of this visit important?	311	74.22	63	15.04	43	10.26	2	0.48	410	100.00

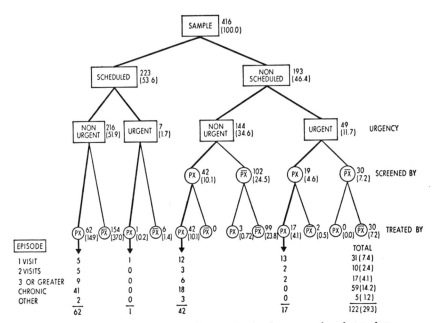

FIG. 1. Composite classification. Number to right of node: top—number of visits; bottom—per cent of 416 visits. PX—physician expander; $\overline{PX}$—not physician expander; Heavy line—non-complex visit; Light line—visit requiring MD screening or treatment.

The final set of nodes in the classification tree partition the sample in terms of the appropriate manpower level for the treatment of the visit. Either the visit, according to the physician's judgment, could have been treated by the physician expander, (PX) or not ($\overline{PX}$).

The heavy lines in the tree lead to subsets that might define the non-complex C visit. The branches include either scheduled or non-scheduled, urgent or non-urgent, screenable by the physician expander, and treatable by the physician expander. This multiple classification accounts for 122 (29.3 per cent) of the sample of 416 visits. This subset excludes only three PX-treatable, non-scheduled visits because they must be M.D. screened.

The bottom of the figure further subclassifies the 122 C visits by the episodic

nature of the illness for which the visit was seen. Thirty-one of the visits were single visit episodes, 7.4 per cent of the total sample. These might be defined as the C visits. The addition of the 10 two-visit episodes to this set increases the percentage to 10 per cent of the total sample. Since the total number of one- and two-visit episodes in the study was 129, the number of C visits is 41/129 (32 per cent). In contrast, the number of visits by chronic cases was 173 in the total sample, of which 59 are classified as C visits, 59/173 (34 per cent).

Discussion

This study is intended to illuminate the process of rendering medical care to patients in an ambulatory care organization. The more specific purpose of this study is to differentiate visits in terms of measures of the intensity of the resources applied to the visit. It has been reasoned that such visit classifications might indicate where changes could take place in the microcosm of ambulatory care, profitable to both the providers and consumers. Traditional medical diagnostic categories may indicate some measure of etiology, appropriate treatment, and prognosis, but do not indicate the appropriate level of manpower, equipment, facility accessibility, etc., for high quality, efficient, personalized care.

The focus has been to define and segregate the C visit and case characterized by non-complexity and modest use of resources. The dominant criterion in this study was the willingness of the physician to delegate the visit to a physician expander. Just under 30 per cent of the visits were so designated. As would be anticipated, there were considerable differences among the physicians in the degree of delegation. In most cases, delegation was fairly complete; there was little need for physician intervention directly or indirectly in the screening and treatment process. Also, the physicians perceived the physician expander as a judge of the disposition of the cases seen by the physician expander but not for the cases seen by the physician. In other words, the screening and treatment were conceived of as a package either delegated to the PX or not. Similar studies should be performed in ambulatory care organizations where care is actually rendered by physician expanders.

The fact that 30 per cent of the visits were deemed treatable by other than a physician is rather significant when one considers that no attempt was made to condition the physicians before the study as to the potential use of physician expanders. If an intensive analysis was made of the sample of visits in light of a detailed knowledge of physician expander skill levels, it is quite probable that the number of visits designated as treatable by the physician expander would be larger. This has obviously important implications for the delivery of ambulatory care. The data suggest that physician expanders will have a role in the C visit where the C visit may be the only visit in an episode of illness or one of many visits in a chronic illness. The attractiveness of the economics of delegating portions of a practice to physician expanders depends upon the volume of visits handled by the practice, proportion of visits or parts of visits delegated, price charged, physician expander salary, etc. However, such innovations as the physician expander cannot be quantitatively costed without a data base for practice (Fig. 1).

The data on episodic nature of visits, treatments, distribution of charges, non-scheduled visits, non-urgent visits, as well as the data on physician expanders, suggest that C visits constitute a significant proportion of the demand in the practice studied. The question then arises: Is there a particular organizational plan to accommodate the C-type demand? Care for the C case or visit need not necessarily be a free standing, specialized delivery organization. What is implied is design for convenience: maximized access without elaborate scheduling, optimal use of physician expanders, absence of extensive facilities for tests and procedures, a record system to preserve continuity of care, and a low risk system of referral for other types of patients (A,B,D) who present to this organization.

Conclusion

Planning for innovations in ambulatory care services should take into account the quantitative and qualitative characteristics of resource utilization in the existing system of care. Data from the evaluation of a private internist group practice are presented to illustrate the importance of relating manpower, equipment, and facility resources quantitatively to patient visits. The analyses suggest that, for the practice studied, innovations such as physician expanders are appropriate. For ambulatory care evaluation, what is needed are cost benefit analyses of patient visits in which benefits are related to the management of different classifications of patient problems with alternate constellations of resources—manpower, equipment, and facilities.

References

1. Garfield, S. R.: The delivery of medical care. *Sci. Am.* 222:15, 1970.

2. Jacobs, A. R., and Gavett, J. W.: Ambulatory Case Classification and Ambulatory Care Planning. Systems Analysis Program Working Paper Series No. F-7021. The Graduate School of Management, University of Rochester, 1971.

3. Weinerman, E., R., et al.: Effects of medical triage in hospital emergency services. *Public Health Rep.* 80:389, 1965.

4. White, K. L.: Organization and delivery of personal health services—public policy issues. *Milbank Mem. Fund Q.* 46:225, 1968.

Chapter 22

Assessing Health Quality—The Case for Tracers

David M. Kessner, Carolyn E. Kalk and James Singer

Abstract A set of specific health problems — called tracers — were selected by a set of criteria. The tracers include otitis media and associated hearing loss, visual disorders, iron-deficiency anemia, urinary-tract infection, essential hypertension, and cancer of the cervix. When one tracer is used in a hypothetical community served by a neighborhood health center, data can be developed that demonstrate the application of the tracer method — the center, for example, is shown to care for only 11 per cent of the estimated population of hypertensive adult males in the community, and drug therapy is found not to meet minimal criteria in 30 per cent of the treated patient sample. By evaluation of the diagnostic, therapeutic, and follow-up processes of the set of tracers and the outcome of treatment, it is possible to assess the quality of routine care provided in a health-care system.

THE question is no longer whether there will be intervention in health services to assure quality, but who will intervene and what methods they will use.

Almost 40 years ago, Lee and Jones[1] defined quality of medical care by eight "articles of faith": scientific basis for medical practice; prevention; consumer-provider co-operation; treatment of the whole individual; close and continuing patient-physician relation; comprehensive and co-ordinated medical services; co-ordination between medical care and social services; and accessibility of care for all people. Today, these unarguable goals have greater active support than when they were first stated. The focus of health-policy makers and consumers is shifting from concern over the bald costs of care to concern for getting their money's worth. Indeed, if anything, the raising of the public consciousness in health matters has hardened the goals; the "accessibility of care" is giving way to the "right to care," and the right to care implies the right to quality care.

During the past decade and a half, the conceptual issues in evaluating health care have been stated and restated many times.[2-11] The basic requirements for a pragmatic evaluation method include a statement of the objectives of the program; standards to define quality of care; data on delivered care that can be compared to standards; careful attention to the nature of the measurement units; assessment of the reliability of the analysis; consideration of the cost of the method; and a plan for integrating evaluation into the organization of health services.

The last requirement is most critical. Evaluation can neither assure quality nor improve care unless it is part and parcel of the delivery system, an ongoing agent for change when change is necessary and a tool for educating providers and consumers alike to the strengths and weaknesses of the system.

In July, 1969, the Institute of Medicine (than called the Board on Medicine) of the National Academy of Sciences undertook a program — entitled "Contrasts in Health Status"—to evaluate health services received by different groups of people in our population. In developing a method for assessing health-care status, the Institute focused on the premise that specific health problems could serve as "tracers" in analyzing health delivery. When combined into sets, they provide a framework for evaluating the interaction between providers, patients, and their environments. They also would yield easily understood data to be fed back into the health-delivery system.

THE TRACER METHOD

The tracer concept was borrowed from the formal sciences. Endocrinologists, for example, use radioactive tracers to study how a body organ such as the thyroid gland handles a critical substance such as iodide. They measure how the gland takes up a minute amount of radioactive iodide, and assume that the organ handles natural iodide in the same manner.

For measuring the functions of a health-care system, the tracers needed are discrete, identifiable health problems each shedding light on how particular parts of the system work, not in isolation, but in relation to one another. The basic assumption remains the same namely, how a physician or team of physicians routinely administers care for common ailments will be an indicator of the general quality of care and the efficacy of the system delivering that care.

The use of specific health problems to analyze health services is not new. In a study of the medical clinic of a university hospital in the early 1960's, for example, Huntley et al.[11] analyzed charts for completeness of patient work-up and proportion of abnormalities that were not followed up. More than ¼ of the patients with a diastolic blood pressure of 100 mm of mercury or

From the Health Services Research Study, Institute of Medicine, National Academy of Sciences, 2101 Constitution Ave., Washington, D. C. 20418, where reprint requests should be addressed to Dr. Kessner.

The opinions and conclusions stated in this paper are those of the authors alone and do not necessarily reflect the policy of the Institute of Medicine or the National Academy of Sciences, or their members.

Supported by grants from Carnegie Corporation of New York, the Fannie E. Ripple Foundation, Association for the Aid of Crippled Children, and the John Hancock Life Insurance Company and by contracts with the Office of Health Evaluation, Deputy Assistant Secretary, Evaluation and Monitoring, Department of Health, Education, and Welfare (Contracts HEW-OS-70-130 and HEW-OS-167) and with the Office of Planning, Research, and Evaluation, Office of Economic Opportunity, (Contract B1C-5243).

Some of the material herein was presented at the annual meeting of the Medical Care Section of the American Public Health Association, Minneapolis, Minn., October 11, 1971.

Printed with permission from *The New England Journal of Medicine*, Vol. 288, pp. 189-192, January 25, 1973.

higher were given no special tests relevant to hypertension, and approximately ½ of these patients had no diagnosis related to the cardiovascular system.

Other analyses using specific diseases include those by Ciocco et al.,[15] and Morehead and their co-workers,[16, 17] Brook[18] and Payne.* These studies all used specific health problems as indicators of either process or outcome variables, or a combination of process and outcome, in the delivery of ambulatory health services.

The tracer methodology developed by the Institute of Medicine differs from previous efforts in several ways. These include the manner in which tracers were selected and combined in sets; specification of criteria for care; and, in application, concurrent assessment of the health professional, the community that he serves, and the people to whom he delivers services.

The tracer method measures both process and outcome of care, which we consider important in any evaluation scheme. It is impossible to pinpoint the strengths and weaknesses of process without knowing the outcome, but outcome alone can be misleading if the patient receives unnecessary diagnostic tests or inappropriate therapy.

SELECTING TRACERS

The first important difference from previous methodologies is that tracers are selected and combined according to criteria. In an attempt to give a rational and uniform basis for selecting the tracers, six criteria were established that would screen out health problems that are not appropriate tracers. In order of importance, the criteria are as follows:

1. *A tracer should have a definite functional impact.* The over-riding purpose of the tracer approach is to focus on specific conditions that reflect the activities of health professionals. Conditions that are unlikely to be treated and those that cause negligible functional impairment are not useful.

2. *A tracer should be relatively well defined and easy to diagnose.* Dermatologic conditions have a clear functional impact. The difficulties, however, of defining clear-cut pathologic entities lessen their utility as tracers. In contrast, it is relatively easy to identify a population of patients with a hematocrit below a specified level and further to diagnose those with iron-deficiency anemia.

3. *Prevalence rates should be high enough to permit the collection of adequate data from a limited population sample.* If an adequate number of cases cannot be studied, it is difficult to evaluate even the most important variables in relation to the set of tracers.

4. *The natural history of the condition should vary with utilization and effectiveness of medical care.* Ideally, in evaluation of a delivery system, the conditions under study should be sensitive to the quality or quantity (or both) of the service received by the patient. It is inappropriate to use conditions

*Cited by Brook.[18]

for which health services do not alter the progress of the disease.

5. *The technics of medical management of the condition should be well defined for at least one of the following processes: prevention, diagnosis, treatment or rehabilitation.* There is danger in using tracers to look at the process of care if minimal standards for medical management cannot be agreed upon.

6. *The effects of nonmedical factors on the tracer should be understood.* Social, cultural, economic, behavioral and environmental factors can influence the prevalence and distribution of many diseases. Thus, the epidemiology of the tracer should be relatively well understood and the population at risk easy to identify.

We screened 15 candidate tracers and selected a set of six — middle ear infection and hearing loss, visual disorders, iron-deficiency anemia, hypertension, urinary-tract infections and cervical cancer — that met the specified criteria. As a set, the six tracers can be used to evaluate the ambulatory care received by a cross-section of the population; the set provides at least two individual tracers relevant to both sexes and four age groups (Table 1).

The activities of a health-service delivery organization are categorized in five major groups (see Table 2). Each major activity is required for management of at least two tracers. This allows us to sample the varied activities of a delivery system from multiple perspectives and thereby strengthens the validity of extrapolating from the analyses of the tracer set to the delivery system as a whole. For example, if there is little or no screening for four of five tracers that require screening, the concordance of this finding suggests that this medical process needs improvement.

CRITERIA FOR CARE

A critical requirement for evaluating health services is the establishment of criteria against which services delivered can be compared. Without formal criteria, objective evaluations and analyses are impossible. Yet establishing criteria has an inherent danger — that of the risk of locking the medical profession into a rigid mode of practice.

We believed criteria for treating the tracer conditions could avoid rigidity if they were formulated on three premises: they should outline minimal, or base-line, care; they should be pragmatic, taking into account unavailability of sophisticated diagnostic equipment; and they should be periodically revised and updated.

Also, in formulating the criteria, we recognized that no single plan could cope with the variation in clinical presentation that the practicing physician faces. Thus, the criteria should be viewed as a plan broadly applicable to populations of patients not as a management formula for individual patients. We made no attempt to rank the importance of various processes involved in delivering care. It is naïve to suggest that a history is more or less important than a physical examination or appropriate laboratory tests. Accurate diagnosis depends on integrating critical historical, physical and laboratory data.

Minimal-care criteria for hypertension in adults — applicable to urban or suburban practice — are shown below.* They were formulated by practicing family physicians and specialists.

To illustrate the application of the tracer methodology, we have outlined a hypothetical community served by a hypothetical neighborhood health center. We will assume that the community is located in the central city and its 42,000 citizens are predominantly blacks, with a median family income of $5,000 per year

---

A MINIMAL-CARE PLAN FOR HYPERTENSION

I. Screening
  A. *Method.* The systolic pressure is recorded at the onset of the first Korotkoff sound, and the diastolic at the final disappearance of the second or the change if the sound persists.
  B. *Criteria.* An individual patient is judged in need of evaluation for elevated blood pressure if the mean of three or more systolic or diastolic pressures exceeds the age-specific criteria specified below:

MALES & FEMALES	SYSTOLIC	DIASTOLIC
	mm Hg	
18-44 years	140	90
45-64 years	150	95
65 or older	160	95

II. Evaluation
  In the evaluation of elevated blood pressure, the history and physical-examination data listed below should be obtained early in the evaluation.
  A. *History.* (1) Personal and social history; (2) family history of high blood pressure, coronary-artery disease, or stroke; (3) previous diagnosis of high blood pressure (females, toxemia of pregnancy or pre-eclampsia) and time of first occurrence; (4) previous treatment for high blood pressure (when started and when stopped, and drugs used); (5) chest pain, pressure, or tightness; location, length of symptoms, frequency of symptoms, effect of deep breathing, description of feeling (crushing, smothering, strangling), symptom temporarily curtails activity, and pain radiates into left shoulder, arm, or jaw and is accompanied by nausea, shortness of breath or fast or fluttering heart beat; (6) shortness of breath; (8) patient awakens wheezing or feeling smothered or choked; (9) patient sleeps on two or more pillows; (10) prior history of kidney trouble, nephrosis or nephritis; (11) history of kidney infection; and (12) prior x-ray examination of kidneys.
  B. *Physical Examination.* (1) Weight and height; (2) blood pressure — supine and upright; (3) funduscopic; (4) heart — abnormal sounds or rhythm; (5) neck — thyroid and neck veins; (6) abdomen — standard description,

including abdominal bruit; and (7) extremities — peripipheral pulses and edema.
  C. *Laboratory.* (1) Urinalysis; (2) hematocrit or hemoglobin; and (3) blood urea nitrogen or serum creatinine.
  D. *Other Tests.* (1) Electrocardiogram; if the patient is less than 30 years of age or if diastolic pressure is 130 mm of mercury or greater; and (2) rapid-sequence intravenous pyelogram.
III. Diagnosis
  A. *Essential Hypertension.* As described in above under I B (Criteria) provided there is no evidence of secondary hypertension.
  B. *Secondary Hypertension.* Hypertension secondary to renal, adrenal, thyroid, or primary vascular disease.
IV. Management
  All drugs are prescribed in acceptable dosages adjusted to the individual patient, contraindications are observed, and patients are monitored for common side effect according to information detailed in AMA Drug Evaluations 1971 (first edition). Fixed-dosage combinations should not be used for initial therapy.
  A. *Mild Essential Hypertension (Diastolic Pressure of 115 Mm of Mercury).* (1) Initial treatment with thiazides alone in a diuretic dose; (2) if pressure is not reduced by 10 mm of mercury or to lowest level that patient can tolerate without symptoms of hypotension in two to four weeks, alpha-methyldopa, reserpine or hydralazine is added to thiazide.
  B. *Moderate Essential Hypertension (Diastolic Pressure of 115 to 130 Mm of Mercury).* (1) Initial treatment with thiazide and alpha-methyldopa, reserpine, or hydralazine; (2) if no response after two to four weeks, change to thiazide-reserpine-hydralazine or thiazide-guanethidine combination.
  C. *Severe Essential Hypertension (Diastolic Pressure of 130 Mm of Mercury or Keith-Wagener Grade III or IV Funduscopic Changes).* Refer to specialist or hospitalize (or both).
  D. *Secondary Hypertension.* Treat, or refer for treatment of, primary condition.
  E. *Undetermined Etiology or No Response to Treatment.* Hypertension of undetermined cause or not responding to treatment regimens above requires further evaluation, to include: (1) determination of serum sodium and potassium; and, if not previously performed, (2) rapid-sequence intravenous pyelography.

EVALUATION BY TRACER

Tracers can be used to evaluate health-service organizations — such as neighborhood health centers — which have responsibility for providing care to a defined population; they can also be used by an individual physician to evaluate his own practice.

and a median educational attainment among adults of 11 years of completed schooling. Some of the data in the illustration are real (developed in pretests of the tracer method); some are not. The latter represent, rather, our generalized experience and "best guesses" in constructing a situation typical of those likely to be found by evaluators of urban health-delivery systems.

Services in a Hypothetical Community

Because we have selected a neighborhood health center for our evaluation, the first thing we will want

*For criteria for the set of 6 tracers order NAPS Document 01997 from National Auxiliary Publications Service, c/o Microfiche Publications, 305 E. 46th St., New York, N.Y. 10022; remitting $1.50 for each microfiche-copy reproduction or $5 for each photocopy. Checks or money orders should be made payable to Microfiche Publications.

Table 1. Age-Sex Groups Represented by Accepted Tracer Conditions.

AGE (YR)	TRACER CONDITION						
	MIDDLE-EAR INFECTION	HEARING LOSS	VISUAL DEFICIENCY	IRON DEFICIENCY ANEMIA	HYPERTENSION	URINARY TRACT INFECTION	CERVICAL CANCER
Female:							
<5	+			+			
5-24	+	+	+				
25-64				+	+	+	+
≥65				+	+	+	
Male:							
<5	+			+			
5-24	+	+	+				
25-64				+	+		
≥65				+	+	+	

to know is how well the center reaches the at-risk populations among those whom it was designed to serve. For this analysis we will need current census figures of demographic and socioeconomic characteristics of the community population, and the age and sex distributions of the persons enrolled in the neighborhood health center.

When we examine the age distributions of the residents, we find more than 40 per cent of the population is under 25 years of age, almost 70 per cent under 45, and about 10 per cent 65 or older. By sex, 54 per cent of all residents are females, but the distribution varies with age from 51 per cent females in the group under 45 years to 65 per cent females in those 65 years and over.

These characteristics are crucial to our selection of tracers. For tracers, we will want to use common ailments treated by the health system; we will want to examine routine, not unusual or exotic, care provided by the health center. And without knowing the predominant age and sex distributions of community residents,

Table 2. Aspects of the Process of Primary Ambulatory Health Care Highlighted by Accepted Tracer Conditions.

PROCESS ACTIVITY	TRACER CONDITION						
	MIDDLE-EAR INFEC-IRON	HEARING LOSS	VISUAL DEFIC-IENCY	IRON-DEFIC-IENCY ANEMIA	HYPER-TEN-SION	URINARY-TRACT INFECT-ION-IRON	CERVICAL CANCER
Prevention	+		+				
Screening	+	+	+	+			+
Evaluation:							
History & physical examination	+			+	+	+	
Laboratory			+	+	+	+	
Other testing	+						
Management:							
Chemotherapy	+			+	+	+	
Health counseling	•	+	+				+
Specialty referral	+	+	+			+	+
Hospitalization				+	+	+	+
Follow-up case	+	+		+	+	+	+

we cannot estimate the prevalence of the tracer diseases or judge their suitability for analyzing routine care.

To find out how well the center serves the community, we need only compare the current census data with a similar analysis of persons enrolled in the health center. In an actual evaluation, we would compare community residents to the center's 9000 enrollees for each age-sex group. In this example, however, we will focus on two groups: all persons under 15, and men 25 to 64 years of age.

Table 3 shows that the health center serves about ⅕ of all community residents. It is used to different extents, however, by the two age groups that we have selected. Nearly ⅓ of the children under 15 years of age but less than 15 per cent of the men 25 to 64-years old are enrolled. This simple analysis clearly points out a segment of the population — young to middle-age men — that has been underserved, an important finding for our assessment of the center's effectiveness.

The Quality of Care

To assess the quality of care given to men 25 to 64 years old we will need to select tracers and apply them to a sample of medical records. The tracers that we select are critical to the evaluation; ideally, they should consist of a set of two or more tracers for each age-sex group. In that way we can view the services provided to the group from two or more perspectives and avoid the risk of isolating anomalous conditions. For simplicity, however, we will use only one tracer, hypertension, in this illustration and will focus on screening and diagnostic and therapeutic processes.

A review of the literature indicates that the prevalence of hypertension in black men of this age is about 23 per cent.[19] When we extrapolate from the community census, we can estimate that there will be approximately 2300 men with hypertension in the community.

Next, we review a sample of the medical records of this age-sex group according to our treatment criteria for hypertension. Performing the review are persons, not necessarily professionals, who are familiar with the medical-care process and who have received two weeks' intensive training. It is assumed that about 78 per cent of the enrolled men have been screened, and 250 cases are identified — for a prevalence rate of 23 per cent in the screened population. From this analysis we can state that more than ⅕ of the enrolled men were not screened, high-risk persons had not been pinpointed for screening because prevalence rate among screened

Table 3. Comparison of Community Population with Selected Health-Center Enrollees.

GROUP	COMMUNITY POPULATION	HEALTH-CENTER ENROLLEES	% OF COMMUNITY POPULATION ENROLLED
Total population	42,000	9,000	21.4
Males & females, 0-14 yrs of age	9,200	2,900	31.5
Males, 25-64 yrs of age	9,900	1,400	14.1

patients was the same as would be expected among a randomly selected sample of enrollees, and the center is caring for only 11 per cent of the estimated hypertensive men in the community.

It is possible, of course, that some of the 300-plus unscreened men actually were screened, but that the findings were not recorded or that appropriate follow-up examination was carried out but not indicated on the chart. Implicit in the use of the tracer method, however, is the assumption that good medical records are a requisite for good medical practice.

In evaluating therapy given to the 250 identified patients with hypertension, we select and abstract a random sample of their medical charts according to the treatment criteria. The abstracts are recorded on a precoded form for ease in processing. It is assumed that this analysis finds that in 30 per cent of the cases fixed-dosage combination drugs were used in initial therapy. Information such as this concerning the process of medical care is critical in assessing the quality of health services. It does not substitute for measures of outcome, such as whether or not the blood pressure actually declined, but provides important information concerning appropriate treatment.

IMPACT OF EVALUATION

There are three purposes to evaluation: to support good medical practice by identifying its efficacious and efficient elements, to indicate areas of practice in need of improvement, and to provide ongoing education to physicians about their own practices. But these purposes are not served if the evaluation results are not fed back into the delivery system and acted upon.

The results should enter the decision-making process at the point where standards are set for acceptable levels of care. We have not attempted to impose our judgment in standard setting. Decisions concerning an acceptable level of performance in, for example, history taking (should the required minimal history be taken for 20 per cent or 80 per cent of the potential hypertensive patients?) must be made by the individual physician, the physicians as a group, or the consumer-physician governing board.

In our hypothetical health center, 23 per cent of the enrolled high-risk population had not been screened for hypertension, and only 11 per cent of the estimated morbidity in the community had been identified. There may also be some question about the adequacy of the center's medical records. Certain remedial actions should be considered: institute case finding among a small sample of community males to estimate the number of persons with high blood pressure who are receiving care elsewhere in the community; restructure health-center procedures to obtain blood pressures on all high-risk enrollees; and consider use of structured medical records to obtain a minimal data base on all patients.

The analysis of drug therapy in hypertension provides basic information that physicians, health-center administrators, medical directors, or consumer boards

need to improve care. It points out that something may be amiss in the way a class of drugs — in this case, antihypertensive agents — is prescribed routinely. By implication, it suggests that inappropriate drug therapy may occur in the treatment of other common ailments and that the center's drug-therapy program should be analyzed in greater detail.

CONCLUSIONS

Tracers provide a workable conceptual framework and data base for assessing the quality of health services. Like any system of evaluation, however, this one will need to be adapted to and tested in live, nonacademic practices. In addition, tracer sets and care criteria will need to be developed — for example, to assess care given to the elderly, adolescents, and persons with emotional disorders. It is especially important to note that no system of evaluation, including tracers, can be instituted nationwide immediately to satisfy the emerging political craving for quality assessment. Comparative testing of all evaluation methods is needed first. Such comparative tests can serve, however, as a first logical step to move evaluation from the perpetual research-demonstration-research cycle to utility and problem solving.

We are indebted to Rashid L. Bashshur, who participated in the development of the field test of the tracer method, to John C. Cassel, James K. Cooper, William M. O'Brien, David L. Sackett, and Herman A. Tyroller, who assisted in developing the general methodology for this study, to Drs. Robert A. Babineau, Bradley E. Brownlow, James A. Burdette, Charles S. Burger, Fitzhugh Mayo, Philip G. Sanfacon, and Randall H. Silver, who assisted in developing the medical-care criteria, and to Charles du V. Florey, Edward D. Fries, Herbert G. Langford, Jeremiah Stamler, and Robert L. Watson, who assisted in developing hypertension as a tracer.

REFERENCES

1. Lee RI, Jones LW: The Fundamentals of Good Medical Care: An outline of the fundamentals of good medical care and an estimate of the service required to supply the medical needs of the United States (Publications of the Committee on the Costs of Medical Care No 22). Chicago, University of Chicago Press, 1933
2. Altman I, Anderson AJ, Barker K: Methodology in Evaluating the Quality of Medical Care: An annotated selected bibliography, 1955-1968. Revised edition. Pittsburgh, University of Pittsburgh Press, 1969
3. Donabedian A: Evaluating the quality of medical care. Milbank Mem Fund Q 44(3):166-206, 1966
4. *Idem:* Promoting quality through evaluating the process of patient care. Med Care 6:181-202, 1968
5. *Idem:* The evaluation of medical care programs. Bull NY Acad Med 44:117-124, 1968
6. *Idem:* A Guide to Medical Care Administration. Vol II. Medical Care Appraisal   Quality and Utilization. New York, American Public Health Association, Inc. 1969
7. Outcomes Conference I-II: Methodology of identifying, measuring and evaluating outcomes of health service programs, systems and subsystems. Edited by CE Hopkins. Rockville, Maryland, Department of Health, Education, and Welfare, Health Services and Mental Health Administration, 1969
8. Klein MW, Malone MF, Bennis WG, et al: Problems of measuring patient care in the out-patient department. J Health Hum Behav 2:138-144, 1961
9. Kelman HR, Elinson J: Strategy and tactics of evaluating a large-scale medical care program. Med Care 7:79-85, 1969
10. Kerr M, Trantow DJ: Defining, measuring, and assessing the quality of health services. Public Health Rep 84:415-424, 1969
11. Klein BW: Evaluating Outcomes of Health Services: An annotated bibliography (Working paper No 1). Los Angeles, School of Public Health, California Center for Health Services Research, University of California, 1970

Chapter 23

The Tracer Concept Revisited

David M. Kessner, James Singer, Carolyn K. Snow, Barbara Stewart
and Colette Thomas

Methodologies to evaluate the quality of patient care have come under
increasing scrutiny since the enactment in 1972 of PL 92-603, which mandated Professional Standards Review Organizations (PSROs).[1] The
PSRO legislation has given health professionals and consumers increased exposure to the concept of assessing the quality of care. Although
PSROs now are required to review only the cost and quality of hospital
and nursing home care provided to Medicare and Medicaid patients, it is
reasonable to assume that PSROs will be expanded to include ambulatory care, or that a similar ongoing review organization eventually will
monitor outpatient services.

Previous studies of the quality of ambulatory care have been ad hoc
efforts limited to reviewing care for a given period of time; they have
employed a variety of methodological approaches.[2] The experience from
some of these studies indicates that the inability to collect ambulatory
care data is a limiting factor that may hamper peer review of outpatient
care. A major obstacle in reviewing such data is the inadequacy of the
medical record. In addition, the complexities of a systematic audit of outpatient records often lead to the accumulation of data that are difficult
to analyze and interpret.

Compounding the data limitations and the inherent complexity of outpatient evaluation, the cost of such activities may be so high as to raise
serious questions about their cost-effectiveness. Yet the apparent importance of cost data is not reflected in current literature on ambulatory
care assessment. In the few instances where cost data have been collected
and published, the methods used to arrive at total costs or individual
cost elements that comprise over-all evaluation are not provided.[3]

The tracer concept, as described in the preceding chapter, is one
method to assess quality of care. The work of refining this concept has
continued as part of a series of research projects to develop cost-effective
approaches to quality of care evaluations. Specifically, the first phase of

the project, "Assessing Ambulatory Care: The Use of an Enriched Encounter Form," entails the use of an expanded billing/encounter form as a potential low-cost method that may avoid the inherent weaknesses and complexities of medical record audits. The objectives of this research are to compare the reliability, utility and cost of assessing the quality of medical care from the following data bases: (1) encounter forms; (2) medical records abstracts; and (3) limited interviews and clinical examinations. The results of the first phase of the study using an enriched encounter form have been reported.* This chapter addresses the reassessment of the original criteria for selecting tracer conditions.[4]

SELECTION OF TRACERS

The tracer method as initially described[5] was based on the premise that one can carefully examine selected medical care activities to gain insight into the quality of general medical care that is being received by patients. It is clear, however, that with the exception of preventive services,[6] it is difficult to extrapolate with security from how a set of tracer problems or diagnoses are managed to the quality of general medical care. On the other hand, there is no question that in assessing the quality of medical care, one should address such components as: (1) the kind of preventive care provided; (2) the content of the screening; (3) the adequacy of diagnostic evaluations including history taking, physical examination, and the use of laboratory, X-ray, and other diagnostic tests; (4) the reliability of case finding and diagnosis; (5) the appropriateness of management with regard to drug therapy, counselling, specialty referral and hospitalization; (6) the proper frequency of follow-up and therapeutic adjustments; and (7) the effect, or outcome, of these medical care processes on the well-being of the patients.

If these various activities are considered as subsets of the care process as a whole, one can select a set of tracers or indicators that highlight each major medical care activity using symptoms, problems, diagnoses, drugs or procedures that are common in a given practice or community.

For example, in assessing the appropriateness of drug therapy, the provider faces choices among a variety of available agents; decides the use of multiple single drugs or a single fixed-dosage combination; is aware of contraindications because of other medical problems or potential drug interactions; takes into consideration the dose, frequency and duration

---

*The final report, *Assessing Ambulatory Care: The Use of an Enriched Encounter Form*, is available from the National Technical Information Service, Springfield, Virginia, 22151, by requesting document number PB 251-317.

of therapy; and monitors for side-effects. In selecting a tracer for drug therapy, then, one should choose a symptom, problem, diagnosis or drug that confronts the provider with some or all of these choices. For instance, hypertension was selected as one of the conditions for assessing drug therapy. Management of hypertensive patients requires the provider to choose, based on severity, complications and concomitant diseases, one or more agents among a number of drugs to carefully adjust the dose and frequency of the drug regimen, to decide between multiple drugs and fixed-dosage combinations and to consider contraindications. Another approach to assessing drug therapy is to evaluate all patients prescribed a specific group of drugs, such as tricyclic agents used in the treatment of neurotic depression. Among this population, one might determine whether a diagnosis appropriate to the prescription of these potent drugs had been made and whether the follow-up visits were being scheduled frequently enough to assess the effectiveness of the drug therapy and look for any adverse effects. If, however, one wants to examine the appropriate use of laboratory tests in diagnostic evaluation, the tracer should be one where the results of biochemical, hematological or microbiological tests are important in arriving at a definitive diagnosis in deciding on a course of treatment or in monitoring the impact of treatment. In a disease such as essential hypertension, where the primary diagnostic indicators are derived from the physical examination, laboratory tests are relatively less important. In contrast, the results of a quantitative urine culture are as essential to the diagnosis and treatment of urinary tract infection, as is a glucose tolerance test to the initial diagnosis of diabetes mellitus.

That the tracer should highlight one or more aspects of the medical management activities being evaluated, then, becomes the first criterion for tracer selection and is central to the tracer concept. There are additional criteria that should be met by tracers chosen for use in evaluation. In previous work on developing the tracer methodology for ambulatory care evaluation, eight other criteria were listed that were thought should be met in the tracer selection process.[7] At that time the objectives were not only to measure the quality of care but also the prevalence of disease in different socioeconomic groups based on clinical examinations under the field conditions; the study population was selected at random from a defined community rather than from the patients of a particular medical provider, and the concern was with differences in disease prevalence or health status and adequacy of medical care process by both socioeconomic and medical care factors.

Some of the criteria outlined at that time are not appropriate when the evaluation focuses on the patients of a given medical practice rather than on the population at large. Indeed, in retrospect they may be too restrictive and confining for larger population studies as well. The original criteria have been reassessed and are now viewed from a different perspective.

In recasting the criteria, there has been an attempt to focus on medicine as it is practiced—the patients who are seen and their presenting complaints. The new selection criteria are:

—The tracer should be of significance either in terms of its potential impact on the functional capacity of the patient, the burden on the provider or the potential for treatment resulting in more harm than good. This is a modification of the initial functional significance criterion. It has been expanded to allow inclusion of tracers that have significance other than their functional impact on the patient. For example, even though the common cold is a short-lived, self-limiting condition that would have met few of the original criteria, it results in considerable economic loss to society, accounts for a major portion of patients in primary care practices, and often is inappropriately and overzealously treated.

—The tracer should occur with relatively high prevalence. Thus common symptoms, diseases, drugs or procedures should be selected so that with a reasonable amount of data collection, enough cases can be obtained for analysis. Even though cervical cancer is a relatively rare disease and would not be a good tracer for assessing the appropriateness of specialty referral or hospitalization for patients found to have abnormal Pap smears, the Pap smear is a good tracer for assessing the comprehensiveness of the screening program since the population to be included in the evaluation is comprised of all women at risk for cervical cancer.

—There should be general consensus on medical management *of the particular condition being assessed.* With diabetes, for example, there remains considerable controversy over the use of oral hypoglycemics and, therefore, this condition might not be a good choice for assessing the appropriateness of drug therapy. On the other hand, it might well serve as a good tracer of the adequacy of the diagnostic process by evaluating the procedures carried out to arrive at the diagnosis.

Another important ingredient is the combining of tracers into sets so that wherever possible a particular medical care activity is evaluated by analysis of two or more tracers. Because of the nature of encounter forms, not all medical care activities can be assessed by this method. Those that can be assessed, however, include some of the important activities health providers perform for the benefit of their patients. They are: the use of laboratory, X-ray and other procedures, drug therapy, and follow-up. Each of these activities is related to the diseases associated with the tracers in the examples given below. The tracers may be combined in sets for analyses that meet the needs of the evaluator.

Laboratory Testing: Urine culture (urinary tract infection, blood analyses (anemia, diabetes mellitus).

Drug Therapy: Antihypertensives (hypertension), tranquilizers (anxiety), antibiotics (urinary tract infections).

Follow-up: Scheduled return visit (hypertension, anxiety/depression, urinary tract infection, anemia, obesity).

Other activities, such as assessing the adequacy, appropriateness and completeness of preventive and screening measures, history taking or physical examination can be done only with medical record data. The encounter form cannot be used for such analysis without changing it from a simple, inexpensive, one-page instrument.

MEDICAL CARE CRITERIA

The minimal care plans for each tracer condition, with the exception of neurotic anxiety and depression,* are a modification of previously published care criteria.[8] These criteria are limited to information obtainable from the enriched encounter form (Appendix G). Perusal of the encounter form and the instructions for its use points out clearly the limitations of the data available for quality assessment from the encounter form. For example, because the patient's reasons for the visit and current diagnoses are not rigidly linked to the laboratory tests, X-rays and other procedures, one cannot be definitely certain that the procedures listed were ordered for a specific diagnosis; however, it is reasonable to assume that these procedures were prompted by all of the current problems or diagnoses about which detailed information is given.

---

*These criteria were developed with the assistance of a panel of psychiatrists and primary care physicians. The panel members were Gordon H. Deckert, The University of Oklahoma; Elmer A. Gardner, Washington, D.C.; Samuel B. Guze, Washington University; Robert S. Lawrence, The Cambridge Hospital; F. Patrick McKegney, The University of Vermont; Darius Gray Ornston, Jr., New Haven, Connecticut; David Rosenman, Yale University; Edward C. Senay, State of Illinois Department of Mental Health; Herbert S. Winston, Bethesda, Maryland.

Further, because only generic or trade names of drugs are recorded, assessment of drug therapy cannot encompass the appropriateness of drug frequency, dosage or duration. Lastly, encounter form data, when applied to specific medical diagnoses, allow only for a look at one point on the continuum of the disease process. The problems associated with the use of such cross-sectional data are discussed further in the final report. These limitations do not preclude the use of the encounter form as a tool for initial process-oriented quality assessment but they do limit the kinds of analyses that can be carried out.

Despite the practical utility of using predetermined criteria against which services can be compared, the users of such criteria must be aware of potential dangers inherent in their use. As previously noted:

> Several cautions ... must be emphasized in establishing treatment criteria, or protocols, for the morbidity conditions used as tracers. Of utmost importance is the fact that no single standard can cope with the day-to-day variations faced by the practicing physician. The criteria cannot be assumed to be a rigid formula applicable to each individual patient. They can, and should, however, be applicable to the aggregate of patients. Further, the criteria must take into account not only the best thinking in the medical community regarding treatment of specific conditions, but also the practical constraints of the particular practice to be evaluated. These include availability of ancillary facilities and consultants, physician-population ratios and patient load, and the health status and socio-economic characteristics of the patient population.[9]

Another possible pitfall relates to the impact of predetermined criteria on physician behavior. It is clear that, "establishing criteria has an inherent danger—the risk of locking the medical profession into a rigid mode of practice. Criteria for treating tracer conditions could avoid rigidity if formulated on three premises: they should outline minimal, or base-line care;* they should be pragmatic, taking into account unavailability of sophisticated diagnostic equipment; and they should be revised and updated periodically."[10]

---

*The minimal care plans for the four diagnoses evaluated in this study (essential hypertension, neurotic anxiety/depression, urinary tract infections, and iron deficiency anemia) are presented in *Assessing Ambulatory Care: The Use of an Enriched Encounter Form.* National Technical Information Service, Springfield, Va. Document number PB 25-317.

Notes

1. PL 92-603, Section 249F, 1972.

2. M.A. Morehead, R.S. Donaldson and M.R. Seravelli. "Comparisons Between OEO Neighborhood Health Centers and Other Care Providers of Ratings of the Quality of Health Care," *Am. J. Public Health,* 61: (1971) 1294-1306; O.L. Peterson, L.F. Andrews and L.S. Spain et al. "An Analytical Study of North Carolina General Practice 1953-54." *J. Med. Educ.,* 31: (1965), 1-165, part 2; B.C. Payne and T. F. Lyons. *Episode of Illness Study,* Ann Arbor, University of Michigan (1972): 60-146; B.C. Payne and T.F. Lyons. *Office Care Study.* Ann Arbor, University of Michigan (1972); R.H. Brook and F.A. Appel. "Quality-of-care Assessment: Choosing a Method for Peer Review," *N. Engl. J. Med.,* 288: (1973) 1323-1329; D.M. Kessner, C.K. Snow and J. Singer. "Assessment of Medical Care for Children," *Contrasts in Health Status,* Washington, D.C., National Academy of Sciences, 3: (1974).

3. R.L. Goldstein, J.S. Roberts and B. Stanton et al. "Data for Peer Review: Acquisition and Use. Results in the Experimental Medical Care Review Organization Program," *Ann. Int. Med.* 82: (1975) 262-267; R.H. Grimm, K. Shimoni, W.R. Harlan and E.H. Estes. "Evaluation of Patient-care Protocol Use by Various Providers," *New Engl. J. Med.,* 292: (1975) 507-511.

4. D.M. Kessner and C.E. Kalk. "A Strategy for Evaluating Health Services," *Contrasts in Health Status,* Washington, D.C., National Academy of Sciences, 2: (1973); D.M. Kessner, C.E. Kalk and J. Singer. "Assessing Health Quality—The Case for Tracers," *New Engl. J. Med.,* 288: (1973) 189.

5. Ibid.

6. See Payne and Lyons, op. cit.; Kessner, Snow and Singer, op. cit.

7. Kessner and Kalk, op. cit.; Kessner, Kalk and Singer, op. cit.

8. Kessner and Kalk, op. cit.

9. Ibid.

10. Kessner, Kalk and Singer, op. cit.

Chapter 24

Evaluating the Impact of the Utah MEDEX Program: A Quasi-Experimental Approach

Robert L. Kane and Donna M. Olsen

Problems of program evaluation are readily appreciated by anyone who has tried to do it. The evaluator, frequently called in after the program is well along, is asked to develop a set of measures to assess progress in the absence of suitable baseline data. Because of the need to incorporate the evaluation design into the basic program plan from the beginning, it is useful to describe the history of the Utah MEDEX program,* which started with that goal, and to cite the adaptations necessary as the program evolved. The MEDEX concept was originally developed at the University of Washington in 1969. Medex are physician's assistants with former training as military corpsmen to provide care to civilian populations.

Utah and the surrounding intermountain states shared the problems of physician maldistribution and shortage of primary care services in rural areas. The Medex seemed like a useful way to increase such services by working with the practicing physicians. After preliminary marketing studies among rural doctors and discussions with the Seattle MEDEX staff, the Department of Family and Community Medicine of the University of Utah College of Medicine decided to pursue the MEDEX model.[1] Immediately apparent was that the prior efforts, which were pioneer undertakings launched by advocates, could neither appropriately nor feasibly incorporate an experimental design. The Utah program—the sixth developed and funded by the NCHSR—seemed more appropriate for such a role. The initial program staff had in fact made an explicit part of their funding application the plan to study the effectiveness of this new form of health manpower. If the experiment appeared to be succeeding in that goals set were reached, further funding would be sought.

The ideal design for such an evaluation is not difficult to envision. As a new therapeutic modality, the Medex would best be assessed by some

*Supported by Contract No. HRA 106-74-58, National Center for Health Services Research (NCHSR), PHS, DHEW.

type of controlled clinical trial: a substantial number of physician practices would be recruited to participate; and after an adequate period of baseline measurement, a randomly chosen group would be given a Medex; both experimental and control groups would be followed. In order to measure the effects of adding a Medex, data would be gathered on the type of patients seen, for how long and by whom. At the same time community data would be collected to see how this addition of new personnel affected access to and outcomes of care. Studies of different aspects of the problem leap quickly to mind, each with demands for information on costs, quality, satisfaction, access, retention, interaction, compliance and many other areas. The optimal design had to be abandoned almost from the outset for a number of reasons. This chapter examines some of the causes for this deviation from the ideal and the problems that occur as a program is implemented with evaluation as a principal component.

INITIAL COMPROMISES

An early problem with the Utah MEDEX program was timing. The decision to move ahead to seek funding to establish the program, the subsequent writing of the grant proposal, and its review occurred within a relatively short span. Word was received in May 1970 that limited federal funds were available to start a MEDEX program in Utah if a class could be underway by September. This meant that many compromises would have to be made. A curriculum was adapted from the Seattle model, preceptors had to be recruited quickly and a large pool of student applicants screened. In addition, the evaluation design, only sketched in the grant application, had to be operationalized. The approach chosen was to translate the program's goal statements into a series of more specific objectives with appropriate quantitative criteria. Although most of these were cast in terms of measuring change from a pre-Medex baseline period, the timetable had to be greatly shortened under pressure to get a program underway at once. In the four-month interval between funding and the initiation of classes, the evaluation unit had to convince potential preceptors of the need to provide data as well as to recruit and train observers to gather data and develop all the necessary forms.

OBJECTIVES

The Utah MEDEX objectives had four major areas of concern. Because the program's overall goal was to improve patient access to quality health care services in medically impoverished areas, it was hoped that the project would:

1. Increase satisfaction with health care providers in the target areas.

2. Increase patient satisfaction in these areas by increasing the quality of health care as perceived by patients, by increasing the availability of health care, and by increasing the accessibility of medical care.

3. Improve the efficiency and effectiveness of health care delivery in those areas.

4. Provide the mechanism by which the Medex will become a productive member of the health care team.

These general concerns in turn generated a series of objectives which the evaluation sought to measure. For convenience these have been grouped under four headings. The data collection source, described later, is indicated in parentheses.

1. Physician satisfaction can be considered positive if:
   - Physicians express greater feelings of satisfaction with their practice in terms, for example,
     — perceiving that the quality of care they render has improved, and
     — feeling that they have at least as much or more control over how they spend their time as before the Medex joined their practices. (Questionnaires)
   - With the addition of a Medex, the physician's working day begins to look more like the regular 8:00 a.m. - 5:00 p.m. pattern. (Activity logs)
   - The physician actually works fewer hours per week. (Activity logs)
   - The physician's income increases. (Practice income data)
   - The doctor is able to spend more time at social and community affairs. (Activity log data)

2. Patient satisfaction would be considered positive if:
   - Patients perceive an improvement in the medical care being delivered in terms of
     — the quantity and quality of care available in the community,
     — their satisfaction with their communications with the doctor's office team, including the Medex,
     — their overall satisfaction with the care received at any specific office encounter. (Patient questionnaires)
   - Patients develop positive attitudes toward the Medex and view

him as a valuable addition to the doctor's staff. (Questionnaire data)

3. Effects on the practice itself would be considered positive if:
   - The number of patient visits per time period, e.g. per day, increases. (Actual counts)
   - The task load of the various office staff, including the doctor, shifts to a more appropriate pattern as the Medex is added. (Task inventory data)
     — some tasks relinquished by others are assumed by the Medex;
     — the total hours worked by the office team remain the same or increase with the addition of the Medex.
   - There is a decrease in patient waiting time and queue length in the office. (Network analysis data)
   - The cost of care, as reflected in such figures as operating expense per patient visit, is reduced. The costs, both direct and indirect, of hiring a Medex are offset by increased volume. (Financial data)
   - Quality of care measures or indicators show an increase or a maintenance of former levels. Such indicators might include:
     — rate of appropriate laboratory studies for given conditions,
     — use of appropriate therapies for given conditions, and
     — effectiveness of professional-patient communications as reflected in patient's knowledge of his condition. (Patient contact records and exit interviews)
   - Medex manage patients with similar diagnoses in the same way as do their preceptors. Do Medex see a different subset of patients than do their preceptors as reflected in patient's age, sex, diagnosis? (Patient contact record)

4. Medex integration into the practice unit would be considered positive if:
   - The Medex is able to prove himself as a useful member of the physician's staff and is accepted by the other members of the staff. (Interview and questionnaire sources)
   - He feels satisfied with his role
     — he and his family feel satisfied with their lifestyle e.g., hours of work, location;
     — he is satisfied with his income. (Interview and questionnaire sources)
   - The selection and matching process results in Medex-preceptor teams which persist one or more years after training in at least 75 percent of cases.

Other factors increased the time pressure and demanded further compromise. As plans for the evaluation were being modified, funding agency representatives visiting the project explained that a new system of evaluation called the Uniform Manpower Evaluation Protocol (UMEP) had been developed under a series of government contracts for use in all programs to train new health practitioners of different types. Although many of the areas identified by the evaluation unit were covered, the new system unfortunately approached the problem differently. While the MEDEX approach had begun with a series of questions to be answered and then proceeded to design a data collection system to answer them, the UMEP was presented as a data set without reference to the issues addressed. Since its purpose was to gather data to address generic issues across programs, it lacked specificity for the problems of concern to Utah MEDEX staff or to the intermountain region. While this requirement was resented by the staff, several of the UMEP instruments fitting the needs defined by program objectives finally were adapted or totally adopted.

The original plan called for a randomized controlled design. However, the problem of recruiting a sufficient number of preceptors in a brief time soon proved formidable; barely enough physicians willing to get involved in so new a venture could be found to act as preceptors for the first class of trainees. Because the physician preceptor served as both teacher and employer, it was not clear whether doctors should be recruited on the basis of teaching abilities or of their need for assistance. Rarely were both these criteria met in a single individual. Thus not only were there not enough physicians to provide any controls, but those who did agree to participate became valuable resources to be handled with care. The evaluation data package had to be trimmed to an amount tolerable to the participating physicians. Several steps were taken to meet this problem. Each physician was personally visited by the evaluation team to explain the need for data that addressed relevant questions about the impact of adding this new health professional. The evaluation data package was explained and arrangements made to recruit local data collectors acceptable to the physicians.

DATA COLLECTION

The MEDEX training model originally was developed as a 15-month experience of which the first third was spent in training at the academic center and the remainder in a preceptorship with the physician who would employ the Medex if all went smoothly. Baseline data were collected during the initial three months before the Medex arrived and later compared with changes during the subsequent year. Additional analyses would compare the performance of the Medex with that of his preceptor.

The data collection instruments included both direct and indirect measures of practice. The evaluation tools consisted of the following:

- **Patient Contact Record (PCR)**—The Patient Contact Record was the heart of the evaluation system. This form, designed to be completed on each visit to the physician or Medex for one week each month, recorded demographic data on the patient, type of visit, diagnoses (up to two), laboratory work, treatment, and disposition.
- **Network analysis**—For one week during each quarter of the study period a data collector observed patients in the office to determine how much time was spent with various office staff and in waiting. At the conclusion of the time-and-motion study, the patient was interviewed about the visit, his provider and his diagnosis. The responses were compared with the patient's PCR, thus allowing verification.
- **Mailback questionnaire**—The observer gave each interviewed patient a self-addressed, postage-paid questionnaire better answered outside the office. Items included the identity of the patient's regular doctor, other sources of care, perceptions of care in the community and attitudes toward Medex.
- **Activity log**—Each preceptor and the Medex were asked to complete a log of activities by checking off the major activity each performed. This also served as the major source of information on services provided outside the office.
- **Task inventory**—The physician and his office staff completed inventories on the various tasks they performed before the Medex arrived and one year later. Medex filled out the inventory at quarterly intervals after beginning their preceptorships.
- **Cost analysis**—Information on practice revenue and costs was gathered for each practice from income tax records for two years prior to the Medex and annually after the Medex entered the practice.
- **Patient count**—To get a better temporal picture of the effect of the Medex on the volume of patients, total numbers of patients seen per week were obtained from the office appointment books. Patient visits for one week every other month of the preceptorship year and two previous years were counted. These weeks corresponded to those when PCRs were collected for validation.

The system was designed to permit the establishment of computer files on each practice and to link a portion of patient contact records with subsets of corresponding network analysis and patient mailback data, while maintaining the anonymity of the patient. A method of not identifying staff and patients by name had been planned deliberately to assure full confidentiality, but in many practices the office staff wrote the patient's name on the form anyway to facilitate their own handling of it.

The data collectors, mostly local housewives, were recruited by the physician but employed by the project and served as the point of contact between the evaluation staff and each office. Before the evaluation began, they were brought to the University for several days of training and orientation to the project. The data collector was responsible to see that forms were filled out on time and mailed in, as well as to gather the observational data on patient activity. These observers became key individuals in the project especially because the practice sites might be as far as 250 miles from the evaluation staff during the first class and up to 500 miles away with later classes. They also provided the evaluation staff with informal data on how the Medex was being received in the practice and in the community.

Early Problems

The problems which plagued the initial evaluation alerted the study group to the need to initiate preparatory activities for subsequent classes much earlier. However, circumstances made this virtually impossible. Perhaps one of the most useful lessons from this experience is the inherent contradiction between a desire for a careful evaluation of a new project cycle and the problems associated with planning on the basis of annual funding cycles. On the one hand it is obvious that annual planning cannot accommodate a project which requires fifteen months of data collection, to say nothing of preparation and analysis time. More important, the uncertainty of funding, both the level and the actual support, prohibits active planning and necessary preparatory activities. With both the second and third classes, the same scenario was repeated. The decision about funding was not made until near the end of the fiscal year. The interval between the decision to have another class and the beginning of that class increased only slightly. The recruiting of preceptors each time was completed only just before, and sometimes even after, the orientation of the new group of students. The only saving of time possible was from the efficiency that came from previous experience with the study design.

Baseline data collection for each class was restricted to that obtained during the three months or so when Medex students were trained at the academic center. The analyses possible were thus based on the extent to which changes observed during the subsequent year of preceptorship training met the criteria derived initially from 3 months of data collected prior to the arrival of the Medex. These essentially descriptive data compared changes in the overall practice over time or compared the performance of the Medex to that of his physician preceptor.

The breadth of the questions necessitated intense data gathering. These data were dependent largely upon the active cooperation of the preceptors and Medex. Certainly the motivation to obtain data was different for the project staff than for the individual participants who often viewed the forms as the price of admission to the program. It seems logical then that the preceptors who experienced disruption would lose enthusiasm for complete and accurate data collection. The data reported here refer to the eight practices in the first Medex class plus two from the second class from which sufficient data were collected.

Of the original twelve students in the MEDEX I class, one was counselled out of the program and a second was not adequately proficient to enter the preceptorship. By the end of the preceptorship two matches had become clearly unworkable and the Medex found other employment. The remaining eight matches yielded the bulk of the data presented. Two of these developed sufficient problems during the post-training year to result in the Medex leaving.

The MEDEX II class appeared to be much more stable. Unfortunately data were not gathered during the final quarter of the 15-month study because of serious communication problems between the evaluation office and the field. Complete data could be obtained from only two practices and partial data from eight practices.

Early Data

By the end of the first two MEDEX classes, with a considerable amount of such descriptive data accumulated, a fairly clear pattern began to emerge. In general, the Medex moved quickly into a provider role seeing a spectrum of patients similar to his preceptor's and working similar hours. As shown in Figure 24:1, the distribution of problems seen by Medex generally paralleled that seen by the physicians except for a disproportionately low number of problems involving the female reproductive system. This exception can be traced to the fears of the program initiators that patients might be less willing to accept the Medex in this role and their decision to deemphasize training in this area.

FIGURE 24:1

The Percentages of the Most Common Diagnoses Found as Seen by
the Physician, Medex and Both

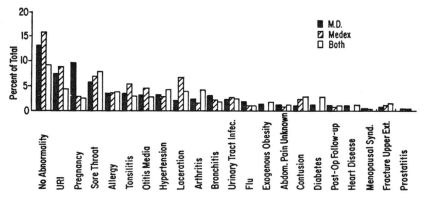

FIGURE 24:2

Patient Care in Provider's Home

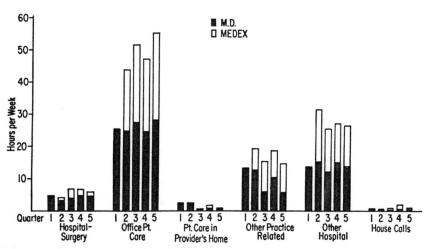

Figure 24:2 shows the hours worked in a typical week during the preceptorship period by both Medex and physicians. In general the patterns of time, as recorded in the activity logs, were quite comparable. The Medex came to assume a pattern similar to his preceptor, while the physician decreased his hours of work only slightly. Little patient care was given by either in sites outside the hospital or office.

While the aggregate data suggest that the patterns across the eighteen practices in the first two classes were uniform, the data from individual practices show marked variations in the effects of adding a Medex. Sample measures of change from the pre-Medex baseline to the final quarter of the preceptorship are displayed in Figure 24:3. Here the variations in effect from practice to practice are clearly evident. The initial assumption that a physician-Medex team was similar to another such team turned out to be in error.

How then does one talk about the effect of the MEDEX program? From the perspective of those sponsoring such training programs it is important to describe the overall impact of adding these new health practitioners to private practices. The aggregate data speak to this issue. But it is equally important to recognize that the impact was not uniform. Different physicians use this new manpower in different ways. Some seek relief from overwork; some see it as a means to provide more service—in fact, some view the Medex as a competitor who spurs them to work harder.

FIGURE 24:3

The Percentage Change in Four Significant Dimensions Following the Arrival of the Medex for Eighteen Physician-Medex Practices

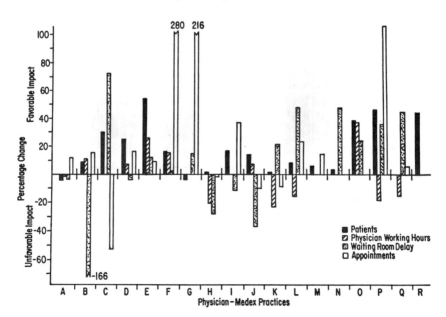

These variations held a particular interest for those operating the training program. They came to view the students and their preceptors as a series of relatively unique pairs and were more comfortable talking about how a particular pair was doing. Where the data from a given practice suggested less than optimal impact, the program staff could explain this failure in terms of individual quirks or environmental effects. The idea of looking at mean values across the program to test the total programmatic impact was viewed as too likely to lose the richness of individual experiences.

Interesting to speculate is whether the program staff would have had the same distrust for aggregate data if these had shown dramatic positive results, which will never be known because descriptive data from the first three classes showed very few, if any, overall effects. Because the descriptive data could be compared only against a predetermined set of expectations, two alternative reactions were possible: (1) The data suggested that the MEDEX program was not as successful as the originators had hoped, (2) The standards set were unrealistic; perhaps the practices taking a Medex had reached their saturation point and just maintaining their current levels of productivity was indeed a noteworthy achievement.

As noted earlier, exigencies of starting each new class had precluded the recruitment of any type of control group for the prospective studies. By the end of the second class there was a clear need for comparison groups matched on the basis of practice size, specialty and location, if not randomly selected controls, to avoid variations in interpreting the findings. With the beginning of the project's third year, sources of archival data were sought that might provide information over time on control practices as well.

The cooperation of the Utah Blue Cross/Blue Shield Plan (BC/BS) fortunately was secured to enable the use of unobtrusive archival measures of impact on hospitalization rates and to a lesser degree outpatient services. Data from the state's Medicaid program were also secured, but only for total volume of service.

Most of the data available for the study were from Blue Shield, i.e., payments for physician services, which provided both number of services and cost. The data were totals for the ten practices studied. Ten control (non-Medex) practices were selected by Blue Shield to match with the ten Medex practices on the basis of town size and number and speciality of physicians in the practice. The services were divided into medical, surgical and obstetrics.

"Matching" has such a bad name in quasi-experimental methodology[2] that a word more needs to be said about the procedures used. The criteria

used do not produce regression artifacts, as they do not plausibly correlate higher with the pre-treatment observations than with the post-treat-
ment observations. The data used in the analysis were not used for
matching, thus avoiding the deceptive matching point pinch in time
series discussed by Cook and Campbell.[3]

The raw data for surgical charges are presented in Figure 24:4A
(charges/quarter for ten Medex and ten control practices). Most obvious
is the large variation between quarters with the Medex and control practices generally parallel in the pre-Medex period, except quarter five. No
consistent seasonal trend is discernible in these data, but a wide oscilla-
tion with no obvious harmonic. During the one year of post-Medex data
the Medex practices show an apparent increase of $4,000 more per
quarter than the controls.

In an attempt to remove some of the variation and permit comparison
of the overall trend for Medex and control practices, the figures were annualized for the three years and the points connected (Figure 24:4B). It
then appears that the Medex practices constantly increased in the dollar
volume of hospital surgery, while control practices continued at the same
volume. This method of analyzing and displaying the data illustrates
how misleading certain methods can be in the presentation of data,
specifically those with much variability.

Regression lines were fitted to the pre-Medex and post-Medex period,
using quarters as data points, to determine if the trends indicated by the
annual figures were valid (Figure 24:4C). This method of displaying the
data presented a picture different from the previous figures. Both Medex
and control practices appear to be decreasing in dollar volume, pre- and
post-Medex. The Medex practices have an apparently higher volume
post-Medex with a rate of decrease less than the control practices. T-tests
on the slopes showed no significant difference pre- to post-Medex for
either the Medex or control practices.

The graphic portrayal of time series data as in Figure 24:4A, provides a
quasi-experimental control as Riecken and Boruch[4] demonstrated with a
wide variety of illustrative graphs. Such portrayals, along with the extended time series of "pretest," helps cut out such plausible rival hypotheses as selection, long-term trends, or effects of changes in general
economic conditions, that would plague a study with only a single pre-
treatment measure. While Figure 24:4A shows convincing effects after
the first quarter under Medex, T-tests on the slopes of the pre- and post-
Medex lines were not significantly different nor were the test $\bar{\gamma}$ at the
changeover point.

The method of presentation and analysis, as seen in Figure 24:4
(A,B,C), can affect greatly the overall interpretation the data, at least for

FIGURE 24:4A

Charges Per Quarter for Surgery in the Hospital

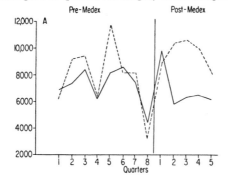

FIGURE 24:4B

Annualized Charges for Surgery in the Hospital

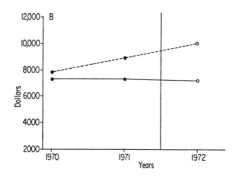

FIGURE 24:4C

Charges for Hospital Surgery: Regression Lines for Pre- and Post-Medex Periods

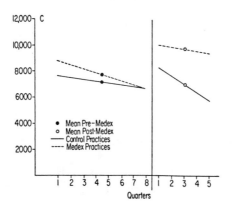

data with such great variability as these. The figures for admissions, length of stay, and number of services for surgery, medical and obstetrics presented a similar pattern.

Changes with MEDEX III

By the third class it appeared that little purpose would be served by repeating the same observational data. The method of data collection was therefore changed. In lieu of the several descriptions of the medical process, the outcomes of the care given by the Medex and his preceptor were compared and less useful data were eliminated or radically changed.

In response to physician and Medex resistance in filling out patient contact records, a system was selected which utilized data gathered directly from the patient by an interviewer. The previous diagnostic coding system used by the provider was replaced with a symptom code developed by Bain and Spaulding.[5] The outcomes were assessed in terms of the degree to which patients presenting with acute complaints regained their usual functional status along a six-point scale from asymptomatic to confined to bed. Usual functional status prior to illness was determined at the time of the visit; follow-up status according to the presenting complaint was assessed by telephone at a predetermined time, the usual interval being six weeks. This technique had been used previously in other ambulatory settings with considerable success.[6] The results of this outcome assessment are seen in Table 24:1. The physicians' results over time appeared to improve slightly. The Medex did almost as well

TABLE 24:1

Measures of Patient Outcome

Percentage Follow-up Status Better than or Equal to Usual Status

Status at Encounter	Pre-Medex	Patients Seen by M.D. Post-Medex Quarter			Patients Seen by Medex Post-Medex Quarter		
		1st	2nd	3rd	1st	2nd	3rd
Performs major activity, not symptomatic	98%	100%	100%	100%	100%	100%	100%
Performs major activity, symptomatic	79	73	89	94	77	75	77
Limited major activity, not limited mobility	69	52	51	59	66	56	58
Limited mobility	35	36	23	47	57	60	64
Bed disabled	79	25	0	100	—	100	50

and on occasion better than his preceptor. It seems possible to conclude that no substantial deterioration in care as measured by functional status resulted from the addition of a Medex.

The data on patient waiting time and contact time with a provider from the first two MEDEX classes showed minimal effects; patient contact time remained about 10 minutes regardless of provider, and waiting time was still about 25 minutes. Moreover, the measures of patient satisfaction collected from the terminal interview had provided relatively little useful data; i.e., patients asked about their satisfaction with care during the pre-Medex period were generally enthusiastic and thus little room for improvement was left. The lack of any significant diminution in their satisfaction was less reassuring when it was noted that many of those who were pleased with the communication between provider and patient could not correctly state their diagnosis related to the appropriate body system. Table 24:2 displays these measures of satisfaction while Table 24:3 shows the degree of agreement between the provider's recorded diagnosis and the patient's impression of the diagnosis.

The results from the original mailback questionnaire were similar. There was a uniformly high level of satisfaction with care in general (see Table 24:4). It was therefore decided to eliminate the exit interview and to change the mailback questionnaire to focus on problems of access to care. The response rate to both types of mailback questionnaires was approximately 50 percent. The second version showed the same general pattern of an initial positive effect with a leveling out as did its predecessor (see Table 24:5).

TABLE 24:2

Patient Satisfaction at Time of Exit Interview

		% Responding Favorably Post-Medex			
	Pre-Medex	1st Quarter	2nd Quarter	3rd Quarter	4th Quarter
Problems listened to fully	95%	96%	97%	97%	96%
Adequate history obtained	94	95	97	93	95
Diagnosis adequately explained	90	94	95	91	93
Overall, problem adequately handled	95	96	98	96	98
(N)	(424)	(374)	(293)	(369)	(334)

TABLE 24:3

Correspondence Between Patients' Description of their Diagnoses and Those Recorded
by Their Physican and/or Medex

	Pre-Medex	Post-Medex			
	4 Qtr. (N= 478)*	1 Qtr. (N= 399)	2 Qtr. (N= 329)	3 Qtr. (N= 397)	4 Qtr. (N= 369)
Percent of exact matches	31%	31%	19%	27%	29%
Percent of diagnostic equivalent matches	2	3	4	3	3
Percent of matches within same body system	18	16	18	17	22
Percent of patients who did not know correct diagnosis	49	52	59	54	47

*More than one diagnosis per patient possible

TABLE 24:4

Patient Satisfaction as Reflected in Mailback Questionnaire Responses
(MEDEX I and II)*

	Pre-Medex Quarter	Post-Medex Quarters			
		1st	2nd	3rd	4th
Which of the following do you most closely agree with?					
A Medex will give doctors more time to see the really sick patients.	58%	84%	88%	90%	85%
A Medex will mean people won't be able to see the doctor as easily.	7	3	4	3	6
I have never heard of a Medex.	35	13	8	6	9
Number of responses	453	399	277	297	221

*Sample size corrected for nonresponse

TABLE 24:4 (Continued)

	Pre-Medex Quarter	Post-Medex Quarters			
		1st	2nd	3rd	4th
Would you say the quality of medical care available in this community is:					
Excellent	29%	29%	30%	33%	24%
Quite good	35	37	37	38	34
About average	25	27	24	23	30
Less than in most places	8	6	6	5	8
Very poor	3	1	2	1	3
Number of responses	452	402	278	297	226
Would you say the amount of medical care available in this community is:					
Excellent	14%	18%	16%	18%	16%
Quite good	32	29	34	38	28
About average	27	32	27	27	31
Less than in most places	20	17	19	14	21
Very poor	6	4	3	4	4
Number of responses	454	406	274	295	225
How do you feel, in general, about the medical care in this community:					
Very satisfied	31%	41%	40%	41%	31%
Pretty satisfied	35	34	33	36	35
So-so	6	10	10	12	12
A little concerned	16	10	13	7	15
Very concerned	12	6	4	4	6
Number of responses	453	403	279	297	224

Studies After Employment

The experience with the initial impact evaluation of the first three MEDEX classes suggested a number of effects. For instance, the study dealt with the training period only, a time during which the practices were under stress because of the introduction of a new type of health professional—the Medex—and the need to devote considerable physician

TABLE 24:5

Patient Satisfaction as Reflected in Mailback Questionnaire Responses
(Medex III)

Mailback responses	Pre-Medex	Post-Medex		
		1st Qtr.	2nd Qtr.	3rd Qtr.
Satisfied with visit	90	90	91	93
Staff spent enough time with patient	91	92	93	94*
Put off visit to doctor because of difficulty getting appointment	35	34	33	33
Waiting time for appointment:				
seen immediately	65	66	66	75*
1-2 days	16	15	13	11
3-6 days	10	10	10	7
1-2 weeks	6	6	7	4
longer	3	4	3	2
(Of those seeing a Medex):				
problem handled competently		99	99	99
willing to see Medex again		97	96	96
(Of those not seeing Medex):				
willing to see one	61	60	60	65

*Differences between pre and 3rd quarter post, significant by Chi-square, at p< .05

time to train and supervise him. Rather than continue the evaluation
process with subsequent classes, it was felt more important to restudy
those on which baseline data originally had been gathered to identify the
effects during the employment period. The decision to restudy the first
three classes of Medex to assess changes between the training and
employment period provided an opportunity to use both the descriptive
approaches of earlier studies and to build on the archival techniques
already explored. To maintain reliability between the previous and the
new observational data, the instruments or the methods of collection
were unchanged. However, those elements were eliminated which had
not proven particularly useful, in order to minimize the data load on participants and on the research team. For this reason the mailback questionnaires and the network analysis were omitted.

Restudying Medex-physician pairs after an interval of one to two years
presented problems in match stability. As might be anticipated, the number of practices which retained the same combination of Medex and
physician decreased with the length of time after MEDEX training.
Although it always had been difficult to obtain usable data from even

those physician-Medex teams matched on schedule, a relatively small number (13) could be compared across time.

With only a small number of practices available for restudy, soliciting their cooperation was done with great trepidation. However, all the practices were very cooperative, which is particularly remarkable because there was now even less control over the situation than during the earlier studies when the Medex had not yet been certified by the training program. This cooperation was a result of self-selection, in that previously noncooperating practices were not even approached for restudy.

One means of expanding the scope of the study lay in the use of archival data. Because archival data used already recorded information, the choice of what could be studied was not so limited; the baseline data would be gathered at the same time as later data. Thus information on hospital services could be included. Moreover, the archival approach provided the opportunity to gain similar information about a control group which would not require extensive observational studies. Three areas were identified for archival study: (1) a measure of hospital services as reflected in Blue Shield data, (2) a measure of patient volume (i.e., the number of patient visits per week) and (3) the changes in physician income and expenses as reflected in income tax returns. Clearly the latter information was highly confidential. Nonetheless both Medex and control practices were willing to make it available with the assurance that no individual practices would be identifiable.

It was gratifying to find a number of practices which would cooperate with this aspect of the study. Even controls who had never benefitted from a Medex were willing to help despite the sensitive nature of some of the material. One advantage of using this type of unobtrusive measure was that the physician, aside from releasing the material, did not need to be actively involved in gathering it. The patient volume data were collected by his/her office staff who were reimbursed for their time by the project. The income tax data were usually provided by the physician's accountant who was similarly reimbursed.

The Blue Shield data presented a special problem. Whereas the original study of the MEDEX I class was confined to Utah for its practices and controls, the expanded study of the first three classes covered sites in six states, each of which had its own separate Blue Shield program. The decision was made to work with those states which had the largest number of MEDEX practices and retrievable computer claim files and to adjust the choice of control practices accordingly. This had the double advantage of limiting the number of Blue Shield plans to be dealt with and avoided a request to review large amounts of data to gain information on only one or two practices. It was determined that three states—Utah,

Colorado and Idaho—could provide sufficient numbers of practices. In each state the plan agreed to provide the necessary data from special runs of existing computer tapes if expenses incurred were reimbursed. Securing the cooperation of the two neighboring plans was in large measure the result of the good offices of the Utah plan. They had previous experience in assisting the study and were able to deal on a collegial basis with their counterparts.

Restudy Data

Although the restudy results have been presented elsewhere in substantial detail, some of the highlights will be noted here to illustrate particular points. The descriptive studies showed that the patterns during employment of the Medex were not very different from those seen during his/her training. The activities of the Medex continued to resemble closely those of the preceptor.[7] Quality of care in terms of both process and outcome showed no signs of deterioration as a result of adding a Medex to the practice.[8] The socialization of the Medex into the physician's practice had often left the Medex in a status different from the other members of the office staff but still clearly subordinate to the physician.[9] The stability of the match was reflected in the degree to which the Medex and his physician agreed in their perception of his role.[10]

The archival studies provided a means for examining if any changes could be attributed to adding a Medex. Using the Blue Shield data as an indicator of shifts in volume of services from the pre-Medex to the employment period, it was possible to compare changes in Medex practices to those in matched controls. Figure 24:5 shows the mean percentage of change in charges per quarter for different categories of service over this time period; in each case the change in the Medex group was larger than that in the controls.

As seen in Figure 24:6, the Medex practices had begun with higher levels of charges in each service category. Nonetheless, the growth in activity, particularly for outpatient and laboratory services was impressive. It should be recognized (a) that this use of third-party data implies an indirect rather than a direct measure of change and (b) the degree of market penetrance for the "Blues" may vary from place to place. There is a marked difference in the amount of billed services between the Medex and control groups. However, the concern here is primarily with relative changes. As long as there is no evidence of a change in the coverage of one group or the degree of reimbursement then this comparison of change over time in payment may be used as an indicator of

FIGURE 24:5

Average Percent Change Pre-Medex to Employment Period in Charges Per Quarter for Various Groups of Services

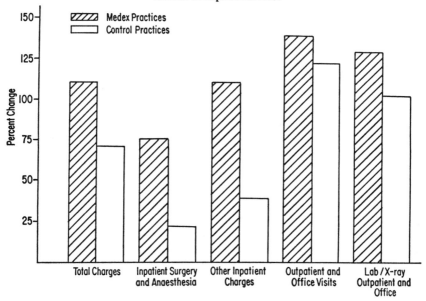

FIGURE 24:6

Charges Per Quarter for Total and Groups of Services

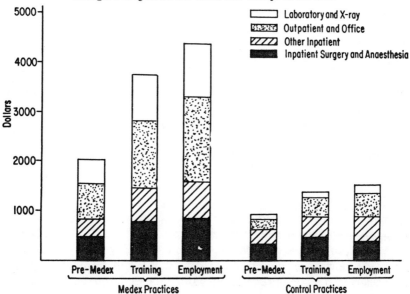

change in volume of service in the two groups. In order to maintain comparable coverage benefits between Medex and control practices, each control was chosen from the same state as the Medex practice and matched on the basis of practice location, size and specialty. All that was required from the physician was his permission to gain access to the data. No patient names were used; even the individual physician identification was not necessary. Thus an archival source of existing data could be tapped to provide an indirect and unobtrusive measure of change over time in which the secular effects are equally distributed across the experimental and control groups.

Data from physician records were also used in this fashion. A group of Medex practices and matched controls were asked to provide copies of a portion of their income tax each year covering the period from two years prior to the arrival of the Medex until the present. Abstracts of these data were then used in conjunction with counts of patient visits taken from appointment logs to look at the changes in revenue, expenses and patient volume. Important effects in the Medex and a matched control group were observed. Effects brought about by the rapid inflation in medical prices and the continued escalation in the demand for care should be evenly distributed across both groups. Figure 24:7 provides one example of how such data can be used. In this case regression lines were drawn and the slopes compared by T-test. Although there were a few significant differences in individual practice pairs, the aggregated data showed no significant differences.

Lessons Learned

Business records from the doctors' own files and administrative records from Blue Cross-Blue Shield, have been of great importance to this study and can be of equally great importance in other studies. Government records from such agencies as the Social Security Administration will in many studies be equally important. The non-defensive cooperation from the Medex and non-Medex doctors, and from the Blue Cross-Blue Shield plans was invaluable inasmuch as cooperation with others cannot necessarily be counted on. With this in mind, a few additional comments are offered.

The cooperating doctors and their accountants were willing to report their data in actual dollar amounts. This degree of openness is not necessary, however, and in general researchers should request only relativized data to indicate deviations from a baseline, but disguising the absolute value. Two procedures may be recommended: (1) The doctor's accountant, paid by the research project as a consultant, may transform data for each period into a percentage of the value at some arbitrary date which

FIGURE 24:7

Changes in Revenues and Expenses for Medex and Control Physicians

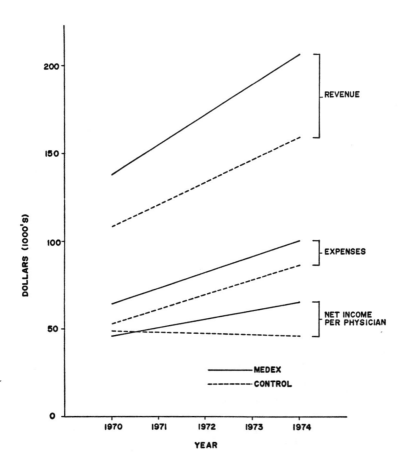

could be the first observational period. Giving that reference date the value of 100, subsequent dates would be expressed in index form from that base. (2) Alternatively, the accountant could multiply all values by an arbitrary multiplier of his own choosing (e.g., .50 or .75 or 1.5 or 2.0, etc.) and report the resulting values without revealing his multiplier. The research team in this case would want to convert all individual practice data into logorithms before averaging. These two transformations would not at all preclude the kinds of inferences as to effects which have been made here. They would, however, require stating results in percentage changes rather than in dollar amounts. Transformations involving additive constants would be likely to distort variances in uncorrectible ways and should be avoided.

The use of the Blue Shield data was made possible because the plan had appropriate data retrieval capacities. Note that the Medex doctors had essential anonymity because their data were pooled before being released to the study. The Blue Shield statisticians could have provided still greater protection by using an index or a multiplier transformation before releasing the data. This, with the permission from the Medex doctors, might have permitted release of identified individual series, so that the practice-by-practice tests for effects would have been done on these data, too. While in this case, Blue Shield quite appropriately did the selecting of control cases, the researchers could have selected them and sent a list as was done for Medex cases, without jeopardizing confidentiality. Campbell, et al.[11] provide a comprehensive review of modes of statistically linking record systems without transferring individual data from one record system to the other. The procedure described here followed their recommendations except for one detail. Were one to anticipate repeatedly negotiating with Blue Cross, utilizing overlapping sets of doctors, he would recommend that on each negotiation Blue Cross randomly delete one person from the list, reporting out the composite data for the remainder, not specifying who had been deleted. This extreme precaution is to prevent identification of one individual's data.

The Blue Cross-Blue Shield may be unique in having offered this research retrieval capacity. They might not be able to do so were requests more frequent, or had searches by illness or by mode of treatment been requested. Medical insurance records have been designed for billing purposes, and present great difficulties for retrieval for other uses. Yet in these files lie the potential for important and definitive evaluations of health delivery and medical treatment options. The interrupted time series are by far the best of the quasi-experimental designs available to health research, as extended time series are not feasible. Given this it should be a top priority goal of HEW to fund each major health record system, public and private, with a statistician, a computer programmer, and clerical assistance, just to develop research retrieval capacity and to service research requests. It is only by having this retrieval and statistical capacity within the primary file that confidentiality can be preserved.

This account illustrates several different approaches to evaluation. Basically one may elect to use descriptive, experimental or quasi-experimental designs. Each has a role to play. As noted, the descriptive approach provides information about what is happening but cannot be used as a basis for making decisions about program impact. Too many factors within and without cannot be accounted for.

There is a natural attraction to the true experimental design where randomization can be applied as the evaluator's cleansing balm to wash away all sorts of contamination. Unfortunately such studies are difficult to establish and to maintain. Too many things crop up to disrupt a prospective design. When experimental studies are conducted, they are often restricted to a small number of atypical sites.

There are occasions when it is not feasible to assign groups or patients at random to create control and experimental groups. One of the most widespread experimental designs in educational research involves an experimental group and a control group both with a pre-test and a post-test, but in which the control group and the experimental group do not have pre-experimental sampling equivalence. Rather, the study and comparison groups constitute naturally assembled patient populations in, for example, two or more similar practices, yet not so similar that one can dispense with the pre-test. This design should be recognized as well worth using in many instances in which randomization is impossible. The more similar the experimental and the control groups, and the more this similarity is confirmed by the pre-test scores, the more effective this control becomes.

The quasi-experimental approach has several immediately obvious advantages in assessing the impact of newly established programs like those involving new health practitioners. To the extent that archival data can be used, it may be possible to sample widely across a variety of settings in an unobtrusive manner.[12] The gathering of such data may often be much better tolerated by the practice involved than would more intensive direct study.

Also important is to recognize that a number of factors may jeopardize the validity of various experimental designs. These factors affect the *internal* and the *external validity* of research findings. *Internal validity* is the basic minimum without which any experiment is uninterpretable: Did, in fact, the experimental treatments make a difference in a specific experimental instance? *External validity* asks the question of generalizability: To what populations, settings, treatment variables, and measurement variables can this effect be generalized? Both types of criteria are obviously important even though they are frequently at odds, in that features increasing one may jeopardize the other. While internal validity is the *sine qua non*, and while the question of external validity, like the question of inductive inference, is never completely answerable, the selection of designs strong in both internal and external validity obviously is an ideal.

In efforts to extend the logic of laboratory experimentation into the field and into settings not fully experimental, an inventory of threats to experimental validity has been assembled, in terms of which numerous experimental and quasi-experimental designs have been evaluated.[13]

Assuming that a pre-test has shown study and comparison groups to have similar characteristics, a pre-test/post-test design can be regarded as controlling for several factors that threaten the validity of the findings. Thus the difference between the experimental group's pre-test and post-test results is more likely to reflect the effect of the experimental treatment or program.

One important threat to internal validity is the extent to which other events may have affected the apparent results of the study. For example, changes in patterns of practice may have as much to do with changes in malpractice coverage or reimbursement policies as with the addition of a Medex. The public's acceptance of the Medex and the reaction of the medical profession will likely be influenced by the availability of the nurse practitioner and the growing emphasis on primary care in medical schools. The function of a Medex will surely relate to regulations determining which services performed by such an individual are legal and reimbursable.

IMPLICATIONS OF RESEARCH FINDINGS FOR POLICY

The United States and other nations should be ready for an experimental approach to social reform in which new programs designed to cure specific social problems are explored, in which it can be known whether or not these programs are effective, and in which they are retained, imitated, modified, or discarded on the basis of apparent effectiveness on the multiple imperfect criteria available. The readiness for this stage is indicated by the inclusion of specific provisions for program evaluation in the first wave of the Great Society legislation, and by the legislation that authorized the experimental nurse practitioner and physician's assistant programs. There have been good intentions in this regard for so long that many may feel that the stage already has been reached when programs are continued or discontinued on the basis of assessed effectiveness. It is generally true that this is not at all so and that most ameliorative programs end up with *no* interpretable evaluation.

Many of the difficulties in evaluation lie in the intransigencies of the research setting and in the presence of recurrent seductive pitfalls of interpretation. This chapter has been devoted to these problems. But the few available solutions turn out to depend upon correct administrative decisions in the political arena and involve political jeopardies that are often sufficient to explain the lack of hard-headed evaluation of effects. It is essential that the social scientist/research advisor understand the political realities of the situation, and that he help create a public demand for hard-headed evaluation. It is important to recognize the political consequences of program evaluation and to identify political strategies that might further a truly experimental approach to social reform. Thus it seems convenient to conclude with some general points about this political nature. It is one of the most characteristic aspects of the present situation that *specific reforms are advocated as though they were certain to be successful.* For this reason, knowing outcomes has immediate political implications. Given the inherent difficulty of making significant improvements by the means usually provided and given the discrepancy between promise and possibility, most administrators wisely prefer to limit the evaluations to those in which they control the outcomes, particularly insofar as published outcomes or press releases are concerned. There is safety under the cloak of ignorance. Even where there are ideological commitments to a hard-headed evaluation, fear of detrimental findings lead to the failure to evaluate social experiments realistically. If the political and administrative system has committed itself in advance to the correctness and efficacy of its reforms, it cannot tolerate failure. The true scientist is able to experiment and advocate without an excess of commitment that negates reality testing. The new health practitioner field is fertile for experimentation and, as a potential social reform, worthy of a courageous examination of the outcomes.

ACKNOWLEDGEMENT

The authors wish to thank Donald T. Campbell, Ph.D., Professor at Northwestern University, for his advice and guidance throughout the evaluation of the Utah MEDEX Program and for his contribution to the present manuscript.

Notes

1. William M. Wilson and C. Hilmon Castle. "The Utah MEDEX Demonstration Project." *Rocky Mt Med J 69,* (1972), 53-56.
2. For a discussion of "matching", see Donald T. Campbell and Julian C. Stanley. *Experimental and quasi-experimental designs for research.* (Chicago, Rand McNally, 1966), p. 15.
3. Thomas D. Cook and Donald T. Campbell. "The Design and Conduct of Quasi-Experiments and True Experiments in Field Settings," in M.D. Dunnette, (ed.) *Handbook of Industrial and Organizational Psychology.* (Chicago, Rand McNally, 1976), pp. 283-84.

4. Henry W. Riecken and Robert F. Boruch (eds.). *Social Experimentation: A Method for Planning and Evaluating Social Innovation.* (New York: Academic Press, 1974), Chapter IV "Quasi-Experimental Designs", pp. 87-116.

5. S.T. Bain and W.B. Spaulding. "The Importance of Coding Presenting Symptoms." *Can Med Assoc J 97,* 1967, 953-959.

6. Robert L. Kane, F. Ross Woolley, Jerry Gardner, et al. "Measuring Outcomes of Care in an Ambulatory Care Population: A Pilot Study," *Journal of Community Health* (in press).

7. Robert L. Kane, Donna M. Olsen, William M. Wilson, et al., "Adding a Medex to the Medical Mix: An Evaluation," *Med Care 14,* (1976), 1000-07.

8. Robert L. Kane, Donna M. Olsen and C. Hilmon Castle. "The Quality of Care of Medex and Their Physician Preceptors," *JAMA 236,* (1976), 2509-25.

9. Robert L. Kane, F. Ross Woolley, Charles C. Hughes, et al., "Communication Patterns of Doctors and Their Assistants," *Med Care 14,* (1976), 348-356.

10. Vaughn L. Pulsipher and Robert L. Kane. "A Model to Predict the Stability of Medex-Preceptor Matches," *The P.A. Journal,* Winter 1977.

11. Donald T. Campbell, Robert F. Boruch, Richard D. Schwartz, and Joseph Steinberg. Confidentiality-preserving Modes of Access to Files and to Interfile Exchange for Useful Statistical Analysis. Appendix A to Anna M. Rivlin, et al. *Protecting Individual Privacy in Evaluation Research.* A report of the Committee on Federal Agency Evaluation Research of the National Academy of Sciences, National Research Council, Washington, D.C. 1975, pp. A-1 to A-25.

12. For examples of "unobtrusive measures", see Eugene J. Webb, Donald T. Campbell, Richard D. Schwartz, and Lee Sechrest. *Unobtrusive Measures: Non-reactive Research in the Social Sciences.* (Chicago, Rand McNally, 1966)

13. For further information, see Campbell and Stanley, op. cit.; Cook and Campbell, op. cit.

Chapter 25
The Social Security Administration Physician Extender Reimbursement Study: Anatomy of a Quasi-Experimental Design

Clifton R. Gaus, Stephen B. Morris and David B. Smith

BACKGROUND

The major objectives of the Social Security Administration's Physician Extender Reimbursement Study are to assess the impact on primary care of employing physician extenders (PEs) and the effects on practice productivity and Medicare expenditures, of alternative methods of reimbursement.

... "to determine under what circumstances payment for services would be appropriate and the most appropriate, equitable, and noninflationary methods and amounts of reimbursement under health care programs established by the Social Security Act for services, which are performed independently by an assistant to a physician, including a nurse practitioner (whether or not performed in the office of or at a place at which such physician is physically present), and—

(i) which such assistant is legally authorized to perform by the State or political subdivision wherein such services are performed, and

(ii) for which such physician assumes full legal and ethical responsibility as to the necessity, propriety, and quality thereof;"...

Section 222(b)(1) subpart (G),
Social Security Amendments of 1972

Ideally, the PE study questions* would be addressed by means of a "true experimental" design involving random assignment of participating medical practices to either treatment or control groups. In order to determine the impact of PE utilization on primary care practice patterns, the treatment group would have a PE placed on its staff while the control group would continue to operate with its original non-PE staff.

---

* See Chapter 9.

Similarly, to determine the impact of experimental reimbursement, PE practices would be assigned randomly to either a treatment group that receives reimbursement or a control group which does not. With this pre-test-post-test control group design, measurements of study variables both before and after initiation of the treatment would allow for analysis of practice pattern changes attributable to the experimental treatment. Potential sources of internal invalidity would be controlled in such an ideal design. However, a practical constraint precluded the use of a true experimental design for the study; it is not feasible to assign PEs randomly to a private medical practice.** It is unlikely that many physicians or PEs would submit to such an imposition and those who might agree would be suspect of selection bias. As a result, established PE and non-PE practices have been assigned to treatment or comparison groups; therefore, the study is not a true experimental design.

The methodology includes identification of eligible PE and comparison practices, collection of baseline data describing current practice patterns, application of the experimental treatment, i.e., reimbursement for PE services and collection of experimental data to compare with baseline data. In addition, substudies of specific issues, including data validation, quality of care, and the cost of employing PEs will be conducted. Baseline data collection was accomplished through ten mailings of survey forms over thirteen months to randomly selected groups of eligible practices. As practices completed the baseline phase, they entered the experimental phase of the study. Practices thus entered the reimbursement serially with data comparable to the baseline again being collected. These "experimental" observations, when compared with the "pre-experimental" baseline formed the analytical base for testing some of the study questions. The study is expected to continue through 1978. The findings of the practice identification survey were made available in September 1976, with the baseline results due in the summer of 1977. Preliminary results of the differential reimbursement experiment—assessing the impact of reimbursement on practice activity and Medicare expenditures—should be available by the end of 1977, with final reports expected one year later.

PRACTICE IDENTIFICATION SURVEYS

The first study activity involved identifying PE and non-PE practices eligible and willing to participate. Brief questionnaires were sent to all

---

** One study conducted by the UCLA PRIMEX FNP program did, in fact, attempt such random assignment, but with fewer than 20 graduates; all assigned randomly to a panel of physicians who had agreed beforehand to hire a Primex.

potential PE participants to solicit information on the location, organization, size and specialty of the practices in which they were employed. A similar questionnaire was sent to a group of 16,500 general practitioners, family practitioners and general internists in order to identify comparison practices similar to the responding PE practices.

In order to participate further in the study, PEs must have completed a formal PE training program no later than July 1975. They must be employed: in a physician-directed office or clinic which is not part of a hospital, in a general or family practice, or in an internal medicine practice. About 1,500 physicians met the eligibility criteria for comparison practices; namely, that they did not employ physician extenders, that they were in general or family practice or internal medicine, and that they were not employed in hospitals. From this group, about 900 comparison practices were identified for participation in the baseline survey. They were selected to represent a similar distribution by location, specialty, size and organization as the PE practices in the baseline survey. Practice identification was completed in June 1976. Since assignment to baseline survey intervals was random, all geographic settings were subject to inclusion in various seasons.

BASELINE SURVEY

The second phase of the study—the baseline survey—which began in January 1976, has involved collection and analysis of cross-sectional data describing current primary care practice patterns in PE and comparison practices. To accomplish this, a self-administered log-diary and questionnaire booklet developed by the Division of Research in Medical Education (DRME) of the University of Southern California School of Medicine were sent to each PE and physician participant. These instruments solicited four types of information: features of the practice organization and participant's background collected by means of the questionnaire; summary data of the participant's weekly clinical encounters and hours worked; daily summary of the participant's major activities (Activity Overview); and a daily log of individual patient encounters in the office, home, hospital or over the telephone.

Baseline data were collected over a 13-month period with PE practices randomly assigned to ten collection intervals of three days each. Comparison practices were assigned to the last five of these ten intervals. In all, about 650 PE practices and 900 comparison practices participated in the baseline survey. Of these, about 350 PE practices and a similar number of comparison practices successfully completed the survey.

The data collected in the baseline survey described differences in practice organization, services rendered, patients seen and practice productivity.

Questionnaire

The information requested by questionnaire expanded on the basic data collected in the practice identification phase. Questions addressed to the PE included the number of hours spent in patient contact in various practice settings during a normal week, the composition of the staff, and a checklist of clinical procedures regularly performed by the PE.

Information requested from the physician included questions on specialty training, continuing education, and teaching activities. Additional questions related to the practice settings in which patients are seen, hospital privileges, practice arrangement, distribution of specialties among practice physicians, type of payment, arrangements for laboratory work, staff composition and size, and a detailed checklist of tasks which the physician delegates to various staff personnel. Much of the data collected by the questionnaires served a descriptive purpose. In addition, detailed practice data allowed detection of possible bias in the practice profile, not apparent during the matching process. The direction of these biases can then be accounted for in the final data analysis.

Patient Encounter Log

Encounter information has been recorded in participating practices for each patient seen by a PE or physician over a three-day period during the baseline phase. Log sheets for each of the three days were provided for inpatient and outpatient visits, telephone contacts, and research/teaching among other activities. All patient care transactions involving study participants were recorded in the log. The data entries on the form included encounter time and location; patient characteristics; and classification of presenting problem by its severity, the affected organ or system and etiology. Diagnostic and therapeutic procedures, as well as the overall complexity of the encounter, were also recorded along with further treatment and charges for the encounter.

Activity Overview

Each participant's activities during the three-day data collection period were recorded for each 15 minute period. Among the major activities thus examined were outpatient and inpatient care, teaching, research, supervision, continuing education, administration of the practice, professional travel, and personal time.

Practice and Patient Encounter Summary

An additional set of data consisted of a weekly summary of practice and patient encounters for the week in which the three-day data collection period occurred. This information was collected to examine whether the three days of major data collection were typical of the practice by showing the degree of variability in the work week.

THE REIMBURSEMENT EXPERIMENT

Initiation of Experimental Medicare Reimbursement

As practices successfully completed the baseline survey, they were included in monthly mailings to the appropriate Medicare carrier for inclusion in the reimbursement experiment. The carrier informed each practice of its eligibility to participate in the reimbursement arrangement. If a practice indicated it would not participate, the carrier notified the SSA stating the reason for nonparticipation, if known.

One of the two agreement forms used to confirm participation in the experiment was signed by the PE's supervising physician. Through this form, the supervising physician agreed to assume full legal and ethical responsibility for the PE's work. The other agreement form was signed by the PE's employer. In this form, the employer agreed to participate and cooperate in data collection activities related to the study, including on-site observations and records abstraction which will be performed as a separate function by SSA in about 100 of the practices participating nationwide.

By signing the agreement forms, the participating practice agreed to assure that claims submitted for reimbursement under the experiment are for services the PE was legally authorized to perform in the State or subdivision in which the services were delivered. A review of the compliance with this agreement will be undertaken by the Social Security Administration's Office of Research and Statistics. The review will include a comparison of claims data with applicable State and local laws and regulations governing the services of PEs.

After receipt of the signed agreements, the carrier assigned an identification number to each PE. This number clearly identified the PE as the provider of services. The carrier sent a letter to the participating practice transmitting the PE identification number and information on the proper claims submittal procedures. The date on this letter served as the first date for which PE services in participating practices could be reimbursed under the experimental authority.

Once the PE identification number is issued by the carrier, practices can begin submitting reimbursement claims for PE services. However, PEs are not reimbursed directly. Rather, claims are recognized only if signed by the physician or designated employer at the time the PE provider number was issued. Since SSA Form 1490 is used for all claims submitted by participating practices to carriers, separate forms which include the PE identification number must be submitted for PE services. Payments for covered PE services are then made at the appropriate rate to the employing practice.

The study does not require any changes in carrier claims processing and data systems related to the 1490-claim form. The use of existing forms during the study period will facilitate a comparison between baseline survey results and data provided by the carriers for the year which preceded experimental reimbursement. Similarly, the claims data for PE and comparison practices can be analyzed both before and after experimental reimbursement.

Two data collection activities will be completed during the reimbursement experiment. First, data similar to those collected in the baseline survey will again be obtained from participating practices to assess possible changes in practice organization and in productivity. Secondary data will be abstracted from claims submitted to Medicare from participating PEs and physicians, as well as from comparison practices. These data will be used to assess: (1) those changes in billing and Medicare payments associated with the experimental reimbursement policy and (2) the financial implications of reimbursement for services, both for the Medicare program and for Medicare beneficiaries.

As an adjunct to the reimbursement experiment, comparison practices which hired an eligible PE during the course of the experiment will be allowed to participate in the reimbursement experiment. These practices will constitute a natural experiment in the effects of Medicare reimbursement on decisions to hire PEs.

After their participation in the baseline survey, comparison practices will be assigned randomly to two groups. One group will be told that it will be included in the reimbursement experiment if the practice hires a PE. The other group will not receive this information. One year after completing the baseline survey, all comparison practices will be surveyed to learn how many PEs were hired in each group. All practices which have hired PEs will then be given the option of participating. For those practices which do so, uniform before-and-after information will be available on practice organization, productivity, charges and Medicare expenditures.

Reimbursement Method

A central goal of the study is to determine the most appropriate, equitable, and noninflationary Medicare reimbursement for PE services. In order to make this determination, the study is providing experimental reimbursement to participating primary care practices for PE services delivered to beneficiaries independent of the supervising physician. Three reimbursement methods are being tested in the study.

Fee-Based Medicare Reimbursement at the Full Physician's Rate

Under this method, Medicare reimburses an employer for a PE service up to the full rate allowed for the supervising physician who delivers the same services. Full reimbursement can be assumed to provide the maximum possible change in many of the variables under study including task delegation and productivity.

Reimbursement at 80 Percent of a Physician's Rate

Under this method, Medicare reimburses an employer for a PE's service up to 80 percent allowed for the supervising physician who delivers the same service. If this rate is greater than the cost to the practice of the PE's time, an economic incentive exists for employing PEs, although a smaller incentive than full reimbursement.

Under partial fee reimbursement, physicians are likely to be paid less for PE services than for their own. However, enough new services such as home and nursing home care may be delivered to increase costs to the Medicare program and to the recipients of care. Questions then can be raised concerning the necessity of these additional services and their effect on the anticipated demand for other types of health care services.

Cost-Related Medicare Reimbursement

Under this method, Medicare reimburses an employer on an average cost basis for the PE's services. The cost for a service is calculated on the basis of the PE's salary including fringe benefits, practice overhead, and physician supervisory time. Two options for cost-related reimbursement are being employed. One is a proportion (62 percent) of the supervising physician's allowable charges which would, on average, meet practice costs for having a PE provide a service without the direct involvement of the physician.

Under the other option, a "lump-sum" payment is made to a participating practice to reimburse the practice costs of PE care provided to Medicare beneficiaries. The size of the lump sum is reviewed periodically throughout the experiment in order to assure an appropriate and equitable level of reimbursement.

Carrier Participation

Thirty of the 64 Medicare carriers (usually insurance companies or Blue Shield Plans) are participating in the study. These carriers were assigned using a stratified random technique to one of the three reimbursement methods so that each method covered an equal number of PE practices eligible to participate in the baseline survey.

In addition, two national carriers were included. One, the Division of Direct Reimbursement of the Social Security Administration, acts as a carrier for federally financed comprehensive health centers, health maintenance organizations and other prepaid group medical practices. Participating practices which are reimbursed through this carrier will use existing cost-related formulae for computing reimbursements for PE services. The second national carrier has been established to administer the second or "lump-sum" option. Participating practices not included in the service areas of the 30 participating carriers will be reimbursed using the lump-sum option.

SPECIAL SUBSTUDIES

Several issues could not be addressed properly through the log diary and questionnaire. These included quality of care, costs of employing a PE and evaluation of the log diary data. These issues were addressed through intensive on-site data collection in about 100 PE and 100 comparison practices participating in the reimbursement experiment. These practices were selected using a stratified random procedure.

Quality of Care

One of the central research questions is whether, with the utilization of PEs, the quality of care delivered by a practice remains constant, increases or decreases. Quality assessment is a difficult task requiring specific data sources and research methods. Given the lack of consensus as to the ideal method for assessing quality of care, several commonly employed measures of quality were taken including:
— opinions of participating physicians
— abstracts of medical records
— field observer evaluation.

Opinions of Participating Physicians

The opinions of supervising and comparison physicians were sought for several reasons. Physician opinion has been used as an indicator of quality in previous evaluation of PE practices, thereby permitting a comparison of findings. Further, since the evaluation of medical quality ultimately relies on physician judgments, physician acceptance and quality are at least conceptually related. Finally, from the point of view of many medical practitioners, peer opinion has a greater face validity as an indicator of quality than many of the other indicators used, and hence, is more convincing.

Abstracts of Medical Records

A sample of medical records was abstracted and evaluated using process measures of quality. While office practices vary considerably in terms of the quality and completeness of such records, it can be argued that quality and completeness are related to the actual quality of care rendered by the practice and, hence, one appropriate source of reasonably valid inferences concerning the quality of care. A tracer approach similar to that used by Kessner and others* seemed to be most appropriate, in which records would be selected from the practice in a systematic way representing common symptoms, diagnoses or treatments for which a fairly well developed list of criteria exists for the evaluation of performance. These records were abstracted and subjected to evaluation by a panel of expert judges who rated the overall acceptability of care provided by a comparison of the evidence supplied in the record abstract with a criterion checklist for that particular symptom, diagnosis or treatment. Through these data interjudge and intermethod reliability are also being evaluated.

Field Observer Evaluation

Those involved in the field data collection were sufficiently knowledgeable about the delivery of primary care and spent sufficient time with a particular practice to make some reasonably valid inferences about certain aspects of the practice related to the quality of care. These observations were structured by a pretested checklist which the field observer completed during the field data collection period. The observers paid particular attention to those aspects of the practice that might be

---

*D. Kessner, C. Kalk, and J. Singer, "Assessing Health Quality—The Case for Tracers," *N.E.J.M.* 288, No. 4 (Jan. 25, 1973), 189-194.

related to access to care (e.g. waiting time) or the effective coordination of services (e.g. scheduling, follow-up). An attempt was made to adapt some of the material and procedures used by the Joint Commission on the Accreditation of Hospitals to evaluate hospital outpatient operations for these purposes. The combination of information from all three of these sources should provide a measure of the relative quality of primary care in the substudy's PE practices.

Costs of PEs to Primary Care Practices

Assuming that quality of care is either the same or improved in PE practices, then costs become an important variable from a variety of viewpoints. Such information helps physicians decide whether to hire PEs for their practices. Also, the Social Security Administration must know how to build into reimbursement arrangements financial incentives which minimize the inflationary impact of such reimbursement both on the Medicare program and on the beneficiary. At the present time, there is little information about the actual costs incurred in hiring a PE and about the circumstances under which financial losses or profits accrue to the physician. This is not in any way to suggest that the only incentive to a physician for hiring a PE is financial. Nevertheless, it is important to know under what conditions a reimbursement policy designed to stimulate the growth and use of PEs makes financial sense from the viewpoint of the consumer and third-party payer who will absorb these costs. Are those conditions presently being met and if not, how can they be met?

Specific information on financial considerations are being collected in the following areas: PE annual salary (or other reimbursement if not a fixed salary); fringe benefits including bonus plans or profit sharing; overhead directly related to PE employment; and physician supervisory time calculated on the physician's hourly wage.

Log Diary Data Validation

Inaccurate, partial or missing information in the log diary could introduce response bias into the production data. Therefore, these data will be validated through on-site review of patient records. The record review serves both to verify the log diary entries and as a quality-of-care component of the study.

ANALYSIS PLAN

The data collected in the study will provide for a cross-sectional analysis between PE and non-PE practices, and among personnel (i.e., physician's assistant, Medex, nurse practitioner). In addition, baseline data will be used as pre-experimental observations against which to compare data collected during the experimental reimbursement period.

The PE Reimbursement Study was designed to address a number of research issues. Those concerning differences in productivity, volume and scope of services between PE and non-PE practices are addressed directly by the baseline data. Issues of quality of care and practice costs are the subject of separate special substudies. All reimbursement-related questions will be examined in the experimentation period which follows the baseline study.

A series of working papers will be developed as data from the various phases of the overall research effort become available:

Working Paper # 1: *Diffusion of Physician Extenders*

The analysis of the practice identification survey data will be presented. The practice size, and geographic and specialty distribution of respondents will be described. Distribution of PEs and physicians will be compared by county for rural-urban differences, poverty levels, and other social indices.

Working Paper # 2: *Physician Extender Practice Activity Patterns*

The analysis of the initial log diary and questionnaire data obtained from the baseline phase will be presented. It will describe the functions carried out by PEs and their supervising physicians prior to reimbursement and compare these activities to those of comparison practices. Practice characteristics related to productivity will be summarized.

Working Paper # 3: *Impact of PE Reimbursement on Medicare Costs*

A time series analysis will be performed on Medicare charge data for the physician extender reimbursed practices and the comparison practices. The analysis will explore the impact of the three levels of experimental reimbursement on cost.

Working Paper # 4: *Impact of PE Reimbursement on PE Practice Activity*

Pre- and post-test data on physician extender reimbursed practices will be evaluated. The analysis will explore the impact of reimbursement on practice patterns, e.g. whether reimbursement produces a tendency to use physician extenders more independently and more productively and whether there are differences in the effect of the different reimbursement methods on practice activity.

Working Paper # 5: *Substudy Analysis*

Results of the field data collection substudy will be summarized. The findings of the substudy will be presented in terms of 1) the reliability of the log diary data 2) the relative quality of care provided by PE practices and 3) the costs associated with PE employment.

A brief final report integrating the findings of the five working papers and policy implications will complete the evaluation effort.

Postscript

The research design had to take into account a number of constraints. The reader may ask why a national mail survey was used to identify participating physician extender practices scattered throughout the United States. From a research or cost standpoint it would seem to make more sense to conduct the study in a limited geographic area, randomly assign the PE practices to a reimbursement or control group and use more extensive field observation rather than less reliable mail surveys.

The decision to conduct a national experiment grew out of a compromise between those who were pressing for change in the present Medicare law to permit reimbursement for PE services and those who were concerned about the cost implications of such reimbursement. The compromise was that any experiment would provide interim Medicare reimbursement to any eligible practice wishing to participate. One may assume that the prospect of receiving interim Medicare reimbursement would have prompted a relatively high response rate to study surveys. Obtaining information from busy primary care practices, however, required major follow-up efforts.

Finally, one may question the limited set of measures for collecting quality-of-care data. However, the complexity of quality assessment and the lack of consensus that presently exists concerning quality definition or measurement placed in-depth quality-of-care evaluation beyond the scope of this study. The quality of care paid for by Medicare as measured by the study will be perhaps the most important aspect of service. Substandard care, no matter how low the charge, is too expensive.

Chapter 26

Methods for Calculating Costs of Educating Child Health Associates

John E. Ott and George Knox

Federal and state governments, associations of medical educators and health policy planners are increasingly interested in determining the cost-effectiveness of training health professionals in order to ensure funding of worthwhile programs and to establish priorities for the number and types of health professionals to be trained. A common method of computing these expenses cannot be found, however, in the literature. Difficulties in comparing costs of different programs arise in general, from variations in the:

— backgrounds and previous educational experience of students,
— prerequisites for admission,
— educational objectives of the programs and methods used to determine whether objectives have been met,
— types of institutions in which the programs are located,
— emphasis on placing students in areas of need which may be geographically distant from the program's location.

In addition, cost factors that make the problem even more complex include:

— identifying sources of income and allocating costs,
— estimating shared or joint costs,
— ascertaining the value of volunteer teaching time,
— evaluating the specific accounting systems used by different institutions.

The cost of medical school education was recently estimated in two major studies. The Association of American Medical Colleges (AAMC) estimated the range of costs in twelve selected medical schools to be $16,000-$26,000/student/year for the 1972-73 academic year.[1] Full- and part-time faculty, housestaff, and other health professionals were asked to record their teaching, research and administrative activities by completing activity logs for a one-week period. All professional activities of the full-time faculty as well as estimated teaching costs of part-time faculty, housestaff, volunteer faculty and allied health professionals who participated in the teaching of medical students on a less-than-full-time basis were considered educational expenses. The Institute of Medicine of the National Academy of Sciences surveyed eighty-two medical schools during the 1972-73 academic year.[2] Using a different methodology, the Institute of Medicine calculated the average cost of undergraduate medical education to be $12,650/student/year with a range of $6,900-$18,650. Their approach was similar to the AAMC study in that they also utilized an analysis of the faculty's activity reports for a one-week period, but different in that the Institute of Medicine estimated the value of time spent in research and patient care with students in attendance compared with time spent in these two activities without students present. The value of this additional time was considered to be an educational expense. The Institute of Medicine study did not include the value of part-time teaching provided by volunteer faculty, housestaff, and other professionals.

Other studies have estimated the cost of preparing nurse practitioners. In 1969, Silver estimated the cost of educating the first pediatric nurse practitioners, who already had a baccalaureate degree when they entered the PNP program at the University of Colorado, at approximately $4,000/student.[3] Yankauer et al. calculated the cost of preparing PNPs in the Bunker Hill Program from 1968-71 at $3,197/nurse.[4] Yankauer included the direct educational and indirect institutional costs but did not include faculty and overhead contributions, start-up and evaluation expenses or informational activities to explain the concept of nurse practitioners.

In 1973, Kahn estimated the expenditures for a similar four-month program to be about $4,000/student.[5] He did not include the cost of instructor preparation of lectures or institutional overhead. Initially no equipment was purchased and other expenses were minimal. Subsequently, additional nursing faculty were hired and audiovisual teaching aids and other equipment were purchased by the program. A 1975 estimate of the cost of preparing and *evaluating* students in this program is $7,000-$8,000/student, and includes tuition, other income, university contributions and federal grant support.[6]

Although one and two-year master's degree nurse practitioner programs are becoming more numerous, there are few published studies about how much these programs cost. Similarly, there are few published studies of the cost of educating physician's assistants. However, one survey of fifteen programs conducted by Andreoli indicated an expenditure of $7,000-$20,000/student/year.[7] The survey did not break down the various expense categories.

A System Sciences study has attempted to determine the costs of training physician's assistants *and* nurse practitioners in forty-four different programs.[8] In this study the costs of basic education per student/per month and per year of training are being estimated for the number of graduates and for all students enrolled in the program, including those who subsequently withdrew. To arrive at valid costs, the study should show that the programs had complete and reliable records of both income and expenditure, used similar accounting systems and assumptions, had equivalent degrees of accounting sophistication and centralized record systems. Unless these factors are taken into consideration, health policy planners may erroneously consider the cost data to be definitive and to make decisions based on limited assumptions.

In this chapter, the costs of training Child Health Associates, capable of carrying out activities traditionally performed by pediatricians, are used as an illustration of how costs might be computed. Explicit categories of expense, including start-up, teaching, administration, deployment, evaluation, and student support costs are defined. The interpretation of the calculated costs of training Child Health Associates is then discussed with potential pitfalls in comparing training costs presented along with recommendations for uniform guidelines to cost accounting to make comparisons among programs more meaningful.

ESTIMATING COSTS OF EDUCATING CHILD HEALTH ASSOCIATES

The costs of educating Child Health Associates in a three-year program leading to a baccalaureate or master's degree from the University of Colorado Medical Center were determined for a seven-year period from July 1968 through June 1975.* The first year of the program was used to design the curriculum and to prepare for and recruit the first class of students who began their studies in July 1969. During this seven-year period, seven classes were enrolled in the program and four classes totalling 47 students graduated.

*Supported by grants from the Carnegie Corporation of New York; the Commonwealth Fund; the National Center for Health Services Research, U.S. Public Health Service, # HS00029-07; Bureau of Health Resources Development, Health Resources Administration U.S. Public Health Service # 1BM 24135; and Bureau of Health Resources Development, Health Resources Administration, U.S. Public Health Service # 231-75-0006.

Actual expenses were analyzed through monthly expenditure summaries which included vouchers, travel statements and other documents. Faculty reports of professional activities covering one year and independent observation of faculty activities provided estimates of faculty time spent in program functions.

Costs were allocated into six categories: (1) start-up, (2) teaching, (3) administration, (4) evaluation, (5) deployment and (6) student support.

Start-up costs were defined as all expenditures during the planning year as well as designing and implementing additional or revised courses. Also included were activities to explain the concept of new health practitioners, participation in the development of accreditation of programs which prepare assistants to the primary care physician and certification mechanisms for graduates.

Teaching costs included payments to both full- and part-time faculty for lectures, laboratories, seminars, clinical teaching and career counseling. In general, teachers were paid for providing an extensive series of lectures for an entire course but not for offering single lectures or for occasional supervision of students in clinical settings. No attempt was made to place a monetary value on volunteer faculty.

Administrative and clerical expenses involved in the overall operation of the program, such as grant administration, minority recruitment, application processing and admission of students were placed in this category. The costs of central university administration and services were designated as overhead expenses. No new construction, equipment or personnel were provided by the university. The space devoted exclusively to the Child Health Associate Program was less than 750 square feet, excluding shared class and laboratory space. No depreciation allowance for physical plant was made. However, a depreciation allowance could be determined by multiplying the number of square feet utilized by the program by the cost of construction per square foot and dividing by the estimated life of the building in years.

Evaluation expenditures included the costs of administering, developing, implementing, interpreting and presenting the results of an evaluation program which determined the appropriateness of the curriculum, the clinical competence of students and graduates, and their impact on clinical practice.

Deployment costs included additional transportation and living expenses incurred by students in the third year of the program during clinical training at distant places. In addition, the estimated value of the time expended by the faculty member who supervised these rotations, as well as travel expenses, were included.

Student support referred to scholarship and loan funds obtained by the program and distributed to students directly or through the university's financial aid office. General university loan or scholarship funds, federally insured bank loans and other external sources of support were not included. Students did not receive salaries, but third year students in the first two classes did receive a small stipend.

METHODOLOGY

Four methods were used to determine the most appropriate means of estimating the costs of training these new health professionals:

Method 1—The first method estimated the cost per month and year of educating all the enrolled students (see Table 26:1). Ninety-two students comprised this group including six students who registered with their entering class but subsequently left the program without graduating, and a class of eighteen students who started the program one week prior to the end of the study period. Start-up costs were amortized over ten years—the time of the program could continue in operation if funds from all sources were terminated at the end of the present funding cycle.*

Method 2—The second approach analyzed the cost per month and year of educating all students who had graduated or who had been in the program long enough that they could be expected to graduate (see Table 26:2). The eighteen students who enrolled in the program one week before the end of the study period were not included in this group, because only a very small fraction of the funds required to train them had been spent during the seven-year study period. As with Method 1, start-up costs were amortized over a ten-year period.

Method 3—The third approach analyzed the cost per month and per year of training all students who had graduated and the full-time equivalent number of students who were currently enrolled and expected to graduate (see Table 26:3). In other words, a student who had completed one year was considered to be one-third of a student, since one-third of the cost of educating the student was expended during the study period. The number of graduate and full-time equivalent students used in this calculation was 61. As with Methods 1 and 2, start-up costs were amortized over a ten-year period.

---

*The Child Health Associate Program is now an integral part of the School of Medicine's budget so continued funding is assured.

Method 4—The fourth approach was to calculate the cost per month and per year of educating each student who actually graduated through June 1975 (see Table 26:4). The total number of students in this group was 47. The costs of developing and implementing the program were amortized over the seven-year study period.

The first two methods understate the costs of training because the monies required to complete the education of students enrolled but not yet graduated by June 1975 are not included. This understatement of costs could be corrected by using the number of full-time equivalent students instead of the actual numbers of students enrolled in the program as shown in Table 26:3. The third method best represents the costs of training Child Health Associates. And the fourth method overestimates the costs of training Child Health Associates because the university legally would be required to continue the program at its own expense until all matriculated students had graduated.

TABLE 26:1

Method 1
Cost of Educating Child Health Associates/Total Number of Students
Enrolled/Month/Year of Training

N = 92

Basic Education Costs

	Per Month	Per Year
Teaching	$212	$2,552
Program administration	44	535
Total Basic Education Costs	$256	$3,087

Other Costs

	Per Month	Per Year
Start-up[1]	$ 48	$ 583
Evaluation	105	1,267
Student support	40	489
Deployment	17	213
Subtotal Other Costs	210	2,552
Overhead	105	1,263
Total other costs	$315	$3,815

[1]Start-up costs were amortized over ten years.

TABLE 26:2

Method 2
Costs of Educating Child Health Associates/Expected Graduate/Month/Year of Training

N = 74

Basic Education Costs

	Per Month	Per Year
Teaching	$264	$3,172
Program administration	55	665
Total basic education costs	$319	$3,837

Other Costs

	Per Month	Per Year
Start-up[1]	$ 60	$ 725
Evaluation	131	1,575
Student support	50	607
Deployment	22	264
Subtotal other costs	263	3,171
Overhead	130	1,567
Total other costs	$393	$4,738

[1]Start-up costs were amortized over ten years.

RESULTS AND DISCUSSION

The basic teaching costs of the Child Health Associate program, which did not include start-up, evaluation, student support, deployment or overhead expenses, ranged from $3,087 to $3,837, $4,655 and $6,042 in Methods 1-4, respectively, per student per year of training. Similarly, evaluation costs ranged from $1,267 per student in Method 1 to $1,575, $1,911 and $2,480 for students in Methods 2, 3 and 4 respectively. Specific training costs are perhaps matched in importance by the methods used to derive the figures. Before the start-up and operational costs can be fairly evaluated for programs for physician's assistants and nurse practitioners, there must be some common agreement about the specific costs which should or should not be included.

Costs Based on Expenditures Versus Income

Costs of training might be studied by reviewing income and anticipated budgets or, as in this study, by evaluating expenditures. Expenditures

TABLE 26:3

Method 3
Costs of Educating Child Health Associates/Graduate and Full-Time Equivalent
Student/Year of Training[1]

N = 61

Basic Education Costs

	Per Month	Per Year
Teaching	$320	$3,848
Program administration	67	807
Total basic education costs	$387	$4,655

Other Costs

	Per Month	Per Year
Start-up[2]	$ 73	$ 879
Evaluation	159	1,911
Student support	61	737
Deployment	26	321
Subtotal other costs	319	3,848
Overhead	205	2,470
Total other costs	$524	$6,318

[1]This table includes only those students who graduated by June 30, 1975.
[2]Start-up costs were amortized over ten years.

were used here because they more accurately reflected the costs of preparing students in the program and the number of variables taken into consideration made an income approach seem less accurate. For example, that portion of income derived from tuition is usually of no direct benefit to the program. Also, some programs are located in medical schools and may receive capitation funds while other programs in schools of allied health or independent colleges do not. Capitation or tuition funds actually spent by the program should be considered part of costs. If the program, however, does not expend this money, the money should probably be listed as a financial credit to the program rather than be considered a training cost. In the present illustration, tuition and capitation funds received by the university, but not directly available to the program, amounted to as much as $75,000 per year. These monies were not reflected in the budget nor credited to the program, but should be taken into account in any final determination of the cost of educating Child Health Associates.

TABLE 26:4

Method 4
Costs of Educating Child Health Associates/Graduate/Year of Training

N = 47

Basic Education Costs

	Per Month	Per Year
Teaching	$416	$4,995
Program administration	87	1,047
Total basic education costs	$503	$6,042

Other Costs

	Per Month	Per Year
Start-up[2]	$ 95	$1,142
Evaluation	206	2,480
Student support	79	957
Deployment	34	416
Subtotal other costs	414	4,995
Overhead	205	2,470
Total other costs	$619	$7,465

[1]This table includes only those students who graduated by June 30, 1975.
[2]Start-up costs were amortized over seven years.

Projected Budgets

There are problems with using projected budgets. Generally, these budgets are prepared one to five years in advance of the time that expenditures are actually made, and changes such as transfers from one expense category to another are frequently necessary. Yet, in the case of federal grants, monies are usually made available on an annual basis. Unexpended funds, due to delay in starting the program or overestimated expenses, are subtracted from the funding for the following year, which results in an overestimate of funds available for the educational program. Federally mandated budget cuts are frequently necessary and cannot be forecast in the original budget estimates. Private foundation grants, on the other hand, are sometimes paid in advance and, if invested, may provide additional income in the form of interest to the program or institution. In the Child Health Associate Program, interest earned on the monies paid in advance to the program were not credited to its account, but would also have been a reasonable inclusion for determining institutional training costs. In addition, smaller foundation grants received after the budgets were constructed were not reflected in the original budget. Accounts usually do not reflect educational costs shared by two or more training programs which would have to be paid if cooperation among the programs were not possible.

Overhead

The overhead percentage allowed for administration of a grant and centrally administered university services varies greatly with the source of funds, whether federal and state, foundation and institutional, tuition and fees. The audited institutional overhead costs allowed for research grants at the University of Colorado during the period under study were 34.5 percent of salaries. In some institutions, the federally permitted overhead is as high as 147 percent. Federal training grants, however, allow only 8 percent of salaries, and private foundations commonly allow 15 percent of the total grant for overhead costs; and neither is adequate to pay the actual costs involved in providing the necessary centrally administered university services.

Historic Costs

Historic costs, as defined here, are the costs of training a specified number of students in a given period of time. This common approach to cost accounting is useful for comparison purposes in well established, relatively stabilized programs. Both the Association of American Medical Colleges and the Institute of Medicine have recommended that costs of educating medical students be computed for a given year and cited as the cost per graduate per year. A drawback to using historic costs is that they underestimate the current cost of training because they are not corrected for inflation.

Replication Costs

Replication costs—the costs of duplicating a program in another setting or at the same institution in a different period of time—might also be considered. These figures are corrected for inflation but tend to be overestimates, since relatively fewer developmental and evaluation expenses are necessary if the replicated program is similar in length and type to the prototype. For example, the historic cost of training the first PNPs in a four-month program was approximately $4,000/student. The cost of duplicating this program today, corrected for inflation, would be at least $7,000/student. An alternative approach to determining replication costs is to ascertain the types of instructors, materials and services needed to reproduce a program and to calculate these costs for a specific geographic location at a given time. The result would be a more accurate estimate of the costs for a given institution, reducing the problems introduced by varying costs in different parts of the country.

Marginal Costs

An economist might also consider the concept of marginal costs which indicates how much additional money would be needed to train one extra student if X number of students can be educated for a given sum. Within the constraints of available physicial facilities and other resources, it is possible to determine the optimum class size for which the cost of training per student is minimized.

Promotional Costs

Since the Child Health Associate Program was the first of its kind, considerable effort was expended to explain the program to medical professionals and the lay public; advising and participating in organizations and regulatory bodies which were developing certification and accreditation mechanisms, regulations and laws; and in developing and implementing an innovative curriculum. Part of these expenses would not be necessary to replicate the Child Health Associate Program or to start a similar new health practitioner program today.

Cost of Prerequisites

The teaching costs cited do not include the cost of taking prerequisite courses for admission. For example, most physician's assistant programs require at least two years of college and up to two years of previous medically related experience prior to admission. The cost of the prerequisite courses varies depending on whether the courses are taken in a private versus a public institution; so that an average estimate is difficult to derive. For example, many nurse practitioner programs require a baccalaureate degree and, frequently, additional nursing experience prior to entrance. According to the Institute of Medicine's study of nursing education, the average institutional educational cost in 1972 of obtaining a baccalaureate degree was $2,500/student/year or $10,000 for a four-year program. Corrected for inflation, the 1976 cost of obtaining such a degree is approximately $13,000.

If nurse practitioner programs accept students with less extensive nursing education, the relative cost of meeting prerequisites undoubtedly decreases. Although difficult to estimate, the cost of prerequisites which duplicate courses included in new health practitioner curricula are an important cost of training new health professionals. These basic biological, physical and social science courses are seldom noted in the expenses of continuing education curricula for nurse practitioners, but are, nonetheless, an integral part of their training. On the other hand, the costs of teaching research methodology and administrative skills are likely to appear in the budgets of master's level nurse practitioner programs but not in other program budgets.

Teaching Costs

Since the type of faculty chosen will determine the salaries paid and the ancillary staff required, the number and types of teachers hired can be the largest cost factor in the students' education. Salary ranges also vary significantly if faculty are permitted supplemental employment as compared with those of faculty rank who are not permitted major sources of outside income. In the example cited, The Child Health Associate Program utilizes physicians and other health professionals who receive a full-time salary. Since the program's courses are structured to use small-group teaching situations, the number of faculty required is larger than if only the lecture method were used. Programs which pay preceptors, rather than relying on volunteers, also have significantly increased salary expenses. If costs among programs are to be compared equitably, the cost of preceptors should be deleted from comparison budgets, or the value of volunteered faculty time should be determined. Programs relying more on nurses or physician's assistants as teachers have lower salary expenses.

The estimation of faculty teaching time, research and administration is dependent largely on the accuracy of their activity reports which are not completely verifiable by independent observation. With a large enough sample of faculty, errors in estimating activity should be random; respondents are understandably reluctant, however, to report their activities in a manner inconsistent with their source of financial support. Because of the small number of faculty in the Child Health Associate Program and the amount of distortion which would have occurred if a typical week were chosen for a work sampling study, an estimate of faculty activities over a year was likely to be more accurate.

Allocating time spent in specific teaching and patient care tasks is extremely complex when instructors teach medical students at the same time they provide patient care. However, determination of the number of hours spent in each activity is less important with full-time Child Health Associate faculty than with undergraduate medical education faculty, because the former do not have primary patient care reponsibilities while they also teach Child Health Associate students. One would expect more shared research, teaching and service tasks in the preparation of academic teachers and medical specialists than in the supervision of primary care providers. Part-time faculty who supervise specialty clinics attended by Child Health Associate students commonly provide patient care as they teach, but the salaries paid by the program for this service constitute a relatively small percentage of the total salaries paid. Nursing school faculty are not usually responsible for patient care at the same time they teach nurse practitioner students.

Evaluation Costs

Because the Child Health Associate Program has undertaken extensive evaluation, those costs have been estimated separately. It is inappropriate to compare total educational costs of new health professional programs with major evaluation components with those having little or no funding available for this purpose. It is also inappropriate to compare evaluation costs of new programs that must document their effectiveness with more established programs. Many medical schools have little funding available for the critical evaluation of medical education.

Scholarships and Loans

Some new health professional programs have also been successful in obtaining stipends, scholarships or loans for their students while others have not. To facilitate comparison among programs, this category of funds should be itemized separately.

SUMMARY

Four methods of computing costs of training have been utilized to determine which method best describes the costs of educating Child Health Associates. Method 1 which calculates the educational costs for each student enrolled in the program without deducting the students who will not graduate, understates the cost of training ($3,087). In the Child Health Associate Program, there was a dropout rate of 8.5 percent; other programs may have higher or lower dropout rates which must be taken into consideration. In addition to those students who left the program without graduating, a class of 18 students entered the program in June 1975, one week before the end of the study period. In the second method, the class which enrolled in June 1975 was omitted, but the class entering the program in June 1974 was included because all of the students passed the first year and were expected to graduate. Including these students in the calculations lowered the estimated educational cost/student ($3,837) to some extent. The third method corrected for the underestimation of costs in the second method ($4,655).

The fourth method of analysis estimates the education costs/graduate/year of training ($6,042) as recommended by the AAMC study of undergraduate medical education.[9] This approach is appropriate for long-established programs with relatively stable numbers of students, but inappropriate for new health professional programs with high start-up costs, rapidly increasing numbers of students and insufficient time to graduate significant numbers. In the Child Health Associate Program, the class size has doubled and 47 students have graduated since the program began. Because of rapidly occurring changes, the identification of a given target year for analysis may greatly distort the findings. The cost/graduate approach overestimates the cost of education because it compresses the start-up costs over an unduly short period of time and does not allow credit for expenses related to students who have not yet graduated from the program. In the case of the Child Health Associate Program, the cost/graduate method of computation yields a significantly higher figure than do more representative methods.

With these limitations in mind, the most representative approach appears to be to figure the cost of training those students who have graduated and the full-time equivalent number of students who are currently enrolled and expected to graduate.

Pitfalls in the comparison of education costs in different programs have been described here and explicit definitions and assumptions drawn to determine the cost of educating Child Health Associates. It should be possible for another program, using similar guidelines, to compute its own costs. This information would be useful for establishing present costs, as well as monitoring changes in costs among programs that result from changes in types of students accepted, alterations in the curriculum, length of time the program has been in existence, and variations in evaluation and procedures for deploying students.

RECOMMENDATIONS

If access to health care is a right, the provision of that care, including the training of health professionals, must be considered a national goal. The costs of reaching this goal should be shared by those who benefit— the federal and regional governments, students and the public. Substantial continued federal support will be necessary until local or regional governments can bear a larger part of the cost of training new health practitioners.

The costs of preparing these professionals reflect varied educational objectives, programs and techniques used to train students of differing backgrounds and interests. Costs will also vary with the type and nature of the institution, its geographic location, number and types of teachers utilized, efficiency of program management, and the expected role and deployment of graduates. It should be clear, therefore, that there is no such thing as an average cost of educating any one or all types of new health practitioners. The costs of no one program should be considered typical; rather, a range of acceptable costs should be identified to leave sufficient flexibility for programs which test innovative ideas, aim at disadvantaged student populations and stress deployment to areas of need. Programs whose costs are higher than usual could then be identified and studied further to determine whether the program's specific characteristics justify their increased expenses.

Extreme caution should be used in comparing the costs of training physician's assistants with nurse practitioners and nurse clinicians, since it has not been demonstrated conclusively that graduates of these programs have similar knowledge, skills or functions. However, since comparisons of the costs of training various types of new health professionals will undoubtedly be used in an attempt to make appropriate policy decisions, it is essential that uniform standards for evaluating costs be established with the cooperation of the federal government, program directors, economists and other health policy planners. These guidelines can then be adapted to the specific accounting systems used by all programs, thereby permitting a more rational approach to cost accounting. The following guidelines are suggested:

- Historic costs may be used as the basic cost determinant, but marginal costs should also be estimated.
- Expenditures from all sources of funds, rather than income or anticipated budgets, should be used to calculate costs.
- Appropriate categories of expense should be determined and applied in a uniform manner. Possible categories might include start-up, teaching, administration, evaluation, deployment and student support.
- Overhead should be eliminated from the calculations because it varies greatly from institution to institution and may include overhead from federal research and training as well as private foundation grants.

- An attempt should be made to estimate contributed or shared costs. Conversely, in comparison studies, the amounts paid to preceptors and sporadic lecturers should be deleted to avoid inappropriate comparisons.
- Uniform methods of physical plant depreciation should be adopted.
- Programs which are located in independent colleges, medical schools and health science centers should probably be considered separately from one another since the resources upon which they can draw are significantly different.
- Tuition and other fees paid by students and capitation monies should be estimated separately, depending on whether or not the program directly benefited from them.
- Until the size of program has stabilized, the cost per student graduated plus the full-time equivalent number of students expected to graduate probably is the most meaningful determination.
- Total costs of training should be determined per unit of time: per student per month or per student per year.

It must be emphasized that determining the cost of training is not the same as evaluating the graduates' cost-effectiveness or the quality of training. Neither lower nor higher costs necessarily indicate a better program. Continued studies of quality of care provided by new health practitioners, patient outcomes and the impact of these professionals on practice settings are needed to evaluate their cost-effectiveness.

Notes

1. "Undergraduate Medical Education: Elements, Objectives, Costs," *J. Med. Educ.,* 49(1974), 103-26; "Financing Undergraduate Medical Education: A Report by the Committee on the Financing of Medical Education of the Association of American Medical Colleges. Supplement," *J. Med. Educ.,* 49 (1974), 1091-1112; and J. E. Koehler and R. L. Slighton, "Activity Analysis and Cost Analysis in Medical Schools," *J. Med. Educ.,* 48 (1973), 531-50.

2. Institute of Medicine, National Academy of Sciences, *Costs of Education in the Health Professions,* Parts I, II, III Washington, D.C. (1974). (Dist. by National Technical Information Services, PB-238-329)

3. Personal communication, H. K. Silver.

4. A. Yankauer, S. Tripp, P. Andrews, and J. P. Connelly, "The Costs of Training and the Income Generation Potential of Pediatric Nurse Practitioners," *Pediatrics,* 49 (1972), 878-87.

5. L. Kahn, "Washington University Pediatric Nurse Practitioner Training Program: Development and Experience," *Missouri Medicine,* 70 (1973), 658-63.

6. Personal communication, L. Kahn.

7. K. Andreoli, *"Costs of Training Physician's Assistants"* Paper presented at the Association of Physician Assistant Programs. (November 1974).

8. System Sciences, Inc., Physician Extender Training and Deployment Study, 1976. (Contract HRA 230-75-0198, HRA, DHEW.)

9. See "Undergraduate Medical Education," Ibid., and "Financing Undergraduate Medical Education," Ibid.

Part V

Issues and Conclusions: The Next to Last Word?

Ann A. Bliss and Eva D. Cohen

The rapid development of the New Health Practitioner movement is largely due to two current crises in American health care: poor accessibility and rising costs. Paradoxically, while increasing resources have been devoted to health care in the past decade, the availability of care to many has declined despite massive allocations of money and manpower. American medicine leads the world in research and development of specialized diagnostic and therapeutic techniques. But it lags behind in actually delivering health care, particularly primary care to those who need it most, the elderly, minorities, the poor, and geographic locations which have no physicians. Even in areas of high physician density, access to primary care is often difficult. Nor does the solution to providing more care lie in simply producing more doctors. Rather, by delegating routine medical care to NHPs, physicians can concentrate their abilities on more serious and complex illnesses, and can extend their services to a much larger group of patients. Economist Rashi Fein has estimated that a 3% increase in physician productivity would provide as much additional care as an entire year's class of medical students.[1] How are NHPs living up to their potential to extend the physician's care?

The first ten years of NPs and PAs have provided sufficient data to sharpen the issues and questions which have arisen as a consequence of this new health manpower phenomenon. Information is available as to the numbers trained, their distribution, performance, certification, quality of care, cost, and legal sanctions.

How Many NHPs are Enough?

NPs and PAs are but two health manpower solutions to the problem of access to medical care. That physicians have been considered the other major solution is reflected in both the increased number of medical schools and growing enrollment of medical students.

In 1967, the first PAs and pediatric nurse practitioners were being graduated. A few new medical schools laboriously and expensively were being established. Increased medical school enrollment had hardly begun. Now, ten years later, the aggregate growth of these three health provider groups over the last decade is significant.

	10 year total since 1967
1,500 nurse practitioners are being prepared every year from over 85 certificate and 50 master's degree programs	7,000
1,000 PAs are being graduated every year from 56 formal programs	5,000
13,000 medical students are graduating yearly from 115 schools[2] (with at least a dozen more schools planned)	110,000
	122,000

In 1967 there were 247,000 MDs providing patient care in the United States. The above tally shows that in a mere ten years an additional 122,000 health workers have been prepared (10 percent of whom are NPs and PAs) for an overall increase of 50 percent in the absolute numbers of medical care providers. This is encouraging to those attempting to increase access to health care by swelling the ranks of providers. However, it can also be alarming when one asks, how many medical care givers are enough? How many does this country need, or can it support? If the presently planned increases in medical schools and students are projected to the year 2,000 there will be a ratio of one physician to every 250 population. This is sufficiently alarming that the Carnegie Council on Policy Studies in Higher Education has recommended that no additional medical schools be built in this country and that of the 13 planned medical schools, only the one in Delaware is actually needed.

Who Should Provide Needed Medical Services and Where?

The issue of sufficient health care immediately moves beyond numbers to more complex considerations of specialty and geographic distribution. The attraction of physicians to specialty practice appears to be holding its own. A growing number of medical school graduates are choosing primary care practices in internal medicine, pediatrics, obstetrics, gynecology, and family medicine. However, the uneven geographic distribution of physicians in urban-suburban areas rather than rural communities remains the pattern. Nearly 85 percent of physicians still practice in urban-suburban rather than rural settings.[3]

The reasons for this vary and include: dispersion of rural patient populations over hundreds of miles of terrain often difficult to travel, the inability of small communities to support a physician, the professional isolation and long hours of rural medical practice, and the socio-cultural preference of the MD's spouse and family for urban-suburban living. Unfortunately, the geographic maldistribution of physicians continues to influence the practice location of nurse practitioners and PAs. To the extent that NHPs remain tied to MDs as their employers, supervisors, and sole source of reimbursement, NHPs risk being maldistributed in the same pattern as MDs, thereby not being able to make their impact in medically underserved areas. This observation is neither new nor profound but disturbingly true despite repeated cautions which have appeared in the literature since 1972.

> Immediately upon graduation, the physician's assistant is in considerable danger of being swallowed whole by the whale that is our present entrepreneurial, subspecialty medical practice system. The likely cooption of the newly minted physician's assistant by subspecialty medicine is one of the most serious issues confronting the PA.

> Although the greatest needs for improved care are in the areas of primary, preventive, and emergency medicine, the PA graduate will be tempted to move into specialty areas. The temptation is largely financial .... The problem is compounded by the fact that the PA's professional role is directly linked to physicians, who are not only poorly distributed, but have paid scant attention to primary and emergency care.[4]

Recommended were multimedia communication links, problem oriented medical record for self assessment as an important reinforcement for PAs working in isolated areas, support of demonstration projects utilizing various economic mechanisms to encourage the location of physician's assistants in areas of medical shortage and the support of demonstration projects that locate health teams in areas of need:

> Maldistribution of services is one of the major problems in health care delivery today. If the physician's assistant movement fails to address itself to maldistribution, its impact will be significantly lessened. In the light of the current financing mechanisms

for health care, we believe there will be strong incentives for graduates of physician's assistant programs (even in primary care) to practice in fields and locations where the remuneration is greatest, namely specialties in suburban and urban centers. A variety of economic incentives could be developed to ameliorate this situation.[5]

In a National Science Foundation study of 1974,

[The] review provided no clear pattern with respect to the location of NHPs or their impact on increasing access to care in areas of manpower shortages. . . . An important policy issue is whether NHPs should be considered a response to physician shortages in specific areas. This issue must be considered within a larger context of the success with which regulations or incentives are able to establish a more equitable distribution of physicians, by specialization and by geographic areas.

Under current practice acts, NHPs must be supervised by physicians. Their impact on increasing access to care in underserved areas is therefore closely tied to the distribution of physicians.[6]

A recommendation contained in that study's Executive Summary Study was that,

Research should examine the relationship between admission of program applicants from underserved areas and their subsequent location and tenure in such areas on graduation.[7]

Yet, in the ten years that nurse practitioners and PAs have been prepared, it is possible to discern trends toward:

- NPs to find employment in HMOs, public health departments, and private physician practices rather than in hospitals.
- PAs to work in hospitals and specialties such as surgery, orthopedics, urology, and emergency care.

However, neither NPs nor PAs appear to be seeking rural practice in significant numbers except in the instance of a few training efforts linked to distribution such as MEDEX; PRIMEX; University of California-Davis Family Nurse Practitioner Program; and Stanford Primary Care Associate Program. It is unfortunate indeed that the original incentive funding for training programs such as PRIMEX and MEDEX tied to distribution has been discontinued in favor of programs without distribution plans. Those interested in the long term survival of either or both NPs and PAs should reexamine their training programs with an eye to making them more responsive to distribution needs.

Are NHPs Bringing About Any Cost Control in Health Care?

When one looks at the cost of health care, trends to federal spending and regulation are apparent. In response to growing inflation and increased demands for relief of the financial burden of health care on consumers, federal funds for training and services have increased to the point that nearly half of health care expenditures are made up of federal dollars. In 1975 alone, public spending for hospital costs and physician fees increased 22 percent compared to a 12 percent increase in 1974.[8]

Accompanying the government's expenditures for health care is strong federal regulation which threatens the free enterprise marketplace of medical care. Problems of controlling hospital costs and physicians' fees have become high priorities. Even greater federal regulation seems inevitable and NHPs are likely to figure prominently as a possible means for controlling costs. NHPs may be especially cost-effective for providing primary care at primary care prices rather than, as is too often the case, primary care being given by specialists at specialists' prices. Federal regulation may yet attempt to determine what services have to be provided, who should provide them and how much they should cost.

What is the Status of the Controversy Between Organized Medicine and Nursing with Regard to NHPs?

The major professional health organizations have been involved on many levels in the evolution of the NHP concept: in the credentialling process, in influencing the scope of legislation, and foremost in accrediting training programs. Endorsement of the NHP concept is sometimes made with encouraging lack of professional jealousy over turf. Indeed, many of the established nursing and medical professional associations have issued statements and guidelines in support of task delegation.

However, a closer look at the medical and nursing organizations which represent NPs and PAs is a study in contrast between diversity and unity. The PAs are as yet, unified under several national organizations, the American Academy of Physicians Assistants (AAPA), the Association of PA Programs (APAP), and the National Commission for Certification of Physician's Assistants (NCCPA). These PA organizations remain closely linked with the American Medical Association (AMA) and the Association of American Medical Colleges (AAMC). So far, so good, but one prospect for PAs which seems certain is the development of specialty groups within AAPA which ultimately will result in subdivisions within the organization. This will be a natural outgrowth of the current increase in specialization among PAs and the forthcoming recertification examinations, which will be specialty oriented.

In contrast, the 7,300 nurse practitioners are without a separate nurse practitioner organization, and are left to rely on the American Nurses Association (ANA). The ANA must represent its 200,000 members and a larger constituency of 850,000 licensed nurses out of the total of 1,400,-000 trained RNs. In consequence, NPs are but a small subgroup of the nursing profession. In addition, NPs suffer further fragmentation by being organized into diverse groups within ANA by specialty—pediatric nurse practitioners, family nurse practitioners, adult nurse practitioners, maternal-infant nurse practitioners, and school nurse practitioners. Some NPs even belong to specialty groups outside the ANA.

For instance, many pediatric nurse practitioners belong to a group called The National Association of Pediatric Nurse Associates and Practitioners (NAP-NAP) which in 1974 broke away from the ANA because it would not approve of conjoint NP certification with the Academy of Pediatrics with which NAP-NAP is closely allied.

Nurse midwives as well have for decades been represented outside the ANA by the American College of Nurse Midwives (ACNM) which is allied with its medical counterpart, the American College of Obstetricians and Gynecologists (ACOG).

Because of the understandable fragmentation among the disparate groups of NPs, they have been slower to achieve the credentialling achieved by PAs. For instance, as yet no entry level certification of NPs is available through the ANA. Over half of NP programs do not offer a degree and are therefore excluded from NLN accreditation. This has necessitated ANA accrediting non-degree continuing education nurse practitioner programs, a process which is just getting underway.

The nurse practitioner movement is beset further with internal philosophical differences. One such dichotomy questions the proper locus of nurse practitioner preparation. Should it remain continuing education, or be moved to the mainstream of nursing education with generalist nurse practitioner preparation taking place at the baccalaureate level and specialist preparation at the master's level?

In addition, NPs experience some resistance from non-NP nurses as well as a new controversy within their own ranks as to the independent versus the collaborative nature of nursing practice. Central to this controversy is the question: Should nurse practitioners practice nursing only, and not pieces of medicine? In the opinion of one group the tools of the physician such as a stethoscope and book of laboratory values should be eschewed. This group maintains that programs which teach physician tasks, use physician tools, and encourage collaborative practice with physicians do not prepare nurses, but are preparing physician's assistants. On the other hand, a few nurse educators who are themselves clinicians advocate strong clinical skills, collaboration with physicians, and open admission to nurse practitioner preparation to a variety of nurses. As one Fellow of the small but prestigious American Academy of Nursing said at the September 1976 Conference on Primary Care held in Kansas City, Missouri, "I believe a nurse should learn to make the best possible assessment of any person for whom she is responsible; however, physician diagnosis involves technical performance and in order to learn this skill it must be practiced under expert supervision again and again. We will misrepresent ourselves to the public if we assume responsibilities for primary care, unable to proficiently carry out the skills that go with the work to be done. Physical diagnosis, rather than a deterrent should be an adjunct to make improved observations, more rational judgements and implement better care of patients." [9]

Given the relative infancy of the NP movement within the much larger and century old profession of nursing it is likely that these questions eventually will be settled. How they become settled may influence for better or worse what is now known as a nurse practitioner.

In 1977, where is the new health practitioner concept going and under what combined auspices does it derive its support?

• A recent Commission report sponsored by the Josiah Macy Foundation addressed itself to the future of medical education and pointed to one alternative of replacing several physician categories with nurse practitioners and physician's assistants. The Commission cited the existing use of nurses in hospital neo-natal and intensive and coronary care units and as the first intervention in an emergency. In addition to recognizing a role for PAs and NPs in primary care, the Commission also submitted that in some hospitals house staff have been replaced with a combination of full-time medical staff and NPs or PAs. The Commission concluded: "and today the PA and NP have firmly established the contributions they can make as health practitioners; every effort should be made to be sure their numbers will increase. Continued success of PA and NP programs will not only have a positive impact on the nation's health care system, but will encourage the development of other practitioners."*

Physicians for the Future: Report of the Macy Commission (New York: Josiah Macy Foundation, 1976). p. 27.

• The legislation which created the National Health Planning and Resources Development Act of 1974 cites as one of ten national health priorities "the training and increased utilization of Physicians' Assistants, especially nurse clinicians." Thus, according to this Act (P.L. 93-641, 93d Congress, January 4, 1975) new health practitioners are viewed as one of the means by which several of the objectives of this act might be achieved: equal access to quality health care at a reasonable cost and the substitution of ambulatory and intermediate care for inpatient hospital care.

• The Nurse Training Act of 1975 (P.L. 94-63) authorizes funding for schools of nursing, medicine and public health as well as hospitals and other institutions to plan, develop, expand or maintain existing nurse practitioner training programs.

• The Health Professions Educational Assistance Act of 1976 (P.L. 94-484) authorizes financial support to meet the cost of new and existing PA training programs.

The Josiah Macy Commission recommendations and the recent legislation may have produced nothing new or startling, but they have achieved one purpose—they give their blessing and backing to a progressive concept of physician substitutability that continues to need support. While the federal government has funded NHP training programs, and can be expected to continue to do so, the extent to which the original intent of the legislation has been met will need to be documented further.

• In 1974 a study was undertaken by the General Accounting Office to determine whether the objectives and congressional expectations of the support for NHP programs were being achieved. This study was undertaken through a GAO review of 19 physician extender programs in 13 states. This report recommended that:

(1) To ensure that physician extenders are trained in the most efficient and economical manner, are granted appropriate and essential professional and legal recognition, and their employers reimbursed equitably for services provided by the extenders, the Secretary of HEW should:

— Study various physician extender programs to determine the best way to train qualified extenders.

— Work with the States to develop legislation clearly defining the role of extenders and providing the necessary framework for them to carry out duties for which they have been trained.

— Work closely with professional organizations and state licensure boards to determine the most appropriate manner of granting official recognition to extenders.

—Conduct expeditiously the study mandated by the Social Security Amendments of 1972 to determine the most appropriate and equitable level of reimbursement for extenders and use the study results as they become available to resolve problems surrounding reimbursement for services provided by extenders under the Social Security Act.

(2) To ensure that physician extender training programs help alleviate the nation's health manpower maldistribution problems and provide the mobility to locate in health manpower shortage areas, the Secretary of HEW should:

—Require as a condition of federal financial support that extender training programs include a method to place graduates in areas where health manpower is scarce.

—Work closely with the States to develop criteria specifying training and experience qualifications acceptable to all states.

• HEW response to the GAO study was to suggest that programs continue to be allowed to vary rather than be standardized in the absence of consensus on the optimal preparation of a physician extender. At the same time HEW supported efforts to determine whether the final product is reasonably standard and whether graduates are prepared with the flexibility to carry out the varied functions and responsibilities agreed to be essential for full performance.

• Among the recommendations of the GAO study were that comparisons be made of the costs of training different types of new health practitioners. In response to the GAO mandate, HEW contracted with System Sciences, Inc. to develop descriptive and comparative data concerning the selection, training and deployment of NPs and PAs. The methodology used existing information from grant and contract files at federal and regional HEW offices, data provided from the training programs and in-depth interviews with the program directors concerning curriculum, clinical skills, program orientation and faculty characteristics. Income and expenditure data were collected from the different training programs and the data on deployment were to be extracted from two other separate studies. This study was to be a descriptive evaluation of the content of training program objectives, education processes, student recruitment and selection, number of graduates, cost and deployment. The major focus was the content and cost of the educational program rather than evaluation of the product of the programs in terms of their performance in subsequent practice. The System Sciences study's final report, *Nurse Practitioner and Physician Assistant Training and*

*Deployment Study** provides a wealth of comparative data on NP and PA programs. The study reports that:

— Program goals and objectives differ, with PA programs oriented toward developing physician support personnel and NP programs oriented toward lesser dependence on physician support.
— NP programs place more emphasis on counseling patients than do PA and MEDEX programs.
— With regard to skills taught in the programs, there are more similarities than differences.
— A higher proportion of NPs work in metropolitan areas than do PAs and Medex.
— Annual median salaries range from $13,500 for a certificate program NP, $14,200 for a Medex, $14,800 for a PA, to $14,900 for a master's degree NP.
— Median unit educational cost per graduate ranged from a low of $5,700 for (adult) certificate NP program graduates to $14,300 per NP master's degree graduate and $15,100 per PA graduate.

Among the recommendations were to (1) standardize reporting requirements for training programs in order to compare them, (2) support research on the demand for NPs and PAs, and (3) examine their clinical impact, quality of care and cost-effectiveness.

Progress is being made toward fulfilling several of the additional recommendations made in the GAO study. Most states by the end of 1976 had passed some form of legislation enabling physician's assistants to practice under medical supervision and expanding the role of the nurse, although legislation in some states still may be too restrictive to permit efficient use of new health practitioners. Certification programs have been initiated as described in previous chapters. The Social Security Administration Physician Extender Reimbursement Study is well underway and is expected to provide data for more informed decision making vis-a-vis federal reimbursement.

A national commitment to substitution of NP and PA services for physician care which could be evidenced through the reimbursement policies recognizing their contribution, is lacking and constitutes the major impediment to fully use these health practitioners.

A reimbursement formula has recently been developed by the American Academy of Physician's Assistants in consultation with members of

---

*Available from the National Technical Information Service, U.S. Dept. of Commerce, Springfield, Virginia, 22161. Publ. No. PB-259 026.

the Senate Finance Committee Staff. The formula would take into account the percentage of Medicare patients seen in the practice, the proportion of Medicare patients seen by PE, costs of physician's supervisory time, and overhead. The final cost was computed so as not to exceed two times the physician extender annual salary.

Other determinants to NHP practice raise issues which remain in need of resolution.

• Hospitals, which increasingly are asked to grant privileges to NHPs employed by private practitioners who have such privileges, need to develop eligibility criteria for staff privileges and carefully specify the functions the NHPs will be allowed to carry out in the hospital under the employing physician's supervision. Ambulatory care clinics and physicians in private practice need to determine whether the NHP merely should triage to determine the severity of a problem, or to diagnose and treat as well. All institutions need to develop policies for the referral of patients to other appropriate providers, be they physician's assistants, nurse practitioners or physicians.

• Minority members still are not entering the NHP professions, despite affirmative action provisions. More aggressive recruiting and student financial aid may make primary care an attractive career for minorities.

Little has been said, as yet, about the consumer's preference for health practitioner. The consumer wants access to care, twenty-four hours per day, seven days per week, and assurance that practitioners at any level have the appropriate skills to deal with their problems and the wisdom to refer those problems outside of their competence to others with the requisite skills. It could be argued that consumers decide through legislation whether or not they wish to receive medical care from NHPs. However, the consumer probably has limited knowledge of the education of NHPs and their capabilities. Training programs, employers of NHPs and the NP and PA professional organizations need to continue to use a variety of media approaches to inform the public about the ability of NHPs to provide preventive, acute and restorative care.

Notes

1. Rashi Fein, "An Economist's View: Medical Manpower—A Continuing Crisis," *JAMA* 201, no. 12 (Sept. 18, 1976): 171-173.
2. W.F. Dube, "Datagram. U.S. Medical School Enrollment, 1969-1970 through 1973-1974," *J. Med. Educ.*, 49 (1974): 302-307. Numbers and estimates of medical school graduates 1975-1977, AAMC, personal communication, January 1977.

3. Charles E. Lewis, Rashi Fein, and David Mechanic, "Table II—Urban and Rural Distribution of Non Federal U.S. Physicians by Major Activity 1967-1972," *A Right to Health: The Problem of Access to Primary Medical Care* (New York: John Wiley and Sons, 1976), p. 103.

4. Alfred M. Sadler, Blair L. Sadler, and Ann A. Bliss. *The Physicians Assistant—Today and Tomorrow.* (New Haven, Conn.: Yale University School of Medicine, 1972), pp. 28-30.

5. Ibid., pp. 144-146.

6. Eva D. Cohen, Linda M. Crootof, Kathleen Keenan, Mieko M. Korper, and Mary Triffin. *An Evaluation of Policy Related Research on New and Expanded Roles of Health Workers,* Prepared for the National Science Foundation Research Applied to National Needs, Office of Regional Activities and Continuing Education, Yale University School of Medicine, October 1974, pp. 121-122.

7. Ibid., Executive Summary, p. 15.

8. HEW Social Security Administration Research and Statistics Note November 21, 1975, DHEW Publication No. (SSA) 75-11701.

9. Elaine McCarty, "Description of Primary Health Care Needs of People," presented to the American Academy of Nursing September 27, 1976, Kansas City, Missouri.

Appendices

Appendix A

Essentials of an Approved Educational Program
for the Assistant to the Primary Care Physician*

Established by

**AMERICAN MEDICAL ASSOCIATION
COUNCIL ON MEDICAL EDUCATION**

in collaboration with

**AMERICAN ACADEMY OF FAMILY PHYSICIANS
AMERICAN ACADEMY OF PEDIATRICS
AMERICAN ACADEMY OF PHYSICIANS' ASSISTANTS **
AMERICAN COLLEGE OF PHYSICIANS
AMERICAN SOCIETY OF INTERNAL MEDICINE**

Adopted by the AMA House of Delegates
December, 1971

OBJECTIVE: The education and health professions cooperate in this program to establish and maintain standards of appropriate quality for educational programs for the assistant to the primary care physician, and to provide recognition for educational programs which meet or exceed the minimal standards outlined in these Essentials.

These standards are to be used as a guide for the development and self-evaluation of programs for the assistant to the primary care physician. Lists of these approved programs are published for the information of employers and the public. Students enrolled in the programs are taught to work with and under the direction of physicians in providing health care services to patients.

●   ●   ●

DESCRIPTION OF THE OCCUPATION: The assistant to the primary care physician is a skilled person, qualified by academic and clinical training to provide patient services under the supervision and responsibility of a doctor of medicine or osteopathy who is, in turn, responsible for the performance of that assistant. The assistant may be involved with the patients of the physician in any medical setting for which the physician is responsible.

The function of the assistant to the primary care physician is to perform, under the responsibility and supervision of the physician, diagnostic and therapeutic tasks in order to allow the physician to extend his services through the more effective use of his knowledge, skills, and abilities.

In rendering services to his patients, the primary care physician is traditionally involved in a variety of activities. Some of these activities, including the application of his knowledge toward a logical and systematic evaluation of the patient's problems and planning a program of management and therapy appropriate to the patient, can only be performed by the physician. The assistant to the primary care physician will not supplant the doctor in the sphere of the decision-making required to establish a diagnosis and plan therapy, but will assist in gathering the data necessary to reach decisions and in implementing the therapeutic plan for the patient.

Intelligence, the ability to relate to people, a capacity for calm and reasoned judgment in meeting emergencies, and an orientation toward service are qualities essential for the assistant to the primary care physician. As a professional, he must maintain respect for the person and privacy of the patient.

The tasks performed by the assistant will include transmission and execution of physician's orders, performance of patient care tasks, and performance of diagnostic and therapeutic procedures as may be delegated by the physician.

Since the function of the primary care physician is interdisciplinary in nature, involving the five major clinical disciplines (medicine, surgery, pediatrics, psychiatry, and obstetrics) within the limitations and capabilities of the particular practice in consideration, the assistant to the primary care physician should be involved in assisting the physician provide those varied medical services necessary for the total health care of the patient.

The ultimate role of the assistant to the primary care physician cannot be rigidly defined because of the variations in practice requirements due to geographic, economic, and sociologic factors. The high degree of responsibility an assistant to the primary care physician may assume requires that, at the conclusion of his formal education, he possess the knowledge, skills, and abilities necessary to provide those services appropriate to the primary care setting. These services would include, but need not be limited to,

---

"Assistant to the Primary Care Physician" is a generic term.
**Approved by Council action, March 15-17, 1974

385

the following:

1) The initial approach to a patient of any age group in any setting to elicit a detailed and accurate history, perform an appropriate physical examination, and record and present pertinent data in a manner meaningful to the physician;
2) Performance and/or assistance in performance of routine laboratory and related studies as appropriate for a specific practice setting, such as the drawing of blood samples, performance of urinalyses, and the taking of electrocardiographic tracings;
3) Performance of such routine therapeutic procedures as injections, immunizations, and the suturing and care of wounds;
4) Instruction and counseling of patients regarding physical and mental health on matters such as diets, disease, therapy, and normal growth and development;

5) Assisting the physician in the hospital setting by making patient rounds, recording patient progress notes, accurately and appropriately transcribing and/or executing standing orders and other specific orders at the direction of the supervising physician, and compiling and recording detailed narrative case summaries;
6) Providing assistance in the delivery of services to patients requiring continuing care (home, nursing home, extended care facilities, etc.) including the review and monitoring of treatment and therapy plans;
7) Independent performance of evaluative and treatment procedures essential to provide an appropriate response to life-threatening, emergency situations; and
8) Facilitation of the physician's referral of appropriate patients by maintenance of an awareness of the community's various health facilities, agencies, and resources.

ESSENTIAL REQUIREMENTS

I. EDUCATIONAL PROGRAMS MAY BE ESTABLISHED IN

A. Medical schools
B. Senior colleges and universities in affiliation with an accredited teaching hospital.
C. Medical educational facilities of the federal government.
D. Other institutions, with clinical facilities, which are acceptable to the Council on Medical Education of the American Medical Association.

The institution should be accredited or otherwise acceptable to the Council on Medical Education. Senior colleges and universities must have the necessary clinical affiliations.

II. CLINICAL AFFILIATIONS

A. The clinical phase of the educational program must be conducted in a clinical setting and under competent clinical direction.
B. In programs where the academic instruction and clinical teaching are not provided in the same institution, accreditation shall be given to the institution responsible for the academic preparation (student selection, curriculum, academic credit, etc.) and the educational administrators shall be responsible for assuring that the activities assigned to students in the clinical setting are, in fact, educational.
C. In the clinical teaching environment, an appropriate ratio of students to physicians shall be maintained.

III. FACILITIES

A. Adequate classrooms, laboratories, and administrative offices should be provided.
B. Appropriate modern equipment and supplies for directed experience should be available in sufficient quantities.

C. A library should be readily accessible and should contain an adequate supply of up-to-date, scientific books, periodicals, and other reference materials related to the curriculum.

IV. FINANCES

A. Financial resources for continued operation of the educational program should be assured for each class of students enrolled.
B. The institution shall not charge excessive student fees.
C. Advertising must be appropriate to an educational institution.
D. The program shall not substitute students for paid personnel to conduct the work of the clinical facility.

V. FACULTY

A. Program Director
  1. The program director should meet the requirements specified by the institution providing the didactic portion of the educational program.
  2. The program director should be responsible for the organization, administration, periodic review, continued development, and general effectiveness of the program.

B. Medical Director
  1. The medical director should provide competent medical direction for the clinical instruction and for clinical relationships with other educational programs. He should have the understanding and support of practicing physicians.
  2. The medical director should be a physician experienced in the delivery of the type of health care services for which the student is being trained.
  3. The medical director may also be the program director.

C. **Change of Director**
If the program director or medical director is changed, immediate notification should be sent to the AMA Department of Allied Medical Professions and Services. The curriculum vitae of the new director, giving details of his training, education, and experience, must be submitted.

D. **Instructional Staff**
1. The faculty must be qualified, through academic preparation and experience, to teach the subjects assigned.
2. The faculty for the clinical portion of the educational program must include physicians who are involved in the provision of patient care services. Because of the unique characteristics of the assistant to the primary care physician, it is necessary that the preponderance of clinical teaching be conducted by practicing physicians.

E. **Advisory Committee**
An Advisory Committee should be appointed to assist the director in continuing program development and evaluation, in faculty coordination of effective clinical relationships. For maximum effectiveness, an Advisory Committee should include representation of the primary institution involved, the program administration, organized medicine, the practicing physician, and others.

VI. STUDENTS

A. **Selection**
1. Selection of students should be made by an admissions · committee in cooperation with those responsible for the educational program. Admissions data should be on file at all times in the institution responsible for the administration of the program.
2. Selection procedures must include an analysis of previous performance and experience and may seek to accommodate candidates with a health related background and give due credit for the knowledge, skills, and abilities they possess.

B. **Health**
Applicants shall be required to submit evidence of good health. When students are learning in a clinical setting or a hospital, the hospital or clinical setting should provide them with the protection of the same physical examinations and immunizations as are provided to hospital employees working in the same clinical setting.

C. **Number**
The number of students enrolled in each class should be commensurate with the most effective learning and teaching practices and should also be consistent with acceptable student-teacher ratios.

D. **Counseling**
A student guidance and placement service should be available.

E. **Student Identification**
Students enrolled in the educational program must be clearly identified to distinquish them from physicians, medical students, and students and personnel for other health occupations.

VII. RECORDS

Satisfactory records should be provided for all work accomplished by the student while enrolled in the program. Annual reports of the operation of the program should be prepared and available for review.

A. **Student**
1. Transcripts of high school and any college credits and other credentials must be on file.
2. Reports of medical examination upon admission and records of any subsequent illness during training should be maintained.
3. Records or class and laboratory participation and academic and clinical achievements of each student should be maintained in accordance with the requirements of the institution.

B. **Curriculum**
1. A synopsis of the current curriculum should be kept on file.
2. This synopsis should include the rotation of assignments, the outline of the instruction supplied, and lists of multi-media instructional aids used to augment the experience of the student.

C. **Activity**
1. A satisfactory record system shall be provided for all student performance.
2. Practical and written examinations should be continually evaluated.

VIII. CURRICULUM

A. The length of the educational programs for the assistant to the primary care physician may vary from program to program. The length of time an individual spends in the training program may vary on the basis of the student's background and in consideration of his previous education, experience, knowledge, skills and abilities, and his ability to perform the tasks, functions and duties implied in the "Description of the Occupation."

B. Instruction, tailored to meet the student's needs, should follow a planned outline including:
1. Assignment of appropriate instructional materials.
2. Classroom presentations, discussions, and demonstrations.
3. Supervised practice discussions.
4. Examinations, tests, and quizzes — both practical and written — for the didactic and clinical portions of the educational program.

C. General courses of topics or study, both didactic and clinical, should include the following:
1. The general courses and topics of study must be achievement oriented and provide the graduates with the necessary knowledge, skills, and

abilities to accurately and reliably perform tasks, functions, and duties implied in the "Description of the Occupation."

2. Instruction should be sufficiently comprehensive so as to provide the graduate with an understanding of mental and physical disease in both the ambulatory and hospitalized patient. Attention should also be given to preventive medicine and public health and to the social and economic aspects of the systems for delivering health and medical services. Instruction should stress the role of the assitant to the primary care physician relative to the health maintenance and medical care of his supervising physician's patients. Throughout, the student should be encouraged to develop those basic intellectual, ethical, and moral attitudes and principles that are essential for his gaining and maintaining the trust of those with whom he works and the support of the community in which he lives.

3. A "model unit of primary medical care," such as the models used in departments of family practice in medical schools and family practice residencies, should be encouraged so that the medical student, the resident, and the assistant to the primary care physician can jointly share the educational experience in an atmosphere that reflects and encourages the actual practice of primary medical care.

4. The curriculum should be broad enough to provide the assistant to the primary care physician with the technical capabilities, behavioral characteristics, and judgment necessary to perform in a professional capacity all of his assignments, and should take into consideration any proficiency and knowledge obtained elsewhere and demonstrated prior to completion of the program.

IX. ADMINISTRATION

A. An official publication, including a description of the program, should be available. It should include information regarding the organization of the program, a brief description of required courses, names and academic rank of faculty, entrance requirements, tuition and fees, and information concerning hospitals and facilities used for training.

B. The evaluation (including survey team visits) of a program of study must be initiated by the express invitation of the chief administrator of the institution or his officially designated representative.

C. The program may withdraw its request for initial approval at any time (even after evaluation) prior to final action. The AMA Council on Medical Educa-

tion and the collaborating organizations may withdraw approval whenever:

1. The educational program is not maintained in accordance with the standards outlined above, or

2. There are no students in the program for two consecutive years.

Approval is withdrawn only after advance notice has been given to the director of the program that such action is contemplated, and the reasons therefore, sufficient to permit timely response and use of the established procedure for appeal and review.

D. **Evaluation**

1. The head of the institution being evaluated is given an opportunity to become acquainted with the factual part of the report prepared by the visiting survey team, and to comment on its accuracy before final action is taken.

2. At the request of the head of the institution, a reevaluation may be made. Adverse decisions may be appealed in writing to the Council on Medical Education of the American Medical Association.

E. **Reports**

An annual report should be made to the AMA Council on Medical Education and the collaborating organizations. A report form is provided and should be completed, signed by the program director, and returned promptly.

F. **Reevaluation**

The American Medical Association and collaborating organizations will periodically reevaluate and provide consultation to educational programs.

X. CHANGES IN ESSENTIALS

Proposed changes in the *Essentials of an Approved Educational Program for the Assistant to the Primary Care Physician* will be considered by a standing committee representing the spectrum of approved programs for the assistant to the primary care physician, the American Academy of Family Physicians, the American Academy of Pediatrics, American Academy of Physicians' Assistants, the American College of Physicians and the American Society of Internal Medicine. Recommended changes will be submitted to these collaborating organizations and the American Medical Association.

XI. APPLICATIONS AND INQUIRIES

Applications for program approval should be directed to:

Department of Allied Medical
Professions and Services
Division of Medical Education
American Medical Association
535 N. Dearborn Street
Chicago, Illinois 60610

Appendix B

Guidelines for Nurse Practitioner Training Programs

Federal support for nurse practitioner training is tied to adherence to the HEW Guidelines for the Nurse Training Act of 1975. Title IX regulations authorize the Secretary of Health, Education and Welfare to award grants to public or nonprofit private schools of nursing, medicine, and public health, public or nonprofit private hospitals, and other public or nonprofit private entities to meet the costs of projects to (1) plan, develop, and operate, (2) significantly expand, or (3) maintain existing programs for the training of nurse practitioners. This Act included certain criteria to be used by HEW in evaluating applications. The following guidelines for nurse practitioner training programs were outlined:

The guidelines set forth below have been prescribed by the Secretary after consultation with appropriate educational organizations and professional nursing and medical organizations, as required by Section 822(a) (2)(B) of the Public Health Service Act.

A. *Definitions.* 1. "Program for the training of nurse practitioners" or "nurse practitioner training program" means an educational program for registered nurses (irrespective of the type of school of nursing in which the nurses received their training) which meets the guidelines prescribed herein and which has as its objective the education of nurses (including pediatric and geriatric nurses) who will, upon completion of their studies in such program, be qualified to effectively provide primary health care, including primary health care in homes and in ambulatory care facilities, long-term care facilities, and other health care institutions.

2. "Nurse practitioner" means a registered nurse who has successfully completed a formal program of study designed to prepare registered nurses to deliver primary health care including the ability to:

a. Assess the health status of individuals and families through health and medical history taking, physical examination, and defining of health and developmental problems;

b. Institute and provide continuity of health care to clients (patients), work with the client to insure understanding of and compliance with the therapeutic regimen within established protocols, and recognize when to refer the client to a physician or other health care provider;

c. Provide instruction and counseling to individuals, families and groups in the areas of health promotion and maintenance, including involving such persons in planning for their health care; and

d. Work in collaboration with other health care providers and agencies to provide, and where appropriate, coordinate services to individuals and families.

3. "Primary health care" means care which may be initiated by the client or provider in a variety of settings and which consists of a broad range of personal health care services including:

a. Promotion and maintenance of health;
b. Prevention of illness and disability;
c. Basic care during acute and chronic phases of illness;
d. Guidance and counseling of individuals and families; and
e. Referral to other health care providers and community resources when appropriate.

In providing such services (i) the physical, emotional, social, and economic status, as well as the cultural and environmental backgrounds of individuals, families, and communities (where applicable) are considered; (ii) the client is provided access to the health care system; and (iii) a single provider or team of providers, along with the client, is responsible for the continuing coordination and management of all aspects of basic health services needed for individual and family care.

B. *Organization and administration.* 1. A nurse practitioner training program shall have active collaboration with nurses and physicians who have expertise relevant to the nurse practitioner role and primary health care, to assist in the planning, development, and operation of such a program. In addition, where the institution or organization conducting the program is other than a school of nursing, medicine, or public health, such collaboration shall be with nurses and physicians who are affiliated with either a collegiate school of nursing, school of medicine, or school of public health.

2. Co-program directors from nursing and medicine are recommended.

C. *Student enrollment.* 1. A nurse practitioner training program shall have an enrollment of not less than eight full-time students in each class.

2. Registered nurses who have received their initial nursing preparation from a school of nursing as defined in section 853 of the Public Health Service Act and who are currently licensed to practice nursing are eligible for enrollment.

3. The policies for the recruitment and selection of students shall be consistent with the requirements of the sponsoring institution and developed in cooperation with the faculty responsible for conducting the training. Admission criteria shall take into consideration the educational background and work experience of applicants.

D. *Length of program.* A nurse practitioner training program shall be a minimum of one academic year (or nine months) in length and shall include at least four months (in the aggregate) of classroom instruction.

E. *Curriculum.* 1. A nurse practitioner training program shall be a discrete program consisting of classroom instruction and faculty-supervised clinical practice designed to teach registered nurses the knowledge and skills needed to perform the functions of a nurse practitioner specified in the definition of that term as set forth in these guidelines. The curriculum shall be developed and implemented cooperatively by nurse educators, physicians, and appropriate representatives of other health disciplines. The following are examples of broad areas of program content which should be included: Communications and interviewing (history taking); basic physical examination including basic pathophysiology; positive health maintenance; care during acute and chronic phases of illness; management of chronic illness; health teaching and counseling; role realignment and establishment of collaborative roles with physicians and other health care providers; and community resources. The program content, both classroom instruction and clinical practice, should be developed so that the nurse practitioner is prepared to provide primary health care as defined in these guidelines.

2. The curriculum may include a preceptorship, in which the student is assigned to a designated preceptor (a nurse practitioner or physician) who is responsible for teaching, supervising, and evaluating the student and for providing the student with an

environment which permits observation and active participation in the delivery of primary health care. If a preceptorship is included, it shall be under the direction and supervision of the faculty.

F. *Faculty qualifications.* A nurse practitioner training program shall have a sufficient number of qualified nursing and medical (and other related professional) faculty with academic preparation and clinical expertise relevant to their areas of teaching responsibility and with demonstrated ability in the development and implementation of educational programs.

G. *Resources.* 1. A nurse practitioner training program shall have available sufficient educational and clinical resources including a variety of practice settings, particularly in ambulatory care.

2. Clinical practice facilities shall be adequate in terms of space and equipment, number of clients, diversity of client age and need for care, number of students enrolled in the program, and other students using the facility for training purposes.

3. Where the institution or organization conducting the program does not provide the clinical practice settings itself, it shall provide for such settings through written agreements with other appropriate institutions or organizations.

4. Where the institution or organization conducting the program is other than a school of nursing, medicine, or public health, it shall provide for sufficient educational expertise through written agreements with a collegiate school of nursing, school of medicine, or school of public health.

FEDERAL REGISTER, VOL. 41, NO. 16—FRIDAY,
JANUARY 23, 1976

In addition, federal requirements include the collection, evaluation and availability of program data for HEW on the number of student applicants and students enrolled, their characteristics and student performance in classroom work and clinical practice. Information will also be requested by HEW on the number of graduates per class, the attrition rate, employment after graduation (including setting and location) and utilization and performance of graduates (including employer assessment).

Appendix C
Criteria for the Appraisal of Baccalaureate and Higher Degree Programs in Nursing*

DEFINITIONS OF TERMS

Criterion. The committees that developed these criteria defined the term *criterion* as meaning a dimension of quality along which there might be gradation and upon which a judgment might be made. They agreed that to be of value, the criteria should be stated clearly and their nature should be such that the school can produce relevant evidence that the criteria are being met. It is the responsibility of the school of nursing to present evidence as to how the criteria are met. It is the responsibility of the Board of Review for Baccalaureate and Higher Degree Programs to apply the criteria judiciously in the appraisal of the educational program(s).

School of Nursing. The term *school of nursing* as used in these criteria means a department, a school, a division, or other administrative unit in a senior college or a university that provides a program or programs of education in professional nursing leading to a baccalaureate or higher degree.

ORGANIZATION AND ADMINISTRATION

I. The school of nursing's statement of philosophy and purposes is consistent with the philosophy and purposes of the parent institution.

II. The school of nursing is organized in accordance with the structural plan of the parent institution with regard to:

A. Relationships with the central administrative authorities.

B. Relationships among educational, administrative, and service units of the institution.

C. Faculty and student representation on central councils and committees of the institution.

---

* Reproduced by permission from "Criteria for the Appraisal of Baccalaureate and Higher Degree Programs in Nursing." New York: National League for Nursing, 1972. Copyright © 1972 by National League for Nursing.

III. The school receives financial support commensurate with the financial resources of the institution and appropriate to the needs of the school.

IV. The personnel policies for faculty members of the school are those in effect for other faculty members in the institution in regard to appointment, responsibilities, academic rank, tenure, salaries, promotion, and recognition of professional competencies.

V. The administrator of the school of nursing, with the participation of the faculty, is responsible for:

A. Faculty appointment and review.

B. The educational program(s).

C. The preparation and administration of the budget.

VI. The school is administered by a nurse educator who holds a doctoral degree.

VII. The administrator of the school of nursing makes provisions for:

A. Facilitation and coordination of student and faculty activities related to organization, curriculum development, personnel policies, evaluation, and budget.

B. Involvement of faculty and students in the improvement of health care and the strengthening of nursing as a profession.

C. An environment conducive to intellectual and creative pursuits.

D. Involvement of community agencies as partners in the educational enterprise.

E. Liaison with the central administration of the institution and with other faculties in the institution.

STUDENTS

I. Qualified applicants are admitted without discrimination in regard to age, creed, ethnic origin, marital status, race, and sex.

II. The general policies in effect for students in nursing are consistent with those policies that are common to all units of the parent institution; policies specific to students in nursing are developed jointly by students and faculty of the school of nursing, provided that the policies are justified in terms of the nature and purposes of the program(s).

III. Accurate and clearly stated information about admission, progression, and graduation requirements is available.

IV. Students' rights and responsibilities are established and available in written form and are implemented through student-faculty-administrative relationships.

 A. Exercise of the liberty to discuss, inquire, and express opinions is encouraged.

 B. Channels for the receipt and consideration of student views and grievances are clearly defined.

 V. Although ultimate responsibility for the development and conduct of the educational program(s) in nursing rests with the faculty, channels are provided for student involvement in:

 A. The development of criteria for admission, progression, and graduation.

 B. Curriculum planning and evaluation.

 C. Evaluation of teaching effectiveness and faculty selection and promotion.

FACULTY

 I. Faculty members are academically and professionally qualified in that they:

 A. Meet the institution's requirements for faculty appointment.

 B. Have graduate preparation relevant to their areas of responsibility and have demonstrated leadership in those areas.

 C. Represent specialty areas in nursing appropriate to the goals of the program.

 D. Continue to improve their expertise in the areas of their responsibility.

 II. The school encourages continued academic study and seeks to increase the number of faculty who hold doctoral or other advanced degrees appropriate to their responsibilities.

III. Faculty carry out the following responsibilities:

 A. The development, implementation, and evaluation of the curriculum.

 B. Participation in academic guidance and counseling.

 C. Participation in academic activities of the total faculty of the institution.

    D. Participation in professional and community activities for the purpose of bringing education, service, and research together for the improvement of health care.

    E. The encouragement of peer and student evaluation of teaching effectiveness.

IV. Faculty rights and responsibilities are established and available in written form and are implemented through student-faculty-administrative relationships.

    A. Exercise of the liberty to discuss, inquire, and express opinions is encouraged.

    B. Channels for the receipt and consideration of faculty views and grievances are clearly defined.

CURRICULUM

I. The following criteria are applicable both to programs that lead to the first professional degree and to those that lead to advanced professional degrees.

    A. The curriculum implements the philosophy, purposes, and objectives of the program(s) and reflects:
        1. The contribution of nursing and other disciplines toward meeting the health needs of society.
        2. The present and the emerging roles of the professional nurse.
        3. Critical thinking and the synthesis of learning.
        4. The need of individuals to develop as contributing members of society.

    B. The objectives of the program(s) interpret the purposes in specific terms. If more than one program is offered, the objectives clearly distinguish between them.

    C. The curriculum plan is based on a conceptual framework(s) consistent with the stated philosophy, purposes, and objectives of the program(s).

    D. There is a rationale for the organization of the nursing major and for the allocation of credit for the nursing courses.

    E. The learning experiences and the methods of instruction are so selected as to fulfill the purposes and objectives of the program(s).

    F. Opportunities for independent study are provided.

G. The learning experiences are sufficiently flexible to permit students to develop in accordance with their individual talents and needs.

H. Opportunities for learning experiences with students and/or practitioners of other health-related disciplines are provided.

I. The liberal education courses are shared with students in other units of the institution and are an integral part of the curriculum.

J. Provisions are made for students to take electives.

K. The curriculum permits entry at appropriate levels and provides for individual differences among students.

L. The curriculum is evaluated systematically by faculty and students in reference to the stated purposes, objectives, and conceptual framework.

M. The process by which curricular change occurs is clearly outlined and provides evidence of ongoing student and faculty involvement.

II. The following criteria are applicable to the curriculum that leads to the *first professional degree.*

A. The curriculum focuses on the theory and practice of nursing and draws on relevant arts and sciences.

B. The liberal and professional education requirements are organized so that knowledges, understandings, and skills are progressively developed throughout the program.

C. The major in nursing is concentrated at the upper-division level.

D. The learning experiences include opportunities for decision-making and the development of independent judgment.

E. The research process and its contribution to nursing practice is emphasized.

F. Both theory and practice provide for the development of leadership skills.

III. The following criteria are applicable to curriculums that lead to *advanced professional degrees.*

A. The courses are built on the curriculum leading to the first professional degree in nursing.

B. The focus of the curriculum is on the theory and practice of nursing.

C. The learning experiences are relevant to the area of specialization and to the student's needs.

D. The learning experiences include the development and testing of nursing theories.

E. Research techniques are used in studying problems and/or participating in research projects.

F. Opportunities are provided to develop increasing competence in solving problems confronting society, especially as they affect the field of health care.

G. Provisions are made for delineation of roles of practice and choice of relevant courses and experiences to prepare for the role selected.

RESOURCES, FACILITIES, AND SERVICES

I. The resources, facilities, and services of the institution are available to and used by the school of nursing.

II. The physical facilities of the institution are adequate to the needs of the program(s). They include:

A. Offices for the administrator, faculty members, and staff.

B. Classrooms, laboratories, and conference rooms.

C. Space as required for research.

D. Comprehensive and up-to-date library resources.

E. Space for equipment and instructional materials.

F. Space for noninstructional activities of faculty and students.

III. Other resources and facilities essential to conducting the program(s) meet the following requirements:

A. The agencies or services are approved by the appropriate accrediting or evaluating bodies if such exist.

B. The facilities and resources for learning experiences include the variety needed for the purposes of the program(s).

C. Secretarial services and other supporting services are sufficient to the needs of the program(s).

D. Instructional materials are adequate.

IV. The faculty conducts periodic evaluation of its resources, facilities, and services.

Appendix D

Summary of Statutory Provisions Governing Legal Scope of Nursing Practice in the Various States

Virginia C. Hall

If Additional Acts Amendment, Criteria and Conditions Stated

State	Type of Definition	Definition Includes Prohibition Against Acts of Diagnosis and Prescription	Rules and Regulations	Professional Opinion	Education and Training	Physician Supervision	If new Definition, based on New York's	Prohibition of Practice of Medicine in Nurse Practice Act	Exception for Nursing in Medical Practice Act
Alabama	Traditional	Yes	—	—	—	—	—	No	No
Alaska	Traditional & Additional Acts Amendment	Yes (Applies to "medical" acts only and additional acts not subject to prohibition)	Yes*	—	—	—	—	No	No
Arizona	Traditional & Additional Acts Amendment[1]	No	Yes*	Yes*	Yes	No	—	No	Yes (Under physician supervision)
Arkansas	Traditional	Yes (Applies to "medical" acts only)	—	—	—	—	—	No	Yes (Also separate exemption for nurse acting under physician supervision)
California	New	No	—	—	—	—	No	No	Yes (For persons lawfully practicing another profession)
Colorado	New & Additional Acts Amendment	No	Yes**	No	Yes	No	Yes	No	Yes (Also separate exemption for persons acting under physician supervision)
Connecticut	New	No	—	—	—	—	Yes	Yes	Yes (Under physician supervision)

If Additional Acts Amendment, Criteria and Conditions Stated

State	Type of Definition	Definition Includes Prohibition Against Acts of Diagnosis and Prescription	Rules and Regulations	Professional Opinion	Education and Training	Physician Supervision	If new Definition, based on New York's	Prohibition of Practice of Medicine in Nurse Practice Act	Exception for Nursing in Medical Practice Act
Delaware	Traditional	Yes	—	—	—	—	—	No	No
District of Columbia	No Definition	—	—	—	—	—	—	No	Yes
Florida	Traditional	No	—	—	—	—	—	No	Yes (Under physician supervision)
Georgia	No Definition	—					—	No	Yes (Also separate exemption for persons acting under physician supervision)
Hawaii	Traditional	Yes (Applies to "medical" acts only)	—	—	—	—	—	No	No (?)[2]
Idaho	Traditional & Additional Acts Amendment	No	Yes (Applies to "medical" acts only and additional acts not subject to prohibition)	No	No	No	—	No	No
Illinois	Traditional	Yes (Applies to "medical" acts only)	—	—	—	—	—	No	Yes (For persons lawfully practicing another profession)
Indiana	New & Additional Acts Amendment	No	Yes***	No	No	No	Yes	No	Yes
Iowa	Traditional	No	—	—	—	—	—	Yes	Yes
Kansas	Traditional	Yes	—	—	—	—	—	No	Yes (Also separate exemption for persons acting under physician supervision)

State	Type of Definition	Definition Includes Prohibition Against Acts of Diagnosis and Prescription	If Additional Acts Amendment, Criteria and Conditions Stated				If new Definition, based on New York's	Prohibition of Practice of Medicine in Nurse Practice Act	Exception for Nursing in Medical Practice Act
			Rules and Regulations	Professional Opinion	Education and Training	Physician Supervision			
Kentucky	Traditional	Yes (Applies to "medical" acts only)	—	—	—	—	—	No	Yes
Louisiana	Traditional	Yes (Applies to "medical" acts only)	—	—	—	—	—	No	No
Maine	Traditional & Additional Acts Amendment	No	No	No	Yes	Yes	—	No	No
Maryland	New & Additional Acts Amendment	No	Yes**	Yes°	Yes	No?(?)	No	No	Yes (For persons lawfully practicing another profession)
Massachusetts	Traditional & Additional Acts Amendment	No	Yes*	Yes°°	Yes	No	—	No	Yes (Applies only to nurses performing "Additional acts")
Michigan	Traditional	Yes (Applies to "medical" acts only)	—	—	—	—	—	No	Yes (For persons lawfully practicing another profession and separate exemption for persons acting under physician supervision)
Minnesota	New	No	—	—	—	—	No	No	Yes (For persons lawfully practicing another profession)

If Additional Acts Amendment, Criteria and Conditions Stated

State	Type of Definition	Definition Includes Prohibition Against Acts of Diagnosis and Prescription	Rules and Regulations	Professional Opinion	Education and Training	Physician Supervision	If new Definition, based on New York's	Prohibition of Practice of Medicine in Nurse Practice Act	Exception for Nursing in Medical Practice Act
Mississippi	Traditional & Additional Acts Amendment	Yes (Applies to "medical" acts only and additional acts not subject to prohibition)	Yes*	No	No	No	—	No	No
Missouri	Traditional	No	—	—	—	—	—	No	Yes
Montana	Traditional	Yes	—	—	—	—	—	No	Yes
Nebraska	Traditional	No	—	—	—	—	—	No	Yes (For persons lawfully practicing another profession—not applicable to prescription or administration of drugs)
Nevada	Traditional & Additional Acts Amendment	Yes (Applies to "medical" acts only and additional acts not subject to prohibition)	Yes**	Yes°	Yes	No	—	No	Yes
New Hampshire	Traditional & Additional Acts Amendment	Yes (Additional acts not subject to prohibition)	Yes*	Yes°°	Yes	No	—	No	Yes
New Mexico	Traditional	Yes (Applies to "medical" acts only)	—	—	—	—	—	No	Yes (Plus separate exemption for nurse practitioners in certain settings)
New Jersey	New	No	—	—	—	—	Yes	No	Yes (Under physician supervision)

State	Type of Definition	Definition Includes Prohibition Against Acts of Diagnosis and Prescription	If Additional Acts Amendment, Criteria and Conditions Stated				If new Definition, based on New York's	Prohibition of Practice of Medicine in Nurse Practice Act	Exception for Nursing in Medical Practice Act
			Rules and Regulations	Professional Opinion	Education and Training	Physician Supervision			
New York	New	No	—	—	—	—	Yes	Yes	Yes (For persons lawfully practicing another profession)
North Carolina	Traditional & Additional Acts Amendment	Yes (Applies to "medical" acts only and excepts acts under supervision of physician)	Yes*	No	No	Yes[4]	—	No	Yes (For nursing and those acts "otherwise constituting medical practice" which are permitted by regulations of medical and nuc boards)
North Dakota	Traditional	No	—	—	—	—	—	No	No
Ohio	Traditional	Yes (Applies to "medical" acts only)	—	—	—	—	—	Yes	Yes (For nurse anesthetists only, under physician supervision)
Oklahoma	Traditional	Yes	—	—	—	—	—	No	Yes (Under physician supervision)
Oregon	New & Additional Acts Amendment	No	Yes**	Yes[5]	Yes	No	Yes	No	Yes
Pennsylvania	New & Additional Acts Amendment	Yes (Applies to "medical" acts only and additional acts not subject to prohibition)	Yes*	No	No	No	Yes	Yes	No
Rhode Island	Traditional	No	—	—	—	—	—	No	No
South Carolina	Traditional	Yes (Applies to "medical" acts only)	—	—	—	—	—	No	Yes
South Dakota	Traditional & Additional Acts Amendment	No	No	No	Yes	Yes	—	Yes	Yes

If Additional Acts Amendment, Criteria and Conditions Stated

State	Type of Definition	Definition Includes Prohibition Against Acts of Diagnosis and Prescription	Rules and Regulations	Professional Opinion	Education and Training	Physician Supervision	If new Definition, based on New York's	Prohibition of Practice of Medicine in Nurse Practice Act	Exception for Nursing in Medical Practice Act
Tennessee	Traditional	Yes (Applies to "medical" acts only)	—	—	—	—	—	No	Yes (Plus separate exemption for nurses under physician supervision)
Texas	Traditional	Yes (Applies to "medical" acts only)	—	—	—	—	—	Yes	Yes
Utah	Traditional	Yes	—	—	—	—	—	No	Yes
Vermont	New & Additional Acts Amendment	No	No	Yes	Yes	No	Yes	Yes	Yes (Under physician supervision)
Virginia	Traditional	No	—	—	—	—	—	No	Yes (Includes specific reference to certain procedures, which must be performed under orders of physician, plus separate exemption for nurses acting under physician supervision pursuant to rules and regulations of Boards of Nursing and Medicine)
Washington	New & Additional Acts Amendment	No	Yes**	Yes°	Yes	No	Yes	No	No
West Virginia	Traditional	No	—	—	—	—	—	No	Yes
Wisconsin	Traditional	No	—	—	—	—	—	No	Yes (Under physician supervision)[6]

| State | Type of Definition | Definition Includes Prohibition Against Acts of Diagnosis and Prescription | If Additional Acts Amendment, Criteria and Conditions Stated | | | | If new Definition, based on New York's | Prohibition of Practice of Medicine in Nurse Practice Act | Exception for Nursing in Medical Practice Act |
			Rules and Regulations	Professional Opinion	Education and Training	Physician Supervision			
Wyoming	Traditional	No	—	—	—	—	—	No	Yes (Under physician supervision)

[1] Arizona's additional acts amendment, unlike any other, describes substantively one such act: the dispensing of prepackaged, labelled drugs under certain limited, specific circumstances.

[2] Hawaii has a delegation provision which applies to "any physician-support personnel" and which could be construed as including nurses.

[3] Although Maryland's additional acts amendment does not mention physician supervision, the amendment could be interpreted as subordinate to the definitions general description of nursing as consisting of "independent" nursing functions and "delegated" medical functions, in which case any medical acts within the additional acts amendment would have to be delegated acts.

[4] North Carolina's additional acts amendment does not mention physician supervision, but it appears in a separate section from the definition and would appear to be subordinate to that provision of the definition which prohibits acts of medical diagnosis and prescription except under physician supervision.

[5] Oregon alone among the states with additional acts amendments which refer to professional opinion speaks only of nursing opinion, as opposed to medical and nursing opinion.

[6] Wisconsin's law in this regard is somewhat oblique, but it would appear that not only nurses but any persons are authorized to "assist" physicians.

*By Boards of Nursing and Medicine.
**By Board of Nursing.
***By Board of Nursing or "in collaboration with" Board of Medicine.
°Cumulative with rules and regulations.
°°Independent of rules and regulations.

Appendix E

Analysis of Legislation for Physician's Assistants in 38 States

State	Type of Law	Regulatory Agency	Power to Make Rules	Approval of PA	Job Description	Activities Prohibited	Certification Renewal	PAs per Physician	Education Program Approved	Approval of MD	Report to Legislature
Alabama	Regulatory authority, 1971	Board of medical examiners	Yes	Yes	Yes	Optometry	—	—	Yes	Yes	—
Alaska	Regulatory authority, 1974	Board of medical examiners	Yes	Yes		Regulations to be developed				Yes	—
Arizona	Regulatory authority, 1972	Board of medical examiners, board of osteopathic examiners	Yes	Yes	—	Chiropractics, dentistry, optician's services, naturopathy, optometry, pharmacy	—	—	—	—	—
Arkansas	General delegatory, 1971	—	—	—	—	Optometric services	—	—	—	—	—
California	Regulatory authority, 1970	Board of medical examiners	Yes	Yes	Yes	Dentistry, dental hygiene, optometry	Annual	2	Yes	Yes	1972
Colorado	General delegatory, 1963	—	—	—	—	—	—	—	—	—	—
Colorado	Regulatory authority, 1969	Board of medical examiners	Yes	Yes	—	Pharmacy	Annual	1	Yes	Yes	1977

State	Type of Law	Regulatory Agency	Power to Make Rules	Approval of PA	Job Description	Activities Prohibited	Certification Renewal	PAs per Physician	Education Program Approved	Approval of MD	Report to Legislature
Connecticut	General delegatory, 1971	—	—	—	—	Dentistry, dental hygiene, optometry	—	—	—	—	—
Delaware	General delegatory, 1971	—	—	—	—	Optometry	—	—	—	—	—
Florida	Regulatory authority, 1971	Board of medical examiners	Yes	Yes	Yes	—	Annual	2	Yes	Yes	1973
Georgia	Regulatory authority, 1972	Board of medical examiners	Yes	Yes	Yes	Pharmacy	—	2	Yes	Yes	—
Hawaii	Regulatory authority, 1973	Board of medical examiners	Yes	Yes	—	Optometry	—	—	Yes	—	—
Idaho	Regulatory authority, 1972	Board of medical examiners	Yes	Yes	—	Pharmacy, dentistry, dental hygiene, optometry	—	—	Yes	Yes	—
Illinois	Regulatory Authority 1976	Department of Registration and Education	Yes	No	—	Optometry	Biennial	1	Yes	—	1980
Iowa	Regulatory authority, 1971	Board of medical examiners	Yes	Yes	Yes	Optometry	Annual	2	Yes	Yes	1973
Kansas	General delegatory, 1964	—	—	—	—	—	—	—	—	—	—

State	Type of Law	Regulatory Agency	Power to Make Rules	Approval of PA	Job Description	Activities Prohibited	Certification Renewal	PAs per Physician	Education Program Approved	Approval of MD	Report to Legislature
Maine	Regulatory authority, 1973	Board of Registration in Medicine	—	—	—	Optometry	—	—	Yes	—	—
Maryland	Regulatory authority, 1972	Board of medical examiners	—	—	—	—	—	—	—	—	—
Massachusetts	Regulatory authority, 1973	Board of Approval and Certification of PA Programs	Yes	—	—	Chiropractics, dentistry, dental hygiene, optometry, ophthalmology, podiatry	—	2	Yes	—	Annual
Michigan	Regulatory authority, 1973	Department of Health	Yes	—	—	—	—	—	Yes	—	Annual
Montana	General delegatory, 1970	—	—	—	—	—	—	—	—	—	—
Nebraska	Regulatory authority, 1973	Board of medical examiners	Yes	Yes	Yes	—	Annual	2	Yes	Yes	Annual
Nevada	Regulatory authority, 1973	Board of medical examiners	Yes	Yes	—	Chiropractics, dentistry, optometry, podiatry, hearing aid specialists	—	1	Yes	Yes	—
New Hampshire	Regulatory authority, 1971	Board of medical examiners	Yes	Yes	—	Optometry, optician's services	—	—	—	—	—
New Mexico	Regulatory authority, 1973	Board of medical examiners	Yes	Yes	—	Optometry, podiatry	Annual	2	—	—	—

State	Type of Law	Regulatory Agency	Power to Make Rules	Approval of PA	Job Description	Activities Prohibited	Certification Renewal	PAs per Physician	Education Program Approved	Approval of MD	Report to Legislature
New York	Regulatory authority, 1971	Commissioner of health, commissioner of education	Yes	Yes	—	—	Biennial	2	Yes	—	—
North Carolina	Regulatory authority, 1971	Board of medical examiners	Yes	Yes	—	—	Annual	2	Yes	Yes	—
Oklahoma	Regulatory authority, 1972	Board of medical examiners	Yes	Yes	—	Optometry	—	—	Yes	—	—
Oregon	Regulatory authority, 1971	Board of medical examiners	Yes	Yes	Yes	Optometry, nursing, dentistry, dental hygiene	Annual	1	Yes	Yes	1973
South Carolina	Regulatory authority, 1974	Board of medical examiners	Yes	Yes	—	Optometry	—	—	—	—	—
South Dakota	Regulatory authority, 1973	Board of medical examiners	Yes	Yes	Yes	Chiropractics, dentistry, dental hygiene, optometry, pharmacy, podiatry	Annual	—	Yes	Yes	1981
Tennessee	General delegatory, 1973	—	—	—	—	—	—	—	—	—	—
Utah	Regulatory authority, 1971	Medical association	—	—	—	—	—	—	Yes	—	—
Vermont	Regulatory authority, 1972	Agency of human services	Yes	Yes	—	—	—	—	—	—	1975

State	Type of Law	Regulatory Agency	Power to Make Rules	Approval of PA	Job Description	Activities Prohibited	Certification Renewal	PAs per Physician	Education Program Approved	Approval of MD	Report to Legislature
Virginia	Regulatory authority, 1973	Board of medical examiners	Yes	Yes	Yes	Pharmacy	Annual	2	Yes	Yes	—
Washington	Regulatory authority, 1971	Board of medical examiners	Yes	Yes	Yes	Optometry, dentistry, dental hygiene, chiropractice services, chiropody	Annual	1	Yes	Yes	—
West Virginia	Regulatory authority, 1971	Medical licensing board	Yes	Yes	Yes	Pharmacy, optometry	Annual	—	Yes	Yes	—
Wisconsin	Regulatory authority, 1973	Board of medical examiners	Yes	Yes	—	Chiropractics, dentistry, dental hygiene, optometry, podiatry	Annual	—	Yes	—	Biennial
Wyoming	Regulatory authority, 1973	Board of medical examiners	Yes	Yes	Yes	Optometry	—	2	Yes	Yes	1975

Source: Winston J. Dean. "State Legislation for Physician's Assistants—A Review and Analysis." *Health Serv. Rep.*, 88, no. 1 (January 1973), 3-12. Updated by the editors in 1976.

Appendix F

Algorithms—A Tool for Training of or Treatment by Physician Extenders

Gerald Sparer, Joyce Johnson, Megan McDonald and Alan Berkowitz

---

The findings from a study of four algorithm development projects are presented here. These four projects either are currently or have been engaged in algorithm development, physician extender training coupled with algorithms, and health care delivery based on the use of algorithms.

AN ALGORITHM DEFINED

An algorithm or, as it is sometimes called, protocol is a set of unambiguous step-by-step instructions for solving or managing clinical problems. The algorithm system generally has four components, a triage process, the algorithm, a corresponding checklist and an audit process. These four components can be combined in various ways.

The triage process usually precedes the use of an algorithm and/or is incorporated into the body of the algorithm. It is a process which attempts to identify patients with serious or life threatening illnesses or injuries which require the immediate attention of the physician rather than the physician extender.

The algorithm itself is based on branching binary logic. A portion of the Dartmouth-PROMIS upper respiratory infection algorithm is illustrated in Table 1. Algorithms indicate the specific history, physical examination and laboratory data to be obtained for specific complaints or symptoms. The data collected and the subsequent therapeutic steps taken are individualized according to each patient's characteristics.

The checklist complements the algorithm and is not only used to collect data and indicate the action taken but can be audited as well. The checklist can be distinct from the logic as in Table 2 or it can be incorporated into the logic as is the case with the Ambulatory Care Project's algorithms.

---

*The project on which this is based was performed pursuant to a contract (106-74-144) with the Bureau of Health Services Research, Health Resources Administration, Department of Health, Education, and Welfare.

The audit systems vary from project to project. They can be complex computer and physician reviews using the checklist as a basis or simple review of the checklist.

It is important to emphasize that the term "physician extender" is used for distinct provider categories, e.g., nurse practitioners and physician's assistants.

OVERVIEW

The study was initiated by staff of the National Center for Health Services Research early in 1974. For several years prior the Center had supported the training of physician extenders in the use of algorithms for the delivery of health care as had the Veterans Administration and the Department of the Army. Representatives of these three organizations had met periodically and exchanged information regarding the progress of their projects. Out of these meetings grew an interest to test the impact of the algorithm on the health care delivery system. It became apparent, however, that neither a thorough understanding of the similarities and differences in these projects nor the internal capacity to do a detailed description and comparison of the projects existed to provide the data base on which to build an impact study. Consequently, prior to considering more sophisticated analyses on algorithm-trained physician extenders and their impact on health services delivery systems, a descriptive study was outlined to provide the data base for the design of more intensive studies. Four test projects which were thought to be the major innovators in algorithm development and use were selected for this study.

This study, conducted during a nine-month period under a contract funded by the National Center for Health Services Research and awarded to System Sciences, Inc., was completed within the initial time and cost estimates. The Project Director for the study was Mr. Joseph Romm who provided expert leadership to the core team of three System Sciences, Inc. staff members.

The major objective of the study included:

— an analysis and comparison of the various algorithms developed by four programs;
— a description of the training processes by which physician extenders were trained to use algorithms;
— a description of the operational characteristics of health care delivery modes where algorithm-trained physician extenders were used;
— a review of evaluative studies of algorithms;
— an annotated bibliography, and

—the development of an experimental design to assess the impact of algorithms on the health care delivery system.

In many respects the study was designed to define the state-of-the art of algorithms, from development through training and application to health care, and finally to impact analysis. Certainly, all of the initial steps were needed in order to develop a feasible experiment to measure algorithm impact. In other respects, the study provided a mechanism and a baseline to facilitate the collaboration of those in the algorithm development field.

Neither all of our findings nor all of the data can be presented here. However, for those interested in the complete study, copies may be purchased through the National Technical Information Service.

METHODS

Three methods were used to collect the data presented here. Data were extracted from existing documents, both published and unpublished. Visits were made to the sites engaged in the development, training and use of the algorithms where both interviews and observations and record reviews were made. The nature of the study was descriptive, and existing documents and sources were used as much as possible.

The projects included in the study are as follows:

Project AMOS, a nationwide Army-sponsored project
—Fort Belvoir, Virginia
—Fort Sam Houston, Texas
— Fort Ord, California
— Fort Hood, Texas

Dartmouth-PROMIS Laboratory/MEDEX-New England Program in New Hampshire
— Matthew Thornton Health Plan, New Hampshire
— Project Headquarters, Hanover, New Hampshire

Ambulatory Care Project (ACP) in Boston
— Beth Israel Hospital, ACP Headquarters, Massachusetts
— Beth Israel Hospital, Walk-In Clinic, Massachusetts
— Boston City Hospital Diabetes Clinic, Massachusetts

San Francisco Veterans Administration Hospital, California

FINDINGS

Training at Four Study Projects

Training characteristics of the four study projects are summarized in Table 3. While training is structured around the algorithm, it is influenced most significantly by the level of competence of the trainees and by the operational mode in which the algorithm-trained physician extender is to practice.

The AMOSIST Training Program is designed for personnel with minimal health care experience, although many experienced technicians receive training. The AMOSIST's scope of care in the Army acute minor illness clinics is limited to presenting complaints covered by the algorithms. The AMOSISTs perform two functions, triaging patients either to physicians or other AMOSISTs and treating patients with acute minor illnesses. Both functions are performed through the use of algorithms. The patient population served by the AMOSIST is general population adults currently or previously in the military service or dependents of active or retired military personnel.

Training is short and structured, consisting of two full-time weeks of didactic training and ten weeks of closely supervised on-the-job experience. During the 12-week training period, three groups of exams are given.

The Beth Israel Ambulatory Care Project has two different approaches, one to deal with inexperienced health assistants using chronic illness maintenance algorithms in the Boston City Hospital Diabetes Clinic, and the other for experienced health care providers (usually registered nurses) using acute minor illness algorithms in an institutional setting. For the health assistants, training consisted of 80 hours of semistructured class time during a four to six-week period, followed by six months of close on-the-job supervision. For the experienced providers, training was essentially an orientation to algorithms and their use. Since 1969 the project's focus has been on algorithm research rather than physician extender training.

The health assistants are trained to serve primarily diabetics and hypertensives while the experienced health providers are trained to serve general population adults with acute minor illnesses.

The MEDEX program at Dartmouth (using algorithms developed by the PROMIS Lab) is directed at personnel with at least two years of patient contact experience although most MEDEX students have more. The structured twelve-month training cycle consists of three months of formal classroom and practical instruction followed by nine months of physician-supervised, on-the-job training. Qualifying tests and preceptor ratings lead to MEDEX certification. The graduates are situated in the New England area in both rural and urban sites serving a general practice population.

The San Francisco Veterans Administration Hospital (SFVAH) program was an experimental demonstration over a two-year period and is no longer operational. It was directed at personnel with varied experience and enabled them to use simple algorithms designed essentially to acquire data rather than to diagnose. All patients were to be seen by a physician following the data acquisition by the health technician. Twelve months of semistructured training took place, consisting of three months in the classroom and nine months on-the-job with close supervision. After training, the health technicians worked in a drop-in clinic and in a part of the general medical clinic of the hospital. Obviously, the population served was made up of older males.

Table 3 presents some of the differences among the four projects. Both the MEDEX and the Veterans Administration Hospital programs provide 12 months of training as compared to 12 weeks (or about three months) by AMOS and two weeks by ACP. The training emphasis on algorithms spans a broad range. At the extremes are Project AMOS, which teaches AMOSIST students only as much as they need to know in order to follow the algorithms only as tools to assist in the broad medical training of physician assistants. The SFVAH and ACP training programs fall between these two extremes with ACP closer to Project AMOS in its training philosophy and the SFVAH closer to the MEDEX program. It should be noted, however, that the ACP was designed primarily as an algorithm development program and not as a training program.

Algorithms in Practice

Again, the operational mode and the level of competence of the physician extender govern how algorithms are used in practice and the degree of independence exercised by the physician extender in the delivery of health care services.

In the high volume Army acute minor illness clinics, representing only a small part of high volume Army general hospitals, the AMOSIST treats only those patients who present complaints covered by the algorithms in use. All other patients are seen by the physician. The AMOSISTs are required to use the data collection sheets, and therefore the algorithms, for each patient seen. There is frequent consultation with the physician (at least one in every five patients) and little audit of the algorithm data collection instruments. This is consistent with the narrow range of independence of the AMOSIST and the simplicity of the algorithms.

A sample composed of several days of completed algorithm data collection sheets was taken in December 1974 at two acute minor illness clinics. The sample indicated that the predominant algorithms in use were those for upper respiratory infection/otitis, urinary tract infection, dermatology problems, viral gastroenteritis and extremity pain.

In the Boston City Hospital Diabetes Clinic, the ACP health assistants use several chronic disease algorithms, the principal one being the diabetes algorithm. All procedures for maintenance of the diabetic are performed by the health assistants and reviewed by a supervising nurse. All patients are then routed to the physician before leaving. The structure of the algorithm, which is repetitive and complete, is in accord with the health assistant's narrow range of independence. Audit is accomplished by a visual review of the data collection sheets and medical records.

In the walk-in-clinic at Beth Israel Hospital the registered nurse is essentially an independent health care provider, seeing 70 percent of her patients without consulting the physician. She uses the ACP acute minor illness algorithms (a hospital requirement), all of which are audited by computer. The single most frequent patient complaint at the clinic during a two-week sample period in September 1974 related to urinary tract infection and vaginitis 18 percent of the time. Complaints related to upper respiratory infections, cough and ear problems comprised the second highest proportion of all complaints, 15 percent.

During the nine months of preceptor-supervised, on-the-job training the MEDEX trainees use algorithms which are reviewed by physicians and then audited by both the PROMIS-Lab staff and by computer. The extent of algorithm use is unknown; however, at least five algorithm data collection sheets per week must be submitted during this training period. On completion of training, formal use of the algorithm appears to end (data collection sheets are not used) although the algorithm logic is probably retained and used by Medex. In both solo practices and group practices or health centers, Medex appear to provide a significant proportion of the care independently which is consistent with both the level of training and the complexity of the algorithm.

A summary of the data collection sheets submitted for audit by the trainees indicates that the upper respiratory infection data collection sheets comprised over 50 percent of the total, with ear problems, cough and laceration algorithm data collection sheets accounting for most of the remainder.

The health technicians trained at the SFVAH did not operate independently. Algorithms were used in all instances to classify complaints and obtain appropriate patient data and served only as referral or triage mechanisms, with all patients referred to physicians.

Comparative Analysis of Algorithms Developed by Three Study Projects

A comparative analysis was completed of the structural features of the algorithms developed at three projects. The time and scope of the study precluded analysis of the medical content, logic and documentation of the various algorithms. The analysis addressed the complexity of the algorithm, its scope in terms of diagnosis and treatment, and the relative independence of the physician extender who is trained and is using the algorithm.

Five parameters were selected for comparison:

— Number of instructions, decision points or items of information;
— Number of logical branch points;
— Number of physician referral points;
— Number and types of illnesses physician extenders can treat and/or diagnose;
— Number and types of procedures physician extenders can perform and/or order.

The SFVAH algorithms were not included as they were developed as data acquisition tools, not as tools to assist in diagnosis and treatment. The three remaining projects have a total of 23 different algorithms which are listed in Table 4. The projects have only three algorithms in common—upper respiratory infection (URI), back pain, and headache. There are six other algorithms which two of the development sites have in common.

Because of space limitations, only those algorithms developed at two or more sites are compared in Tables 3 and 4. There were significant differences among the algorithms. Table 5 indicates that, in most cases, the Dartmouth algorithms have significantly more logical branch points than those at other programs. Further, when looking at the number of physician referral points as compared to the number of instructions, decision points or items of information, the Dartmouth algorithms stand out as being the most detailed and complex with the least physician intervention. This is a logical finding when one looks at the differences in training and objectives among the programs.

Similarly, Table 6 shows that the Medex diagnoses and/or treats more illnesses and performs more procedures than physician extenders trained at the other programs—again, not a surprising finding considering the program differences.

A comparison of the URI and URI-related algorithms is used to illustrate the specific type of differences among the three projects. The ACP URI algorithm is the most limited. It allows diagnosis and/or treatment of streptococcal sore throat, sinusitis, otitis externa, otitis media, URI and mononucleosis. The AMOS URI algorithm (which also includes as a component a headache algorithm), in addition to ACP's algorithm, enables the physician extender to identify and treat furuncle of the ear, pharyngitis, labyrinthitis, chest wall syndrome, rhinitis, tracheobronchitis, laryngitis and differentiates serous otitis from eczematoid otitis externa. The Dartmouth URI algorithm does not cover eczematoid otitis externa or furuncle but it enables the physician extender to diagnose and/or treat, in addition to both the AMOS and the ACP algorithms, epiglottitis, peritonsilar abscess, pneumonia, and bronchitis. If Dartmouth's ear algorithm is included, Meniere's disease, mastoiditis, otosclerosis, cholesteatoma, perforated tympanic membrane, foreign body and impaired hearing can also be diagnosed and/or treated.

Not only does the Dartmouth algorithm cover a much greater range of illness, but the Medex relies much less on the physician for referral. For example, Dartmouth's URI algorithm makes referrals to the physician 17 times while diagnosing 11 diseases as compared to the ACP URI algorithm with 21 referral points and six diseases and the AMOS algorithm with 34 referral points and 15 diseases.

Similarly, as shown by the comparison of the ear algorithms, the Dartmouth algorithm diagnoses ten diseases and refers ten times to the physician while the AMOS algorithm makes six diagnoses and refers to the physician at 15 points. Dartmouth's ear algorithm has 26 logical branch points versus 30 for the AMOSIST. Quite different knowledge and skills are required of the Medex than of the AMOSIST. ACP's URI algorithm, which includes ear problems, is the least complex and most restrictive for the physician extender.

The procedures performed or ordered by the physician extender also vary. The ACP health assistant cannot order a chest X-ray while the other URI algorithms permit the physician extender to do this. However, the ACP health assistant may order gram stain of sputum. The Medex does his or her own WBC and differential.

Dartmouth is the only site with a separate cough algorithm. Sinus X-rays may be ordered, Tine test or PPD done, and Zeihl-Neelsen stain and gram stain of sputum performed. Symptom complexes suggestive of tuberculosis, pericarditis, congestive heart failure and chronic obstructive lung disease can also be made using this algorithm. The Medex, with a completely different level of training, competence and experience than the others, is permitted a much greater degree of independent function.

Looking at the URI comparative task analysis, Table 7, some further differences among the URI algorithms can be elucidated. Only the Dartmouth algorithm calls for an examination for epiglottitis and for peritonsillar abscess and looks for obliteration of the jaw angle, although all protocols attempt to adequately identify mononucleosis. ACP's algorithm omits examination of the mastoids. It also does very little with mononucleosis. The posterior cervical nodes are examined, the monospot ordered, but the algorithm does not specify examination for splenomegaly or axillary adenopathy. The AMOS algorithm examines the abdomen but specifics are not given. Interestingly, only the ACP algorithm specifies taking the important smoking history. This is covered by the Dartmouth cough algorithm but ignored by the AMOS URI algorithm.

This is perhaps a consequence of the concept of episodic medical care which does not provide continuity between patient and practitioner over time. Concern with such habits as smoking tends to get deemphasized when treatment is oriented to the single illness episode. It is the impression of the authors that this kind of system does not give adequate attention to the patient with, say, both chronic lung disease and a URI. The AMOSIST does not know the significance of the former, and for the ACP nurse this depends strictly upon her additional experience, which at present is quite considerable and sophisticated.

The differences in the ear algorithms highlight some additional points. The AMOS algorithm does not (and of the three, most needs to) specify taking a past medical history including regular medications and allergy. Further, only the Darmouth algorithm deals with tinnitus through valsalva and neurological exam (including Weber and Rinne tests).

However, one must be extremely cautious about making comparative value judgments. These differences reflect conscious, often empirical decisions by algorithm developers at each site concerning the advantages to be gained by each procedure. These decisions were governed by many parameters including both individual physician taste and, perhaps most important, the gross lack of empirical evidence supporting the necessity for many procedures.

The Audit Mechanisms

The audit systems, as with the algorithms, differ greatly among the three projects and reflect the values, needs, medical care structure and cost benefit to the three projects.

Project AMOS currently uses a simple nonautomated audit system which requires that 2.5 percent, or every fortieth chart, be sequentially audited each week. The system depends on a weekly "self-audit conference" in which each AMOSIST and physician review and score several charts according to criteria developed on a "self-audit form."

ACP employs a computerized audit system which detects three types of deviations from the branching logic:

— "Extra" data.
— "Missing" data.
— "Wrong" or inconsistent data.

A list of deviations from each algorithm is printed out and returned to the physician extender within a week. While there is no formal mechanism for discussing errors with each physician extender, the ACP staff is quite vigorous in identifying and correcting patterns of error. In addition to the computer audit, manual chart audits are performed in all cases of error as well as from a sample of "perfect" algorithms to assess the possibility of other types of errors not identified by the computer.

The Dartmouth audit system is used during training on a sampling basis and also as a developmental tool for further algorithm refinement. The system recognizes that there is only one correct pathway through the logic of an algorithm for any set of patient data. Any errors in following the logic are detected by a computer program which prints a statement summarizing the pertinent patient data and indicating the nature of the error. This statement can be analyzed by both the physician preceptor and MEDEX staff to determine the significance of the error. Errors in both omission of data and performance of extra procedures are indicated by the printout.

In addition to auditing the physician extender's performance in evaluating individual patients, the system analyzes the Medex's performance in multiple patient encounters in order to detect recurrent errors and tabulate the specific branch points at which the Medex's observations disagree with those of his or her preceptor. For each plan, a computer program indicates the number of times the plan was actually carried out, which includes those instances in which the algorithm had not suggested the plan, and the percent of checklists in which each of these occurred. An item of major interest is the printout in which errors of omission in following the protocol logic are tallied by branch point. Recurrent mistakes at the same branch point are readily detected by this analysis. Part of the printout is a tabulation of those plans "aborted" at the direction of the physician preceptor, either because he or she did not agree with the logic of the algorithm or because the plans generated by the algorithm were inappropriate for an individual patient. This is, in effect, a comparison between the preceptor's judgment about individual patients and the algorithm system's attempt to standardize the medical evaluation of all patients.

As a component of medical audit, the basic criticism of computer audit by itself is simple. It does not permit one to view what goes on between the physician extender and the patient with respect to such areas as the accuracy of the history and physical and the ability to communicate with the patient. Quite a few errors made by AMOSISTs were seen during observation that could not be identified by a computerized audit, although this was not the case at other sites. The factors covered by computerized audits are considered by the authors to be much less important than those they omit. For example, computer audits review the completed data collection sheet rather than the algorithm user or the algorithm user/patient encounter. The all important question of quality of patient care is addressed only indirectly. It is conceivable, for example, that a physician extender who cannot identify an inflamed tympanic membrane can continue indefinitely to treat patients "correctly" on the basis of the algorithm.

While a useful research tool, the computerized audit also directs attention away from the patient and toward the algorithm. Periodic "direct looks" at the physician extender/patient interaction should occur, and less attention and reliance placed on automated audity systems.

SUMMARY AND CONCLUSIONS

In conclusion, the review of four training and operational algorithm programs indicated more differences than similarities. Comparisons were especially difficult to make as the programs differed in their objectives, patients, types of physician extenders and health care delivery modes. Further, the structure and complexity of the algorithms used are different. The findings confirmed, however, the initial belief that an experimental impact study could not have been successfully undertaken without the descriptive baseline data, which this study has provided.

The algorithm is a small part of a medical care delivery system and must reflect the interests, needs and medical care requirements of the system from which it comes. The great differences in algorithm structure, content and use reflect decisions predicated upon these factors. The authors wish to caution those delivery systems which have, or wish to, import algorithms. The decision to import a specific algorithm must depend on the patient population, the potential practitioner and the other needs of the system. If the algorithm does not meet these needs, it cannot be used effectively or safely.

Further, it is a conclusion of the authors that medical audit should play a strong role in any health care delivery system which uses algorithms. The medical audit should be directed at assessment of the overall quality of care, not just a single episode of illness.

Conclusions can be summarized briefly in the following four statements

— Algorithms are a potentially useful tool for training physician extenders, and probably would be extremely useful for training medical students as well.

— Algorithms provide a basis for standards of ambulatory medical care and are potentially applicable for medical audit, quality of care assessment, and peer review.

— The training and competence of the physician extender using algorithm are critical determinants of algorithm use, and transfer or export of algorithms should take careful account of the characteristics of the health care delivery system in which they will be used.

— Where training and use of physician extenders are limited by a set of algorithms (e.g., in the Army), the triaging must be of high quality to assure that patients with nonalgorithm-related complaints are sent to the physician rather than to the physician extender.

Further research will need to be undertaken to more fully determine the ultimate usefulness of the algorithms. Specifically, three questions should be addressed:

— Does the algorithm-trained physician extender acquire more knowledge about diagnosis and treatment than the nonalgorithm-trained physician extender, i.e., is it a useful training tool in the longer term?

— Does the algorithm-trained physician extender, using the algorithms in treatment, provide more effective and efficient care than the algorithm-trained physician extender who does not continue to use algorithms or the nonalgorithm-trained extender or physician?

— Does the algorithm provide a useful tool for medical audit of ambulatory care that could be applied to a range of health care delivery systems?

These questions can only be addressed by experimental studies which are designed to compare individuals exposed to comparable levels of training and deployed to comparable settings. These will be difficult studies to design. However, the answers to these questions will address the important issues about the value of the algorithms for training, diagnosis and treatment, and medical audit.

TABLE 1

**Dartmouth-Promis Laboratory
Algorithm for Upper Respiratory Illness: Pharyngitis Component**

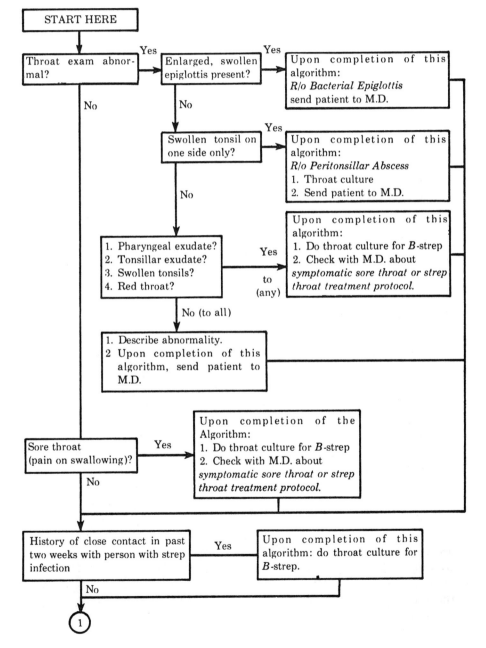

TABLE 2

DARTMOUTH-PROMIS LABORATORY

URI CHECKLIST

User I.D. No: _1_   Patient Name: _John Doe_   Pt. No.: _1_

Today's Date: _1/2/73_   Patient's Birthday: _1/2/40_   Phone Number: _999-1111_

(✓ – PRESENT;   O – ABSENT;   ✗, & – PRECEPTOR DISAGREES WITH FINDING OR PLAN)

SUBJECTIVE DATA:

Chief Complaint: _Sore Throat_   Duration: _2 Days_   Course: _Worsening_

Other description: _Gradual onset. No relief from Aspirin or gargling. Has malaise and is unable to work but is ambulatory at home._

Allergies Present (incl. Medications): _None._   Regular Medications: _None_

✓2 Sore throat/swallowing pain

Right Ear	Left Ear	
o 9	o 10	Pain → Check mastoids
o 11	o 12	Tinnitus
o 15	o 14	Loss of hearing
o	o	lbc of T.M. perforation
56	57	Sx relieved by wax removal
29	29	Ear sx present ≥ weeks

- ✓ 30 lbc of infectious mono
- o 55 lbc of strep exposure
- o 53 Cough present
- ___ 54 Sputum production
- ___ 59 Chest pain present

o 6 Runny nose
o 5 Facial/Dental pain → Check for periapical abscess

Chronic Diseases
- o 90 Heart Disease
- o 91 Chronic Kidney Disease
- o 92 Diabetes
- o 93 Asthma/Chronic Lung Disease
- o 94 High Blood Pressure
- o 95 Chronic Blood Disease
- o 99 Other:

OBJECTIVE DATA: BP: _110/78_   Weight: _163 lbs._   Temperature: _98.4 (p.o.)_

✓1 Abnormal throat exam
- o 18 Enlarged/swollen epiglottis
- o 19 Unilateral swollen tonsil
- ✓20 Exudate✓; Swollen tonsils o ; Red throat ✓
- o 60 Other abn:

o 3 Abnormal nasal exam
- ___ 21 Purulent nasal discharge
- ___ 22 Wet/swollen membranes___; or Non-purulent discharge___
- ___ 61 Other abn:
- ___ 23 Periapical abscess

o 15 Neck swelling so severe as to obliterate angle of jaw

o 4 Sinus tenderness present

	Right	Left	
	—	—	Frontal
	—	—	Axillary

o 16 Cervical lymph nodes enlarged/tender
- ___ 31 Posterior cervical nodes enlarged
- ___ 50 Enlarged spleen___; or axillary nodes___

o 17 Abnormal chest exam
- ___ 32 Localized chest exam abn.
- ___ 58 Temperature ≥ 101°F.

o 7 (R) o 8 (L) Abnormal ear exam

Right Ear	Left Ear	
24	25	Ext. canal abnormal
34	35	Foreign body present
36	37	Otitis externa present before wax removal
38	39	Wax obstruction present
40	41	Wax not removed
42	43	Otitis externa present after wax removal
26	27	Abnormal T.M.
46	47	Perforated T.M.
51	52	Ear discharge present
48	49	Bulging T.M.___; Red T.M.___; no light reflex___; no landmarks___
44	45	Other abn:

28 Mastoid tenderness R___, L___

PLANS:

	Results
___103 Throat Culture	
___104 Throat Culture for ∤ –strep only	
___105 Culture nasal discharge R or L	
___107 Culture ear discharge R or L	
___109 WBC with Diff.	
✓110 Heterophile	
___113 Check with M.D. about Chest X-ray	
___111 Chest X-ray PA and Lat	
___112 Sinus X-ray	
___149 Other plan:	

Protocols
- ✓ 150 Strep Throat Protocol
- ___151 Sympt. Sore Throat Protocol
- ___152 Runny Nose Protocol
- ___ Acute Sinusitis Protocol
- ___154 Otitis Externa Protocol
- ___155 Otitis Media Protocol
- ___157 Cough Protocol
- ___175 Other Rx. given:

Disposition

___102 Sent to M.D. ******

✓174 Pt. discharged with M.D. approval

FINAL DIAGNOSIS:

___054.0 Strep Pharyngitis	___508.4 Epiglottitis	___075 Inf. Mono.	___380 Otitis Externa
___462 Non-strep Pharyngitis	___501 Peritonsillar Abscess	___489 Acute Bronch.	___381.0 Acute Otitis Media
___470 Flu Syndrome	___460 Head Cold	___485 Bronch. Pneum.	___381.9 Serous Otitis Media
	___461.9 Acute Sinusitis	___481.0 Lobar Pneum.	___ Other:

✓101 M.D. performed audit

John Smith/mx
(SIGNATURE)

TABLE 3

Operational and Training Differences

	AMOS	ACP	DARTMOUTH	SFVAH
OPERATIONAL MODE	Acute minor illness clinics	(1) Walk-in clinic; (2) Chronic illness maintenance clinic	Private practitioners	Walk-in clinics
PHYSICIAN EXTENDER EXPERIENCE	Minimal military medical experience	(1) Nurse-registered (2) Inexperienced health assistants	Experienced health care personnel	Minimal medical experience
INDEPENDENCE	Closely supervised; narrow range of independence	(1) Wide latitude, independent; (2) Narrow range of independence, MD sees all patients	Largely independent	Completely dependent, MD sees all patients

TABLE 3 (Continued)

Operational and Training Differences

	AMOS	ACP	DARTMOUTH	SFVAH
ALGORITHMS	Simple, few procedures	(1) Complete, many procedures; (2) Complete, repetitive	Complex, complete, many procedures	Used for data collection only, no patient treatment instructions
AUDIT	Small sample of data collection sheets visually reviewed	(1) All data collection instruments reviewed by computer; (2) Visual review of data collection forms and medical records	Sample reviewed by MD and computer during training period	All seen by an MD
PATIENTS	General population adults	(1) General population adults; (2) Primarily elderly diabetics	General practice population	Primarily male, older
TRAINING TYPE	Structured	(1) No formal training (2) Semistructured	Structured	Semistructured
LENGTH	2 weeks didactic, 10 weeks preceptorship	Part-time 4-6 weeks	3 months didactic, 9 months preceptorship	3 months didactic, 9 months preceptorship
NUMBER TRAINED	259	14	97 graduates	10 graduates

TABLE 4

Algorithms Developed at Three Sites

DARTMOUTH*	ACP	AMOS
1. URI	URI	URI/otitis**
2.	Prenatal	
3. Female GU/Gyn	UTI-Vaginitis	UTI
4. Low Back pain	Low back pain	Back or neck pain
5.	GYN	
6.	Warts/acne	Dermatology
7.	Nausea, vomiting, diarrhea, abdominal pain	
8. Headache	Headache	**
9.	Chest pain	
10.	Arthritis	
11. Male GU	Male GU	
12.	Birth Control	
13.	Diabetes	
14.	Hypertension	
15.	Diabetes-Hypertension	
16.	Cardiovascular	
17. Ear problems		Ear problems
18. Cough		
19. Bone and joint trauma		Extremity pain
20. Laceration		
21.		Conjunctivitis-eye irritations
22.		Eyelid
23.		Breast
TOTAL 9	16	9

*In addition, the PROMIS Lab at Dartmouth was revising five old algorithms which do not appear in this table.

**URI is divided into six algorithms including headache.

TABLE 5

Quantitative Comparative Analysis of Algorithm Length and Complexity for those Developed at Two or More Sites

Algorithm*	Number of Instructions, Decision Points or Items of Information			Number of Logical Branch Points			Number of MD Referral Points		
	DART-MOUTH	ACP	AMOS	DART-MOUTH	ACP	AMOS	DART-MOUTH	ACP	AMOS
URI	78	56	95	45	17	72	17	21	34
UTI-Vaginitis	131 (GU-GYN)	62	18	72	18	13	17	34	10
Low back pain	55	58	10	29	4	5	13	18	4
Dermatology	—	48	55	—	11	17	—	38	14
Headache	42	66	See URI	24	12	See URI	7	30	See URI
Male GU	151	64	—	81	19	—	25	33	—
Ear Problems	46	See URI	35	26	See URI	30	10	See URI	15
Cough	97	See URI	See URI	54	See URI	See URI	24	See URI	See URI
Bone and joint trauma	32	—	12	14	—	7	8	—	6

*General rather than specific names of algorithm per development site are used.

TABLE 6

Comparative Analysis of Number and Types of Illnesses and Procedures Covered by those Algorithms Developed at Two or More Sites

	NUMBER OF ILLNESSES PE WILL DIAGNOSE AND/OR TREAT*			NUMBER AND TYPES OF PROCEDURES DONE/ORDERED BY PE		
	DARTMOUTH	ACP	AMOS	DARTMOUTH	ACP	AMOS
EAR PROBLEMS	1. Otitis externa 2. Otitis media 3. Labyrinthitis 4. Menieres disease 5. Mastoiditis 6. Cholesteatoma 7. Otosclerosis 8. Perforated tymp. mem. 9. Foreign body 10. Impaired hearing	See URI (no separate ear algorithm)	1. Viral labyrinthitis 2. Otitis media 3. Serous otitis 4. Otitis externa 5. Furuncle 6. Eczematoid otitis externa	• Culture of ear discharge • Irrigation of canal • Cerumen removal • Schedule for audiogram	See URI - (no separate ear algorithm)	• Irrigate ears • Culture drainage • Audiometry appt.
COUGH	1. Strep pharyngitis 2. URI 3. Epiglottitis 4. Peritonsillar abscess 5. Sinusitis 6. Tuberculosis 7. Pneumonia 8. Pericarditis 9. Congestive heart failure 10. Chronic obstructive lung disease 11. Acute bronchitis 12. Non-specific cough	See URI	See URI	• Chest X-ray • EKG • Tine test or PPD • TB culture of sputum • Zeihl-Neelson strain of sputum • Gram stain of sputum • Throat culture • Throat culture for B-strep • Culture of nasal discharge • Sinus X-rays	See URI	See URI
BONE AND JOINT TRAUMA	1. Acute strain 2. Laceration 3. Symptomatic Rx 4. Fractures	--	1. Bursitis 2. Tendonitis 3. Muscle ache 4. Sprain 5. Strain 6. Bruise	• Extremity X-rays • Immobilize limb • Splint limb • Sterile drape	--	(0)

*At ACP the PE independently treats all the illness he presumptively or positively diagnoses. Diagnoses handled independently by other physician extenders are underlined.

TABLE 6 (Continued)

Comparative Analysis of Number and Types of Illnesses and Procedures Covered by those Algorithms Developed at Two or More Sites

	NUMBER OF ILLNESSES PE WILL DIAGNOSE AND/OR TREAT*			NUMBER AND TYPES OF PROCEDURES DONE/ORDERED BY PE		
	DARTMOUTH	ACP	AMOS	DARTMOUTH	ACP	AMOS
URI	1. Strep pharyngitis 2. URI 3. Epiglottitis 4. Peritonsillar abscess 5. Sinusitis, acute 6. Mononucleosis 7. Pneumonia (lobar bronchial) 8. Acute otitis externa 9. Acute otitis media 10. Serous Otitis media 11. Bronchitis	1. Strep sore throat (Includes ear and headache algorithms) 2. Sinusitis 3. Otitis externa 4. Otitis media 5. URI 6. Mononucleosis	1. URI 2. Otitis media 3. Otitis externa 4. Furuncle 5. Sinusitis, acute and chronic 6. Pharyngitis 7. Labyrinthitis 8. Chest wall syndrome 9. Serous otitis 10. Eczematoid otitis externa 11. Strep throat 12. Mononucleosis 13. Rhinitis, purulent and allergic 14. Tracheobronchitis 15. Laryngitis	° Throat culture ° Culture for B-strep ° Culture nasal discharge ° Irrigate ear canal ° Remove ear wax ° Culture ear discharge ° Heterophile ° WBC and differential ° Chest X-ray	° Throat culture ° Nasal culture ° Monospot ° Sputum culture ° Gram stain	° Irrigate ears ° Culture drainage ° Audiometry appt. ° Monospot ° Culture throat ° Chest X-ray
UTI-VAGINITIS	1. Pyelonephritis 2. Cystitis 3. Incomplete abortion 4. Cervical carcinoma 5. Enlarged uterus 6. Salpingitis 7. Syphilis 8. Pneumonia 9. Urolithiasis 10. Vaginitis 11. Ovarian enlargement	1. UTI, simple 2. Monilia 3. Trichomonas 4. Nonspecific vaginitis 5. Urethritis	1. Uncomplicated cystitis	° Urinalysis ° Urine culture ° Pap smear ° Pregnancy test ° Culture cervix, rectum for GC ° STS ° Wet prep for trichomonas, yeast forms ° Urine sediment ° Chest X-rays ° Abdominal X-rays	° Urinalysis ° Pap smear ° GC culture ° Gram stain ° Urine culture	° Urinalysis ° Urine culture
LOW BACK PAIN	1. Disc disease 2. Osteomyelitis 3. Vertebral metastases 4. Cauda Aquina 5. Vertebral fractures 6. UTI 7. Low back trauma 8. Hip disease 9. Thoracic disease 10. Abdominal disease	1. UTI 2. Acute low back strain 3. Acute low back strain with possible root involvement	1. Musculospastic back pain 2. Musculospastic neck pain	° Stool hematest ° X-ray ° Urinalysis ° Urine culture ° Prothrombin time	° Urinalysis ° Urine culture	

TABLE 6 (Continued)

	NUMBER OF ILLNESSES PE WILL DIAGNOSE AND/OR TREAT*			NUMBER AND TYPES OF PROCEDURES DONE/ORDERED BY PE		
	DARTMOUTH	ACP	AMOS	DARTMOUTH	ACP	AMOS
DERMATOLOGY	--	1. Warts 2. Acne	1. Dandruff 2. Acne 3. Aphthous stomatitis 4. Herpes labialis 5. Impetigo 6. Contact dermatitis 7. Sunburn 8. Atopic dermatitis 9. Pityriasis rosea 10. Pediculosis 11. Insect Bite 12. Skin fungal infection (4 types)	--	° Liquid nitrogen to lesions	(0)
HEADACHE	1. Acute sinusitis 2. Chronic sinusitis 3. Glaucoma 4. Tension headache 5. Temporal arteritis 6. Vascular headache 7. Non-specific headache	1. Muscular headache 2. Vascular headache 3. Acute sinusitis 4. Chronic sinusitis	See URI	° Orders tonometry ° ESR	(0)	See URI
MALE GU	1. Pneumonia 2. Syphilis 3. Gonorrhea 4. Prostatitis 5. Urethritis 6. Urolithiasis 7. Epididymitis 8. Varicocele 9. Inguinal hernia 10. Pyelonephritis 11. Torsion of testes 12. UTI 13. BPH 14. Neoplasm of testes 15. Neoplasm of prostate 16. Spermatocele	1. GC contact 2. VD checkups 3. GC urethritis 4. Non-specific urethritis 5. Syphilis contact 6. Syphilis	--	° Urinalysis ° Urine culture ° STS ° Post-prostate massage culture ° Culture of prostate secretions ° Gram stain ° Wet preps of secretions ° Obtain names of sexual contacts	° Mid-stream urinalysis ° Stat RPR ° GC smear ° GC culture ° STS ° Culture of urethral discharge ° CBC	--

*At ACP the PE independently treats all the illness he presumptively or positively diagnoses. Diagnoses handled independently by other physician extenders are underlined.

TABLE 7

URI Algorithm Comparative Task Analysis

	DARTMOUTH MEDEX	ACP PE	AMOSIST
Obtains description of chief complaint	X	X	X
Obtains past medical history, allergies, medications used	X	Allergies not specified except for antibiotics	Not specified by algorithm
Obtains history of associated URI complaints (sore throat, pain in face or teeth, runny nose, ear pain, tinnitus, decreased hearing, cough)	X	X	X
Obtains history of exposure to B-strep	X	X	X
Examines ears	X	X	X
Examines throat	X	X	X
Examines nasal passages	X	X	X
Examines chest	X	X	X
Checks for sinus tenderness	X	X	X
Checks for lymphadenopathy (cervical)	X	X	X
Checks for neck swelling (obliteration of jaw angle)	X	No	No
Checks for enlarged, swollen epiglottis	X	No	No
If epiglottis abnormal, refers to MD	X	No	No
Checks for peritonsillar abscess	X	No	Not specified
If possibility, does throat culture	X	X	No
Refers possible peritonsillar abscess to MD	X	No	Not specified
If tonsil swollen on one side only with exudate or red throat, does throat culture for B-strep	X	Cultures all sore throats and swollen glands	Cultures all exudates

TABLE 7 (Continued)

URI Algorithm Comparative Task Analysis

	DARTMOUTH MEDEX	ACP PE	AMOSIST
Treats symptomatic sore throat	X	X	X
If throat examination is abnormal with pain on swallowing does throat culture for *B*-strep	X	X	X
If nasal exam abnormal with discharge and sinus tenderness cultures nasal discharge	X	Cultures without tender sinuses	Does not culture nasal discharge
Treats for acute sinusitis	X	X	X
If nasal exam abnormal with discharge but no sinus tenderness treats for runny nose	X	X	X
If periepical abscess present, sends to MD	X	No - does not make this diagnosis	No - does not make this diagnosis
Does sinus X-ray if nasal exam is abnormal and facial or tooth pain is present	X	No	Yes - refers to MD
Checks for ear abnormality	X	X	X
If foreign body is present in ear, sends to MD	X	Not specified	X
If otitis externa is found irrigates canal with Burow's solution	X	No	X
Treats for otitis externa	X	X	X
If ear was present with tinnitus/pain/hearing loss, wax removed by syringe irrigation	X	No—consults with MD	X
If TM perforated with discharge, cultures discharge	X	No—refers to MD	No—refers to MD
Treats for otitis media	X	X	X

TABLE 7 (Continued)

URI Algorithm Comparative Task Analysis

	DARTMOUTH MEDEX	ACP PE	AMOSIST
Checks for presence of other TM abnormality (redness, bulging, loss of light reflex or landmarks)	X	X	X
If present, treats for otitis media	X	X	X
If ear exam normal, checks for mastoid tenderness	X	No	X
If mastoid tender, refers to MD	X	No	X
If ear pain, tinnitus/loss of hearing present > 2 weeks, refers to MD	X	Not specified	Sends to MD regardless of time
If ear pain, tinnitus/loss of hearing, present with runny nose, treats for runny nose	X	X	No—refers to MD
If neck swelling obliterates angle of jaw heterophile, WBC and differential done	X	Monospot only	No—if postcervical or auricular nodes enlarged, sends to MD, orders mono-spot
Throat culture taken and patient referred to MD	X	X	X
If cervical nodes are enlarged/tender, checks posterior cervical nodes	X	X	X
If these are abnormal, checks for splenomegaly and axillary adenopathy	X	No	Yes (does abdominal exam, axillary nodes not specified)
If these are enlarged, sends to MD	X	No—does not examine abdomen	X

TABLE 7 (Continued)

URI Algorithm Comparative Task Analysis

	DARTMOUTH MEDEX	ACP PE	AMOSIST
If not, does heterophile, WBC and differential	X	No	No
Examines chest (inspection, percussion, auscultation)	X	X	X
If *any* abnormality *localized*, obtains chest PA and Lateral	X	Any abnormality to MD, No X-ray	X
If chest examination abnormal but *no* localization, consults with MD about chest X ray	X	Sends to MD	No, sends to MD
Sends patient to MD	X	X	Cough productive of green sputum
If patient has cough with fever ≥101°F and/or chest pain, sends patient to MD	X	Temperature ≥102°F goes to MD	Temperature > 102°F or present 4 days
If not, treats for cough	X	X	No
All cases are checked with MD before discharge	X	No	X
If MD agrees, patients are discharged with 48-hour follow-up	X	Not specified	Follow-up specified on treatment protocols
Takes history of smoking	No	X	No

ER09el

Appendix G

Encounter Form

ENCOUNTER FORM

PROVIDER NUMBER: _____

PATIENT STATUS:	[1] New patient	PATIENT IDENTIFICATION_____
	[2] Established patient	DATE OF SERVICE_____
		DATE OF BIRTH_____
		MARITAL STATUS

OFFICE VISIT: [1] Brief

[2] Routine

[3] Extended

(Stamped here with addressograph plate or entered by hand.)

PATIENT'S REASON FOR THIS VISIT: (Specify presenting complaints or symptoms)

_____

_____

_____

CURRENT PROBLEMS/DIAGNOSES FOR THIS PATIENT: (Detail two most important)

IF NONE, check here [0]

1. _____

    a. [1] mild [2] moderate [3] severe

    b. [1] initial detection [4] complication
       [2] routine follow-up [5] not treated
       [3] recurrence this visit

2. _____

    a. [1] mild [2] moderate [3] severe

    b. [1] initial detection [4] complication
       [2] routine follow-up [5] not treated
       [3] recurrence this visit

OTHER ACTIVE PROBLEMS/DIAGNOSES

3. _____

4. _____

5. _____

LABORATORY PROCEDURES: (Check and list all ordered this visit)

[0] NONE   [ ] _____
[ ] urinalysis
[ ] hematocrit
[ ] sickle cell prep   [ ] _____
[ ] CBC
[ ] Blood sugar
[ ] BUN   [ ] _____
[ ] creatinine
[ ] uric acid   [ ] _____
[ ] serum electrolytes
[ ] SGOT/SGPT   [ ] _____
[ ] culture _____
[ ] RPR (Hinton)   [ ] _____

X-RAY EXAMINATIONS: (Check and list all ordered at this visit)

[0] NONE
[ ] chest
[ ] UGI
[ ] IVP
[ ] other

OTHER TESTS/PROCEDURES: (Check and list all ordered at this visit)

[0] NONE
[ ] EKG
[ ] Pap Smear
[ ] Tine test
[ ] Immunization _____
[ ] Other _____

DRUGS PRESCRIBED OR CONTINUED THIS VISIT: (List all prescription and nonprescription drugs the patient is now taking)

IF NONE, check here [0]

_____ _____

_____

_____

DISPOSITION: (Check all that apply)

Within

[0] no follow-up planned
[1] telephone follow-up planned
[2] to return if needed, p.r.n.
[3] to return to: [1] M.D. [2] Nurse [3] other
       in: __ days __ weeks __ mos
[4] to see social worker
[5] to see dietician
[ ] other _____

Outside

[ ] referred to specialty clinic

_____

[ ] referred to psychiatrist/psychologist
[ ] admitted to hospital
[ ] other _____

Instructions for Completing Encounter Form

PATIENT AND ENCOUNTER IDENTIFICATION DATA

The information requested at the top of the form is largely self-explanatory. A new patient is one who has never been seen here before *or was last seen before October 1972.* The classifications of length of visit are admittedly subjective but should serve to separate the brief follow-up check from the usual routine visit or the extended initial evaluation or diagnostic work-up.

PATIENT'S REASON FOR THIS VISIT

This should reflect the patient's perception of the *reason(s)* for the visit and not the provider's diagnosis. Thus, complaints such as "nervousness," "shortness of breath," etc. are appropriate. In the absence of prompting symptoms or complaints, other reasons such as routine physical evaluation or a scheduled follow-up for a specific problem are also appropriate.

CURRENT PROBLEMS/DIAGNOSES

Space is available for giving detailed information about two problems or diagnoses. These should be related to the most important problems dealt with during this visit and, in most cases, will also relate to the reason(s) for the visit. If the diagnosis has not been established, indicate diagnoses that are being considered. For example, if the presenting complaint is "weight loss" and the working diagnosis is hyperthyroidism, please indicate "? hyperthyroidism." If the diagnosis is unclear at the time, indicate "weight loss—unknown etiology."

The space for the second detailed diagnosis can be used to relate to the patient's presenting complaint(s) or to another active problem dealt with at this visit. It can also be used to specify another problem not dealt with at this visit. Thus, for the patient with "weight loss" of unknown etiology who does not have other diagnoses related to the reason for this visit, the second space can be used for another active problem such as hypertension, depression, etc.

For patients who present for a routine physical who are found not to have any current problems or diagnoses, please check "NONE" box.

OTHER ACTIVE PROBLEMS/DIAGNOSES

Space is allotted to list up to three additional active problems. These should include the patient's most important other problems or those problems related to the two described in detail above. Thus, if hypertension is one of the two problems described above and the patient also has renal insufficiency or has an anxiety reaction, these should be listed.

LABORATORY PROCEDURES, X-RAY EXAMINATIONS, AND OTHER TESTS/PROCEDURES

List all diagnostic examinations *ordered* at this visit, whether or not they were actually done during the visit. This information should be supplied for patients who are having a routine physical as well as those who present with specific problems. Please check "NONE," when applicable.

DRUGS

List name *but not dosage or frequency* of all drugs prescribed *or continued*, including nonprescription drugs. If the patient is on more than five drugs, indicate this by writing "check chart." The complete list will be obtained later from the medical record and added to the form. If "NONE," please check box.

DISPOSITION

Under section "Within. . .," if a specific return visit has been scheduled it should be indicated as the *next return* to a primary provider. For example, if the patient was seen by the MD at this visit and is scheduled to return to the Nurse in two weeks and the MD in two months, just check "Nurse" and "2 weeks."

Please also indicate referrals to a social worker or dietician; it is not necessary to indicate *when* the patient will see them. If a consultation was held during the visit, indicate this under "other" ("Within. . .") and name specialty.

For specialty referrals or hospitalization, use section "Outside. . . ."

Index

About the Editors

ANN A. BLISS

Mrs. Bliss is Assistant Professor at the Yale University School of Medicine and Senior Program Consultant for The Robert Wood Johnson Foundation, Princeton, New Jersey.

Formerly Research Associate in the Yale Trauma Program and Lecturer to The Yale Physician's Associate Program, she has also taught psychiatric nursing and sociology in the baccalaureate and master's degree nursing programs at SUNY at Buffalo and Niagara University. In addition to having clinical nursing experience, she is a psychiatric social worker whose clinical practice includes psychotherapy of children and adults.

Coauthor of *The Physician's Assistant Today and Tomorrow,* she has been Managing Editor of *The PA Journal—A Journal for New Health Practitioners* and recently joined the Editorial Boards of *JEN* (The Journal of Emergency Nursing), and *The Nurse Practitioner.*

Mrs. Bliss is a member of The American Nurses' Association, the Academy of Certified Social Workers and is certified by the Connecticut Society for Clinical Social Work.

A graduate of the Grace-New Haven School of Nursing, she received her B.S. from The University of Pennsylvania, and M.S.S. from Bryn Mawr College.

EVA DANIELSSON COHEN

Ms. Cohen is Director of the Office of Graduate and Continuing Education, Yale University School of Medicine and Lecturer in the Department of Epidemiology and Public Health.

She is the principal author of *An Evaluation of Policy-Related Research on New and Expanded Roles of Health Workers*, a study sponsored by the National Science Foundation. Her other recent publications include, "Women in Medicine: A Survey of Professional Activities, Career Interruptions, and Conflict Resolutions," and "The Swedish No-Fault Patient Compensation Program: Provisions and Preliminary Findings." She has served on the Advisory Committee to the DHEW sponsored *Nurse Practitioner and Physician Assistant Training and Deployment Study*.

In addition to her research on the education and employment patterns of health personnel, she currently administers continuing education programs for health professionals.

She is a graduate of the University of Stockholm, Sweden, and received her M.P.H. from Yale University. Ms. Cohen is a member of the American Public Health Association.